UROLOGY

From Antiquity to the 20th Century

UROLOGY

From Antiquity to the 20th Century

By

LEONARD PAUL WERSHUB, M.D., F.A.C.S., D.A.B.

Diplomate of American Board of Urology
Professor of Urology
Curator Medical Memorabilia
New York Medical College
Flower and Fifth Avenue Hospitals
New York, New York

WARREN H. GREEN, INC.
St. Louis, Missouri, U.S.A.

Published by

WARREN H. GREEN, INC.
10 South Brentwood Blvd.
St. Louis, Missouri 63105, U.S.A.

Library of Congress Catalog Card No. 71-78017

Printed in the United States of America
5-A (170)

For

Miriam Enid Wershub
Loyal and True Companion in
Triumph and in Tribulation

There is dead medical literature, and there is a live one. The dead is not all ancient, the live is not all modern. There is none, modern or ancient, which, if it has no living value for the student, will not teach him something by its autopsy.

Oliver Wendell Holmes

Preface

THE history of urology from antiquity to the 20th Century has had an ecumenical dissemination. It is a heritage richer today than ever before, for it includes the contributions of Hippocrates, Aristotle, Avicenna, Rhazes, Maimonides, Galen, Paracelsus, Vesalius, Ambroise Paré, Leonardo da Vinci, Morgagni, Gustave Simon, Rudolf Virchow, Louis Pasteur and many others. Together, they embraced the knowledge of their predecessors thus subsequently making the heritage richer than ever before.

Will and Ariel Durant in *The Lessons of History* write, "History is a fragment of biology: the life of man is a portion of the vicissitudes of organisms on land and sea. Sometimes, wandering alone in the woods on a summer day, we hear or see the movements of a hundred species of flying, leaping, creeping, crawling, burrowing things. The startled animals scurry away at our coming; the birds scatter; the fish disperse in the brook. Suddenly, we perceive to what a perilous minority we belong on this impartial planet, and for a moment we feel, as these varied denizens clearly do, that we are passing interlopers in their natural habitat. Then all the chronicles and achievements of man fall humbly into the history and perspective of polymorphous life; all our economic competition, our strife for mates, our hunger and love and grief and war, are akin to the seeking, mating, striving, and suffering that hide under these fallen trees or leaves, or in the waters, or on the boughs."

I fully recognize that much of the field covered in this book belongs of right to the historian, particularly to one well versed with the classics and languages of the middle and far

East as well as with the archaeologist and his associated disciplines. Nevertheless, it has been a pleasing and stimulating adventure and one that has been prepared at odd moments and in the midst of other work requiring time and concentration. Indeed, a good deal of it has been written during European travel when the only resources were such texts as I had taken along in my luggage and an occasional visit to a local museum, which often proved more confusing than helpful. I mention this with the hope that it may explain some irregularities in the script and in the biographical data supplied. To overcome such inadequacies I may perhaps be forgiven for the insertion of numerous footnotes which at times were deliberately planned.

It is reasonable to assume that man has been afflicted with urological disorders ever since he first roamed the forests and lived in caves. Urology, comprising as it does the diseases of the urinary tract, was perhaps the very first branch of medicine to emerge from the mists of antiquity and ignorance. We can readily appreciate how the male driven by painful, difficult or impossible urination would devise, in desperation, some means of obtaining relief. Thus, over a thousand years before Christ, the Hindus had already invented the catheter to relieve retention of urine, and sounds to dilate strictures of the urethra. The operation of perineal lithotomy was well developed and widely practised by the Hindus long before the procedure reached the European continent.

This book is not a complete or a conventional history of surgery nor is it a textbook of urology. It only deals with diagnosis and treatment from a purely historical point of view, emphasizing that urologic surgery was born long before major abdominal surgery. The history of medicine does not necessarily mean all history of medicine, or for that matter medical history in general. In this presentation of chronologically recorded urological events, attention has been given to the parallel picture of civilization, thus contributing in a meaningful manner to the progress of medicine. To accomplish this, I have tried wherever possible to project certain mores and human activity so closely interwoven in the fabric of any history.

My sincere thanks and appreciation are due to Doctor David D.

Denker. A debt to acknowledge, but difficult to thank, is that of the sincere criticisms and suggestions made by Dr. Elmer Belt concerning the chapter of Leonardo da Vinci; and to Dr. C. D. O'Malley with reference to the chapter of Andreas Vesalius. Both of these scholars, internationally known for their authoritative knowledge of Leonardo da Vinci and Andreas Vesalius, were kind enough to review my meagre chapters dealing with da Vinci and Vesalius. Great credit is due to Mr. Robert Tringali, Director of Graphic Arts at the New York Medical College, for his excellent photography and reproductions. I am greatly indebted to my secretary, Miss Loretta Olsen, and to Miss Doris Hughes for the excellent typing and re-typing of what at one time seemed to be an endless manuscript. I also wish to thank Mrs. Eugenia Dover and Mrs. Judith Myers, of the New York Medical College library for their constant help and untiring efforts in resource material. I also wish to acknowledge the many courtesies extended to me by the Yale Sterling Library and Yale School of Medicine Historical Library, and by the Rare Book Room of the New York Academy of Medicine. And last, but not least, my thanks to my friend Col. N. Henry Josephs for his helpful assistance in the final editing stages of the manuscript.

Much has been omitted in this text, that might have been included; and it is fervently hoped that nothing has been included which ought to have been omitted.

L.P.W.

Contents

UROLOGY

From Antiquity to the 20th Century

Chapter 1

The Beginnings

TIME is relative and in the passage of millenia and out of prehistoric mists there emerged the first species of man, called Homo Erectus. He has been described as hardly impressive looking, with heavy brow ridges, a very flat broad nose, a sloping forehead and a massive jaw. He stood 5 feet tall fully erect. He used a variety of chopping, cutting and scraping instruments and even more important, came upon and learned the use of fire.

From the very beginning of history, there is ample proof that man constantly strove to improve himself. This ancestor of ours ultimately learned* that with the grinding and shaping of stones he could equip himself with a weapon which was of great assistance in hunting for food and for protection, particularly from marauding beasts.

Among the primitives, blood, hair and tears were believed to

---

* Archaeological investigation of the material remains of prehistoric man has shown that a wide variety of cultures flourished in different parts of the world and at different times. For convenience these have been grouped into a series of major cultures based primarily on the nature of the principal material used for implements and sometimes on the technique used in fashioning these implements. The oldest culture in the world was characterized by the use of chipped stone for implements and has been named Palaeolithic culture. Neolithic culture, on the other hand, was characterized by the use of polished stone implements; bronze culture by the use of bronze implements, and so forth . . . accordingly prehistoric times have usually been divided into the following series of periods or ages (beginning with the oldest): *Palaeolithic* (old stone), characterized by chipped stone implements; *Mesolithic* (Intermediate Stone), a transitional period; *Neolithic* (New Stone), with polished stone implements; *Chalcolithic* (Stone and Copper) characterized by the first tentative use of copper implements; *Bronze Age,* with full development of copper and bronze implements; and *Iron Age,* with iron implements,[1]

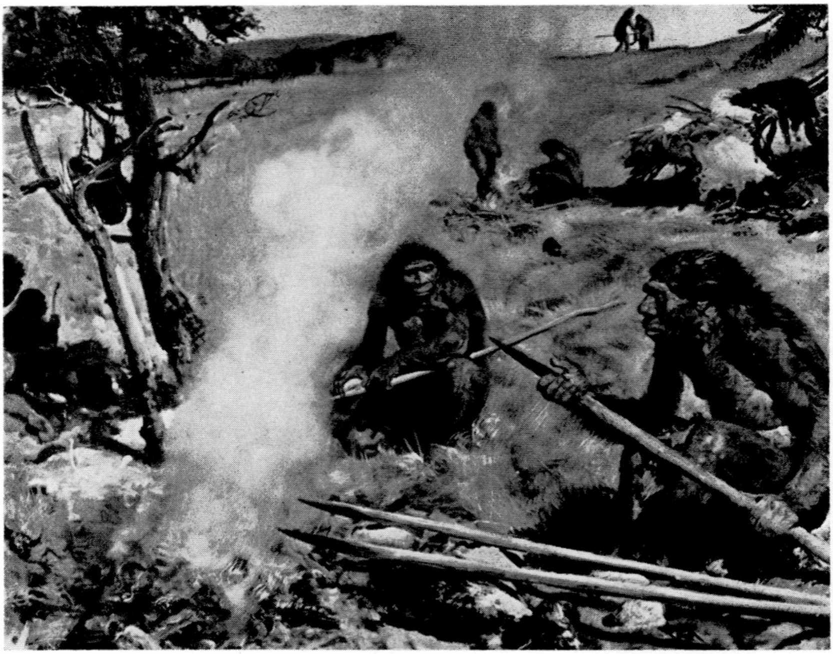

Figure 1. A scene depicting Neanderthal men, the first true members of Homo Sapiens. They were excellent hunters and tool makers and in this scene spears are fashioned from fire-charred saplings that they have sharpened with finely worked stone scrapers. It is believed these ancestors of ours had pondered the nature of death and learned much of the care of disease and illness by close observation of animals under similar circumstances. (Photograph of painting by Z. Burian, courtesy of Paul Hamlin, Ltd., copied by Walter Sanders.)

be imbued with soul substances. For the same reason, urine was used to rub on the body to protect against evil spirits. Some used urine as a poison in sorcery and in witchcraft. Rain was thought to be the urine of a deity and therefore a soul-substance. Young men even urinated on the urine of his beloved, thinking this would make her love him the more.

Throughout most of history, and for most living people, disease has always been present.[2] Sickness is associated with life, and man everywhere endeavors to deal with it as best he can. Studies in paleopathology have shown not only the antiquity of disease, but also that it has always occurred in the same basic forms, such as infection, inflammation, disturbances of development and metabolism, traumatism and tumors. Schistosomiasis,* prevalent in Egypt today, has been found in kidneys 3000 years old, and tuberculosis of the spine has been diagnosed in the skeletal remains of pre-Colombian Indians. Indeed, there is some documentary evidence that suggests the existence in ancient times of poliomyelitis.

The study of the evidences of injury and disease among ancient man and fossil animals is known as *Paleopathology.* This term was first used in the *Standard Dictionary,* Volume 2, 1895, where it is defined as "the science of pathological conditions in the organs of extinct or petrified animals."

Discussing the antiquity of disease, Moodie† states "speculations usually precede discovery. Suggestions and theories precede definite concepts. The first recorded suggestion that there might be considerable antiquity to disease and pathological processes were made by von Walther in 1825. Had von Walther only realized it," writes Moodie, "he had in his possession sufficient evidence to prove a portion of the antiquity of disease, since the bones he studied were of Pleistocene age, representing mammals tens of thousands of years old. Possibly in his opinion

---

* One of the most significant and important contributions to paleopathology made by Sir Marc Armand Ruffer was his discovery of the calcified eggs of *Schistosoma haematobium bilharzia* in the straight tubules of the kidneys of two twentieth dynasty Egyptian mummies. This discovery is of cardinal importance since it rolls back the history of schistosomiasis for three millenia and substantiates the statements in the great medical papyri from ancient Egypt that hematuria was common. Sandison believes this might be regarded as the foundation of a new science of paleoparasitology; "this science has recently been extended by qualitative and quantitative assessments of helminth ova astonishingly well preserved in Medieval cess-pits and latrine deposits."[3]

† Roy L. Moodie (1880-1934), American anatomist and anthropologist, in 1923 published the first comprehensive book on Paleopathology (*Paleopathology, An Introduction to the Study of Ancient Evidences of Disease,* Urbana, University of Illinois Press, 1923). Moodie's book covered the entire field, analyzing and presenting previous works and adding the author's many original observations. This book greatly stimulated studies in paleopathology. For the reader interested in paleopathology, I recommend this book, as well as a short, more popular book also published by Moodie in the same year (1923) *The Antiquity of Disease,* University of Chicago Press.

disease was not disease unless it afflicted the human race. We now know that disease is the same whether manifested in man or in the lower animals."

Thus, it can be said that there is evidence to warrant the geological beginnings of disease. Undoubtedly, the introduction of disease among the early animals was a gradual process with sparse and indefinite evidence completely masking its presence. What has perplexed the paleontologist is his not knowing the specific factors that ultimately led to the extinction of the myriads of organisms, animal or plant, that flourished in the dim past.

Sufficient evidence is available to confirm that the remains of the stone age man of Europe occasionally show evidence of disease and injury. Such studies are confined to the remains of human races which occupied European countries, since no representation of the Neolithic and Paleolithic peoples are to be found in the Western Hemisphere.

The most famous of the skeletal remains representing early (Upper Paleolithic) fossil man are the remains of the skeleton of an extinct species of man found in a cave in the Neanderthal, in the Rhine province of Prussia. Of interest is that the proxial end of the left ulna shows evidence of a healed fracture of the olecranon. The left humerus reveals signs of injury speculated to be the result of weakness in this side as compared to the right humerus.

Of even further speculative deduction is the belief by Virchow (1872) who regarded the shortening of the ulna and humerus as due to rickets. Virchow, in addition to being an extremely keen pathologist, was a distinguished anthropologist as well, and paid much attention to the pathology of fossil bones.

Primitive man knew little of the etiology of disease and because of this ignorance superstitous beliefs as the causative agent were quickly adopted. He could understand injuries resulting from violence, caused by wild animals or by the spear and arrow of hunter or of the enemy and quite early in the history of civilization he learned to treat and give aid to such emergencies. It follows that primitive surgery in the main had to do with removing foreign bodies, setting broken bones, reducing dislocations, stopping hemorrhages, removing arrows, and healing wounds. Moodie[4] reports a specimen of a lumbar vertebra showing a stone arrow embedded deeply in the visceral surface. Apparently, the person was shot through the abdomen and the arrow coming with terrific force since it penetrated the abdominal wall near the umbilicus, plowed its way through the viscera and embedded itself firmly in the body of the vertebra where it remained fixed for thousands of years. From this case, the paleopathologists infer that the individual died of peritonitis, or that he may have died from some other cause such as hemorrhage, but there is no indication that he lived very long after the injury, since there is an absence of *callus* around the wound.

Man learned the basics of medical therapy by watching the curative powers of nature and the practices of animals. He saw cats and dogs using different herbs as emetics and purgatives. He watched the mongoose who, after being bitten by a snake, neutralize and counteract the poison by chewing mimosa leaves. He observed toads bitten by spiders chewed leaves of the plantogo major as an antidote and observed wild goats eat dittany when shot by the poisoned darts of hunters. Animals instinctively alleviate fever by immersion in cold water, routinely and skillfully hunt parasites that torment them and try to lessen the pain of their wounds by licking them. Four-legged animals when a leg is broken, train themselves to go on three legs to immobilize and heal the broken bone with minimum shortening.

Primitive man was swayed by superstitions, myths, sorcery, totemic ordinances, symbolic incantations, and magic. Their ideas about medical supervision, at first seem utter nonsense, but we must bear in mind the extreme antiquity of mankind, and the long years of struggle and trial by error, that was necessary to develop modern theology, ethical, medical and social systems.

All was not even based on empirical beliefs. Herodotus, writing of Pheron, the son of Sesostris, conqueror of Egypt, who was blind for ten years, tells that on the eleventh year of his illness an oracle told him that he would recover his eye sight if he would wash his eyes with the urine of a woman who had intercourse only with her own husband and had known no other man. So, he tried the urine of his own wife, and that of many others, but to no avail, until he was finally cured by the urine of "a woman he took to wife"; all the others he executed.[5]

Primitive man had several beliefs concerning death and in the main that it was produced by revengful gods who inflicted death as a curse because of faulty behavior. For example, the Wachagga, a tribe inhabiting the Kilimanjaro district of Africa had several traditional explanations of the origin of death. According to one of these stories, human mortality is the result of, and the punishment for, the disobedience of man in eating the fruit of a certain tree that the supreme god has forbidden though he had given mankind permission to enjoy the fruits of other trees. Disobedience could only result in the offenders and their descendants being condemned to ultimately die.

According to another tradition, men were told by the messenger of the god that they would cast their skins when old and so renew their youth. A condition, however, was imposed that no eye should witness the act of sloughing. A certain old man, when his skin was partly cast, was imprudent enough to let himself be seen by his granddaughter, and as a result mankind was denied the boon of renewed youthfulness forever. Such beliefs as these are widespread but what is amazing is that traditions common to the primitive man in Africa are prevalent

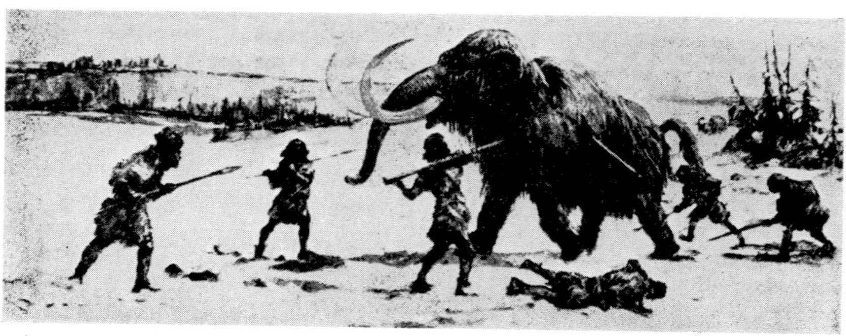

FIGURE 2. It follows that man in his constant dangerous search for food and in defense against his enemies and wild animals would be subject to many traumatic ailments of a urologic nature as well as those of other systems.

amongst the islands of Indonesia, Polynesia and other far-flung countries.[6] Even in the Egyptian medical papyrus, one can find reference to similar beliefs in a magical text, *The Book for Transforming an Old Man Into a Youth of Twenty.*

In many instances, the ingenuity of these people and the resemblance to so-called modern practices is remarkable. For example, among the Ashanti of West Africa, inoculation for smallpox, or against snake bite is successfully practiced. Cupping and bloodletting are widely practiced. Cupping is accomplished by powerful suction with the mouth through a bone tube or similar instrument. Drainage from wounds is accomplished by utilization of sections of bamboo. Foreign bodies are extracted and abscesses opened with a thorn or a sharp-pointed instrument. Montague[7] writes of treatment of ulcers among primitives by cauterization with hot ashes or with heated blades and irons. In the treatment of fractures, splints and occasionally casts made of clay were utilized. Indeed, according to the evidence of skeletal remains, the orthopedic results were excellent. Puschmann[8] clearly portrays the scene and sequence of the combative habits of barbarians, whose favorite pursuits were hunting and war, and as a result of which wounds and injuries were all too common. Such injuries were tended by friends who washed the afflicted areas and placed poultices or other soothing medicaments made from plants, discovered to have healing properties. In this manner, a medical craft originated, and was formed and practiced by those who had remarkable dexterity in healing and knowledge of former successful procedures.

Such skill could not be as easily acquired when it came to the handling of cases afflicted with internal disorders, particularly during severe, devastating epidemics. Under such circumstances, the people turned to the priests, since epidemics and vague sudden ailments appeared dark and mysterious and quite obviously were attributed to supernatural spirits and powers. Thus, with confidence in the priest, or medicine man (a later role among primitives), the afflicted person was subjected to so-called expectant treatment, or *vis medicamentrix.* Or course, since faith, confidence and hope were essential, the priests soon realized that such therapy in certain epidemics was inadequate, and for fear of losing their reputation and position in society, efforts were made to acquire additional medical knowledge, which was transmitted by word of mouth or even by writing. In such surroundings where the priests themselves had to appear to be of essential importance in the treatment of diseases, it followed that they (the priests) made every effort to bind up all therapy with religious ceremonies held in awe by popular superstition.

This class now emerged as a group who combined the knowledge acquired at the Temple Schools with the medical experience of the Empirics. Thus there evolved a school of medicine which treated both internal and external disorders of the body as exemplified by the doctors of the Greek and Roman periods of civilization. During the next thousand years, there was greater diversion or spread of medical knowledge, i.e., from one country to another but little increase in intellectual or pseudo-scientific knowledge.

Looking toward the West, we again see the priests taking over as teachers of medicine. The Roman and German people were ultimately converted to the belief that, "the Christian Church possessed and preserved not only the truths of heavenly life but the knowledge of this world too. . . ." The practice of the healing art had for priests, even then, many inconveniences in store; respect for their Order forbade them to undertake surgical operations, since through their mistakes death might ensue to their patients. In addition, they abstained from the treatment of diseases of women. It was thus possible, that an independent class of practitioners should maintain itself and grow alongside of, but unconnected with, any priestly profession. Puschmann[8] elaborates by including in his group the numerous Jewish doctors who settled in Christian countries and by virtue of their skill and practical ability combined with extensive knowledge were highly respected and sought after. In addition, people living in the South of Europe came under the influence of Arabian medical science, which played a vital part in the subsequent founding of self-supporting medical schools at Salerno and Montpelier.

If I have wandered in recording the above facts of disease

and death, it is primarily to show that out of this determination to thwart hostile powers that the ultimate role of the magician, medicine man, priest and the doctor came into being. No one can deny that medicine had its origin in magic.

What sometimes appears as a superstitious but useful remedy is actually founded on a scientific basis. For example, the use of urine for hygienic or cosmetic purposes is an old-fashioned remedy. In France, the wealthy ladies of Boyle's day took urine baths to beautify the skin. Even today, persons in some rural communities use urine to soften the hands. Among the ancient Romans, urine was used as a mouth wash and prophylactic against dental caries, which is used even among primitive people of today. Pierre Fauchard, "the father of dentistry" recommended "rectified urine," a strongly ammonical solution, as well as sal ammoniac (ammonium chloride), as a dentifrice and toothache remedy. Indeed, the use of fresh or fermented urine as a dentifrice persists in many areas at the present time, and the addition of ammonium compounds and urea to some modern dentifrices echoes this age-old relation of urine to the teeth.

Smith[9] claims that many believe that prior to the use of yeast, urine was used by bakers as a leavening agent, and within relatively recent times it is said to have been used to macerate tobacco leaves in the cigar industry, and to flavor cheese. "I have been told," writes Smith, "that in the Arctic region pots of human urine are used to draw salt-hungry caribou near to human habitations, and I can certify that in California some farmers place pots of urine around fruit trees for a contrary reason—in order to keep away marauding deer."

The history of medicine is rich in myths and magic beliefs since complexes of the primitive mind persists through centuries. Therefore, in the history of this healing art we may find many documents relating to the evolution of myths and their interference with empirical medicine, with religion, and even with experimental science. History of medicine is the history of human reaction to all menaces against man's health, faith, hope, philosophy, on one hand and on the other scientific means, hygienic organization and social laws, are the tools with which successively in the course of centuries, these menaces were combatted. To all these stages, the primitive mind has continuously contributed, sometimes in a positive, sometimes in a negative way. In the history of medicine, the myth plays a remarkable role.[10]

With such a broad premise in mind, let us now turn to that part of the world, the land adjacent to the Mediterranean Sea, which has contributed so much to early medicine and laid the foundation for the ultimate development of the art called medical science.

Chapter II

Mesopotamia

Medical Origins and Urological Fantasies

THE beginnings of medicine are unknown to us since they began at a time when no written records were available and any attempt to reconstruct this era would be purely speculative. But it must be reconstructed. To do this, we go to the records of the earliest civilization, knowing that a medical schema of some sort must have existed. For this reason, we first examine the medical records of Mesopotamia and later turn to Egypt.

Before the Smith papyrus was translated and made available, there existed two views on the general character and early development of Babylonian and Egyptian medicine.[11] One theory, advocated by many historians of medicine, believed that both magical and empirical elements determined the progress of ancient medicine and occurred side by side; whereas the second theory was that the empirical element in Babylonian and Egyptian medicine developed from primitive magic. Subsequently, with the available translation of the Edwin Smith papyrus, many felt that the development of medicine occurred as a purely scientific and rational document without stigma of magical incantations or ritual performances.

"Like Egypt," writes Sigerist,[12] "Mesopotamia is a 'gift of rivers' because without them most of the land would be desert . . . they also flood the land when the snow melts in the mountains of Armenia; the Tigris first, the Euphrates somewhat later, beginning in March and reaching the maximum in May, but unlike that of the Nile their flood is violent and destructive unless it is checked by canals. Hence, canals had to be built. They were constructed to connect the two rivers and drain water from the Euphrates into the Tigris. They irrigated the land, and the larger ones served at the same time as highways of traffic." When Herodotus visited Mesopotamia, he was greatly impressed by these canals and particularly that unlike what he saw in Egypt, the fields were not irrigated by the rivers directly but rather through manual labor working pumps. They would fill the canals with the overflowing water, which was then drained and pumped into the fields.

According to Herodotus, Babylonians had no physicians, but brought their sick into the market-places in order that passers-by might confer with them upon their symptoms in the hope that the patient might elicit from someone who had been similarly afflicted advice as to how to proceed to effect a cure. Whether this is accurate is questionable, since close by, the Assyrians possessed considerable medical information. Sigerist believes that what Herodotus meant was that the Babylonians did not have the kind of physicians such as the specialists, he had met in Egypt.

To the reader of history, the civilization of Mesopotamia appears at times to be closer to us and at times more distant than that of Egypt. The antiquity arises because the Old Testament tells us more of Mesopotamia than it does of Egypt. For example, we read of the tower of Babel and of Nineveh that was to be destroyed. We learn that Abram came from Ur of the Chaldees. Since the middle of the nineteenth century, when Mesopotamia sites were excavated and cuneiform tablets deciphered, it became clear how the Hebrews and other ancient people of the near East were influenced by this culture.

It is quite possible that the dearth of knowledge of Assyrian medicine can be attributed to the scarcity of published Assyrian medical texts. "From their very nature, inscribed as they are in cuneiform characters on brittle clay tablets, these texts are extremely fragmentary and often very difficult to read." Thousands of these clay tablets have been excavated, all containing vast stores of historical, literary, religious, magical, astronomical and medical data of this ancient era. Significantly, there is great similarity between the Assyrian and Egyptian medical texts;

both basically composed of strange mixtures of rational therapeutic treatment with magical spells and incantations.

After thousands of years of neolithic stagnation, the inventiveness of Mesopotamian man is indeed remarkable. For almost three thousand years, Mesopotamia lived as a succession of warring states in contrast to Egypt which maintained an almost continuous dynasty. Because of these many wars, Mesopotamia's physicians gained an empiric knowledge of surgery, including eye operations, phlebotomy, and cupping. In both civilizations, religion and magic was in supreme control and influenced health and medical progress.

The medicine of the Tigris-Euphrates Valley where the Sumerians, Akkadians, Babylonians, and Assyrians lived underwent a peculiar evolution with the development of medical practitioners. From the extant documents, one gathers that these people believed that disease was a punishment inflicted by the gods upon men for some state of impurity or uncleanliness. They believed that the gods allowed demons to take possession of the sick person and each demon entered that part of the body it most desired. Further, if demons were not causing the illness, then the disease was a spell cast by a sorcerer or witch. In short, the sick person had sinned in some manner or other and the first step to be taken was for the seer (diviner) to place the nature of the disorder in the spectrum. Accordingly, after his had been established, the patient might take one of two courses. He might first go to an exorcist, who would prescribe the rites needed to drive out a demon, or propitiate an indignant god. On the other hand, if the illness was deemed to have come from natural causes, the patient could consult a general practitioner, who would undertake treatment resorting to elementary surgery or with drugs. Like all primitive medicinal compounds, the Babylonian *materia medica,* emphasized herbs* and other natural resources, which had previously proven to be of value.

Magic played a great role in the lives of these people just as

* In 1906, R. Campbell Thompsen commenced a systematic study of about 660 tablets in the British Museum, and as a result of these labors, compiled a volume in 1924 entitled *The Assyrian Herbal.* In this work, many identifications were made and a large series of plants identified for the first time.

it did elsewhere at this time in the history of mankind. It was the general belief, and certainly no exception in Mesopotamia, that religion (pagan) and magic provided the means to influence gods and events, and thus prevent evil and disease. Thus, one was required to lead a pure life, observe certain taboos, make the necessary prayers and sacrifices, and resort to what procedure was recommended by one who was vested in the ability to guide and direct. In short, disease was believed to be caused by demons, ghosts and a great variety of so-called evil spirits. Prayers, incantations and sacrifices were the common treatments utilized. Although the literary sources of Mesopotamian medicine are limited, especially when compared to Egyptian sources, a large number of tablets that list symptoms and indicated treatment, are available. The literature on hepatoscopy (see below) is very considerable and there are many literary sources listing and interpreting omens.

The Babylonians had something resembling a medical profession. They were controlled by the celebrated Code of Hammurabi, promulgated over four thousand years ago. It is the oldest extant professional rule book. Its provisions have often been quoted for they indicate a higher regard for the safety of the citizen than for the peace of mind of the practitioner.

"If a physician shall make a severe wound with a bronze operating knife on the slave of a free man and kill him, he shall replace the slave with another slave. If a physician shall make a severe wound with an operating knife on a free man and kill him . . . his hands shall be cut off." Thus, if an operation caused the loss of an eye, the physician's hands were cut off, and if a high born patient died, the physician lost his life. The Draconic laws were most probably a means of protecting against malpractice or lack of skill in physicians.

"The code of Hammurabi, King of Babylon (about 2250 B.C.) was found among the clay tablets of the library of Ashurbanipal. It was first published in Scheil: *Memoires de la Delegation en Perse,* Paris, 1902, 4, 41-162. The code mentions the fees payable to a physician following successful treatment; these varied according to the station of the patient. Similarly, the punishment for the failure of an operation is set out. At least, this shows that in Babylon 4000 years ago the medical profession had advanced far enough in public esteem to warrant the payment of adequate fees.[13]

Singularly, the Assyrian laws (which were stricter than the Babylonian Code) had stringent regulations concerning injury to the genital organs:

> If a woman has crushed a man's testicle in an affray, one of her fingers shall be cut off; and if although a physician has bound it up, the second testicle is affected with it and becomes inflamed or if she has crushed the second testicle in the affray, both her nipples shall be torn off.

In similar vein, a public penalty is imposed on a man who "has struck a lady by birth and has caused her to cast the fruit of her womb." The punishment was a considerably large fine, fifty blows with rods and one month of forced labor for the king. The punishment for abortion was very severe. "If a woman has cast the fruit of her womb by her own act and charges have been brought against her, she shall be impaled and shall not be buried."

The Mesopotamians believed that the liver was the seat of the soul and center of life. Divination was performed in an elaborate and costly ritual before the statue of a god who made his intentions known in the liver of the sacrificed sheep. The ritual was concluded by a post-mortem examination of the liver in which a careful search was made for malformations or other abnormalities. Each real or supposed abnormality was interpreted by the diviner as the god's answer to specific questions. Thus, if the right lobe was shaped like a purse it was interpreted as an omen of disaster. If the common duct tended to go to the right, the patient could be assured he would live. This art of *hepatoscopy* was taught in the temples where clay or bronze models of a liver were used.*

---

* Thus, the Babylonians would ask the patient to breathe into a sheep's nose. Then the sheep was slaughtered and the liver examined to determine the prognosis. Such a liver it was believed would not only register the nature of a disease but also the prospects for recovery.

Hepatoscopy also played a role in the fate of men and nations. Since it was accepted as the seat of all vital functions, it was the obvious means for the gods to reveal their intentions. Thus, a tight sheep's liver meant victory in war, whereas a shriveled one meant defeat.

Physicians were also trained in the relationship between certain celestial movements and outbreak of disease and epidemics. In addition, they would interpret dreams as an aid in prognosis and treatment of a disease. Above all, they knew which gods to invoke for help against the demons of disease; namely *Nabu* the Assyrian God of the Healing Art, or Babylon's *Marduk,* who held the power to overcome all disease.

The Babylonian physician used extracts of hempseeds in menorrhagia, dysmenorrhea and for recurrent fevers, and as a sedative for pain. The Scythians placed the seeds on red hot stones and inhaled the vapors that were given off. This produced a state of intoxication which caused the patient to shout and appear demented. Since the Babylonian physicians believed that like cures like, *similia similibus curantur* (Samuel Hahnemann later claimed this as his original basic homeopathic principle), it is quite probable that this was used as a remedy in cases of imbecility and insanity.

There is a great similarity between the Egyptian and Assyrian medical texts and they resemble each other since both are strange mixtures of rational therapeutic methods and with magic and superstition. Yet, there is a marked difference between an Egyptian prescription and an Assyrian prescription. In the former, the name of the ailment is usually stated in the title, as "prescription for a pain in the head," whereas the Assyrian prescriptions have no distinct titles, but usually convey some notions of the symptoms or diagnosis of the disease in the opening phrase as "If a man's head has a pain, thou shalt do so and so," or "If a man's teeth hurt, thou shalt take" such and such drugs, and so on. Dawson[6] makes note of a further distinction in that the majority of Egyptian prescriptions the exact quantities of each drug to be used are stated whereas this detail is often lacking in the Assyrian texts. Nevertheless, the Assyrians were skilled in the preparation of medicines and even though they resorted to magical incantations as a part of the treatment of disease, the prescribed drugs in the main were wholesome and rational.

Gums and aromatic oils played an important role in prescribed medications. Surviving engraved tablets (stones) tell of oil, of myrrh, pine, turpentine, tar, juniper, resins and many aromatic substances for which modern equivalents have not as yet been found. Fumigation and inhalations are recorded on tablets; hemp, mint, saffron, myrrh, pitch, resins, and many barks were used for fumigating.

Drugs were administered in anal suppositories or in enemas. Occasionally, they were blown into the urethra through a tube. Significantly, potions prepared at night were taken before sunrise on an empty stomach. In the evening, they could only be taken when the stars appeared.

The Babylonians[12] were more systematic than the Egyptians as evidenced by their early codification of their laws, their careful listing of their astronomical observations and astrological findings. Similarly, their medical books were a collection of cases arranged systematically under a specific heading. Classification was determined either symptomatically, etiologically, or clinically, thus a famous book included cases listed under the headings, "If the hand of a ghost seizes on a man," or "If a woman gives birth to a child with . . ."; often, the cases were arranged according to the afflicted organ, as "If a man is affected in the lungs," or "If a man's eyes hurt," or according to the dominating symptom as "jaundice."

Many tablets (and there are still innumerable ones still not deciphered) clearly indicate that the Babylonian doctor was a good diagnostician, who precisely and methodically examined the patient and prescribed the indicated remedies. No references are made to studies or textbooks in anatomy and I find no reference to *uroscopy*.

Numerous references are found in the tablets pertaining to diseases of the genito-urinary organs. For example:

> "If a man in his sleep or in his waking has seminal discharge and he does not know that he went to his wife and his penis and his 'cloth' are full of seminal fluid, thou shalt mix in oil 'clay of the dust of the mountain-stone' and horned alkali. Thou shalt smear a plaster on the point of the man's 'tongue.'

> Thou shalt pour it on the man's sore. And in oil and wine thou shalt mix it. He shall drink it and he will recover."[14]

Singularly, there is no evidence of syphilis, although it is more than likely gonorrhea existed since there are references to urethral discharges, which of course could have been non-specific infections:

> "If a man's urine is like the urine of an ass, that man is sick of gonorrhea; if a man's urine is like beer yeast, that man is sick of gonorrhea; if a man's urine is like wine-yeast, that man is sick of gonorrhea; if a man's urine is like gummy paint (varnish) that man is sick of gonorrhea."[15]

Discharge of blood or of pus and blood are to be found in certain passages:

> "If a man discharges blood from his penis like a woman," or "If from a man's penis blood and pus come forth on him, like the seizure of a jackal. . . ."

In other sections, spermatorrhea, retention of urine, incontinence of urine, impotence and other urological problems are discussed, as well as prescription relative to sexual intercourse and general love charms.

That renal calculi existed among the Mesopotamians is evidenced by several texts which make a distinction between hard and soluble stones. Indeed, the following prescription is both startling and revealing: "Whether it be hard or soluble or soluble stone, or gonorrhea, or strangury, or anus-trouble, or urine coming drop by drop . . ." and the drugs prescribed consisted of black saltpeter, shell of ostrich egg, pine turpentine.

Brown[16] writes: "If we could pay a visit to one of these Babylonian doctors of the scientific class, we should find him a highly cultured gentleman, living in a fine home with gardens and orchards, having an ideal family life, and surrounded with fine objects of art. The doctor is clean shaven on the face and head, and is carefully dressed in flowing robes of colored silk.

He is not a handsome man, but his head and personality denote his culture. He has a friendly disposition and an artistic temperament. His movements show that he is sure of himself;

but we can notice a certain oriental languidness due to the warm climate in which he dwells. The general impression we would gain of the doctor's skill, character and learning would be decidedly favorable."

At the beginning, Babylonian medicine remained primitive. Nevertheless the Babylonians protected society against malpractice of the surgeon by making him liable for his actions. Further, it cannot be denied that not only were abnormalities being recognized, but they were also being treated two thousand years before Christ.

Chapter III

The World of the Pyramids

Egypt

In Egypt men are more skilled in medicine than any of human kind.

HOMER, ODYSSEY, IV, 227

MENES, the founder of the 1st dynasty, united upper and lower Egypt, approximately around 3400 B.C. From 2000 B.C. on, the chronology of Egypt is well established, yet there is no unanimity of opinion for the preceding periods. King Menes welded the country into one kingdom, thereby starting the first of thirty dynasties that lasted for almost 4000 years.* That the country had been inhabited for thousands of years was confirmed by the finding of tools of flint of paleolithic man.† In

* It was a period of great cultural advances of which the most significant undoubtedly was the development of the Egyptian alphabet from pictorial signs, and the development of suitable writing material. The invention of writing affected the social structure and the scribes, those who could read and write, could write a book, compose a document became important to the king.[12]

† Yet much of the country today has made little advancement. The author only recently, after debarking from a plane in a short flight from Cairo to Luxor, was impressed by the primitive and backward status of the natives in this area. Enroute by bus from the air terminal one passes through many narrow, crowded streets, thru small villages, totally lacking in water supply, and sewer systems. The natives could be seen huddled together in their tiny, dark mud-brick houses, surrounded by dirty and dusty streets, with their animals close by. In the smoke of oil lamps and by the light from hearth fires which burned dry dung could be seen many children. Life went on in almost the same routine as that of their ancestors centuries ago. What a contrast to modern Cairo and Alexandria.

addition, villages and cemeteries of a chalcolithic‡ period have been excavated with findings of tools of polished stone, pottery, textiles and objects of copper and gold. These inhabitants learned to till the soil, to domesticate animals, lived in caves and sought protection from illness and misfortune by fetishes or totems.

If we accept the beginning of the First Dynasty of Egypt as around 3400 B.C. we must evaluate the long period of civilization that existed prior to this date. The Egyptians in this earlier era buried their dead in the sands of the desert. Fortunately, they did not bury the dead in the moist soil adjoining the river, for if they had, all records would have ultimately decayed, but by burying the dead in the hot, dry desert sands, records of the pre-dynastic Egyptian era are available and thus the life and culture of that far distant age has been reconstructed. Dawson[6] writes, "Thanks to the dry climate and the preservative effect of direct contact with the sand, so perfectly has nature conserved the remains of these early dwellers in the Nile Valley, that it is possible to examine anatomically the soft and perishable parts of the body, and even to ascertain the nature of the food they ate. . . . The scientific examinations of these specimens has also disclosed some of the methods they used to prepare their food for consumption. Husks of barley were identified in almost every specimen and in a number of cases those of millet were also found. The finding of millet is of great interest because its use in Egypt has been denied, and the species found is not now cultivated except in the East

‡The word Chalcolithic is a term conveniently but loosely used to describe a culture which is still essentially Neolithic in character, but in which the metal *copper* is just beginning to be used, without, however, replacing stone as the principal material for implements. *Chalcolithic* cultures are thus transitional. People in many areas of the world did not pass through this intermediate stage, but obtained their first knowledge of copper directly from other peoples who had already fully developed the art of copper metallurgy. The dates of *Chalcolithic* cultures differ everywhere, depending upon the time which it took for the knowledge of metalworking to spread. The earliest cultures in which copper has been found are in the Near East, and their estimated date is somewhere between 4000 and 3500 B.C. Copper did not appear in Europe much before 2000 B.C.

Indies. Root-tubers and the remains of other plants were found, also metal fish-hooks."

When the kings of ancient Egypt built temples to their gods and pyramidal tombs for themselves, they created monuments from which the modern world was destined to recover, by patient archaeological study, the course and character of early Egyptian history. But there was a long intervening period during which the temples and the pyramids stood with their impressive but often fantastic statues and reliefs, their curious pictures and undeciphered inscriptions, tantalizing every stranger with the mysterious past. Alexander the Great, when he visited Egypt in the 4th Century B.C., could no more read the hieroglyphics than could Napoleon. Later in the Napoleonic era, the Rosetta Stone was deciphered and the key to the ancient writings became available.

Ancient Egyptian medical practice may quite satisfactorily be reconstructed from an analysis of the available sources, particularly the eight papyri known as the Kahun, the Edwin Smith, the Ebers, the Hearst, the Erman, the London, the Berlin, and the Chester Beatly. These documents have been delightfully reviewed by Chauncey P. Leake,[17] and carefully analyzed by the famous Egyptologist, Herman Grapow and many others. Other sources are the many carved stones and statues bearing hieroglyphic historical recordings.

The Ebers Papyrus is the longest and most famous of all the papyri. It was discovered in 1862 in a tomb at Thebes together with the Edwin Smith Papyrus. It is in perfect condition and is now preserved in the University of Leipsig. On the back of this historical document is a calendar which has been of great help to Egyptologists in determining Egyptian chronology. This papyrus was written about 1500 B.C., but according to Dawson and others there is sufficient evidence that it was copied from a series of books many centuries older. "It is stated in the papyrus itself," writes Dawson,[6] "that one passage dates from the First Dynasty (ca. 3400 B.C.) and another prescription is associated with a queen of the Sixth Dynasty. Such statements as these are of no positive value in dating, because it was in Egypt, as elsewhere, a common literary artifice to ascribe to books a very ancient origin in order to enhance their value and authority."

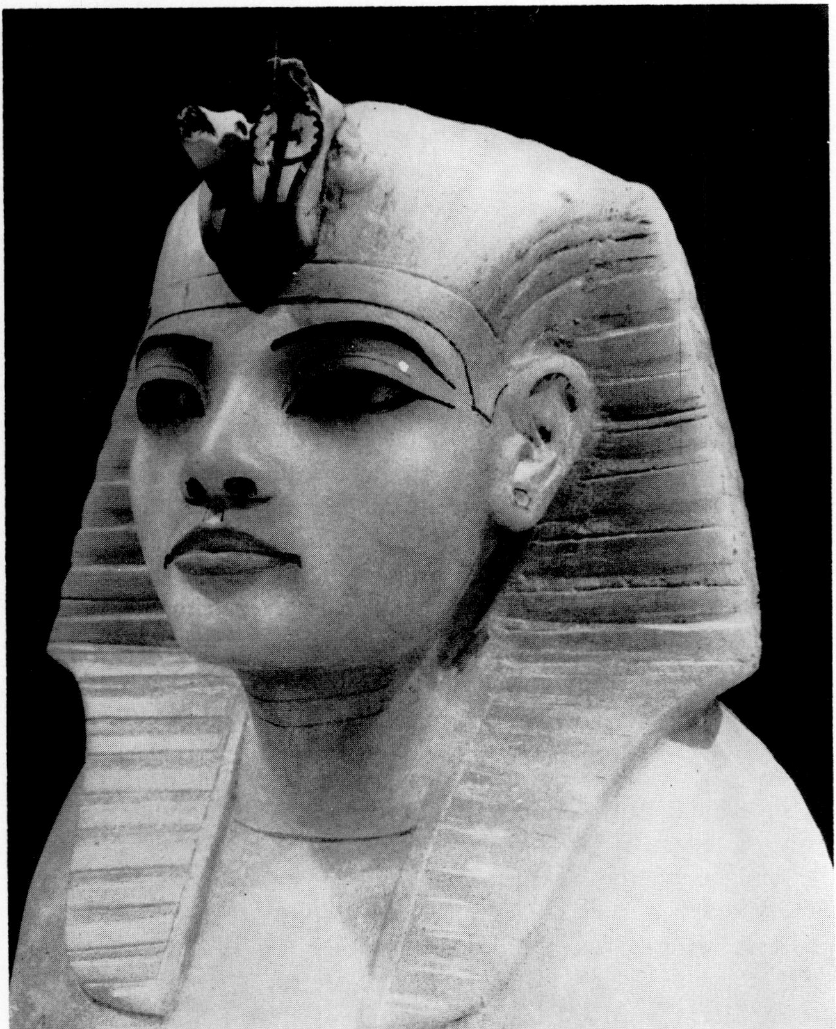

FIGURE 3. Very fine alabaster head from one of the four canopic urns, in the form of Tutankhamen's head, serving as stoppers for the compartments of the canopic chest containing the viscera. (Cairo Museum.)

The Hearst Papyrus was discovered in 1899, by a native, who in 1901 brought it tied up in a head cloth to Dr. Reisner who was then excavating in the neighborhood. It was subsequently acquired by the University of California where it is now preserved. Because of its early rough handling (tied up in a head-cloth), the roll is somewhat damaged along its folds and three columns of writing almost completely obliterated. The rest of the document is in good condition and consists of fifteen closely written columns of writing. It resembles the Ebers Papyrus which dates from the same period.

The Berlin Medical Papyrus is of a somewhat later date than the Ebers and Hearst documents, but like them refers to its more ancient origin. It contains 204 sections, carelessly written. A passage in the back of the roll refers to methods of ascertaining sterility and the sex of the unborn children.

A word about the Kahun Medical Papyrus which was discovered in 1889 by Sir Flinders Petrie. It is one of the oldest of the medical papyri and has been dated as in the period of the Twelfth or Thirteenth Dynasties (ca. 2000-1800 B.C.). It is legible even though the manuscript is in poor condition. Of interest is that it confines itself to one subject, gynecology, and contains 34 sections. The London Medical Papyrus, now in the British Museum is similar to the other papyri, but contains a larger proportion of purely magical matter.

Even though the papyri give much medical information, as an additional source of Egyptian medicine, the medical historian must resort to as many relevant facts as can be gleaned from the sculptures, tomb scenes, religious texts and antiquities preserved in various museums in different parts of the world, with particular emphasis to the Egyptian Museum in Cairo.

Of singular interest is a medical papyrus written in Coptic, the language of the Christian Egyptians of the ninth or tenth century. "This document," writes Dawson,[6] "is entirely purged of magic, but its arrangement and content betray its ancient origin, for it is very similar to the medical books written in the time of the Pharaohs. The groundwork is identical, and it only differs in the fact that many drugs of Greek and Arabic origin had been added to the pharmacopeia." This historical document was discovered in 1892 at Meshaikh, near the ancient Lepidotonpolis in Egypt. It is about two-and-a-half meters in length and contains more than 237 prescriptions, many pertaining to ophthalmological disorders. There are other smaller coptic fragments in the British Museum, in the Berlin Museum, in the John Rylands Library at Manchester (England) and in the Vatican Library.*

Hieroglyphic was used for formal recording by carving on stone. When papyrus was developed with brush-and-ink writing a cursive script evolved which is known as hieratic. This was written from right to left, with red ink for the headings, and black ink for the bulk of the material. From this two-toned system are derived the rubrics of our finely printed books.

Papyrus was made by interweaving split river reeds (cyperus papyrus) and then pounding the crude mats under water, and drying them to form coarse brown sheets. After being written upon with a delicate brush made from a frayed reed, they were glued together at the edges to make a roll. Fortunately, the everlasting dryness of the country has helped to preserve a great number of these valuable papyri, so rich in historical data.

In reviewing the Edwin Smith papyrus, Sigerist[12] calls attention to the picturesque manner in which symptoms were described. Thus a patient was said to be "weak like a breath that passes away"; another "has it on his back like the trouble of one who has been stung," and still another, "face is as if he wept." In the case of a patient with an obstacle in his cardia, the doctor finds that, "his belly is narrow and he is miserable to go like a man suffering from burning in the anus." In still another case, the doctor is examining a patient with an en-

---

* The approximately seven medical papyri extant, containing around 1200 different medical texts, give us a clear picture of a system of medicine partly religious and magical and partly empirical-rational. The rigid diagnoses and prescribed medications tend to show that the Egyptian doctor had relatively little personal freedom of movement within his profession. Despite this, the very specialized education with innumerable specialists made the Egyptian physician outstanding and very much in demand. Thus Herodotus, who traveled to Egypt (in the fifth century B.C.), wrote the Nile country to be a most healthy land, filled with doctors, "one of whom treats only the afflictions of the eye, another, those of the head, the tooth, the abdomen, or the internal organs."[18]

larged gland and he finds it, "like the fruit of colotropis procera, a decaying bubo whose skin is hard but not very."*

The Egyptians never developed a system of uroscopy so popular in Byzantine medicine, and in later Western Medieval Medicine. In the West, it was extremely popular and persisted until the Renaissance, when fortunately it was finally discredited.

Leake,[17] in an analysis of seven of the eight Egyptian medical papyri (omitting the Edman document), writes, "From the evidence available, it would appear that: (1) the ancient Egyptian physicians were relatively keen and accurate observers; (2) they possessed a systematic method of examination; (3) they had an idea of the significance of prognosis, and thus were aware of the natural course of untreated disease; (4) they were exploring the principles of diagnosis; and (5) they had accumulated a large body of tested agents and methods for the treatment and management of sickness. Taken as a whole, the evidence from the papyri indicates a relatively high standard of medical practice in old Egypt."

Rowling[19] has uncovered several interesting health statistics pertaining to urological problems in ancient Egypt. He is firm in the belief that because of age factors the incidence of benign prostatic hypertrophy would be low, that malignant disease of the kidney and prostate would be low, and that stone and infective diseases would be more common. As stated before, there is no evidence of surgical scars on mummies. Since the whole tradition of Egyptian thought hinged on preservation of the body from injury, both in the living and the dead, this may account for the avoidance of surgery. This trend was probably the underlying reason for the preservation of useless and painful carious teeth, rather than extraction.

Equally amazing is the complete absence of reference to catheters and description of catheters comes from Celsus in the first century. The Egyptians were familiar with copper in all

* The Edwin Smith Papyrus has been called the earliest known scientific book, for in addition to describing the treatment of wounds, it also contains comments upon the nature of the wounds and the organs affected by them. It differs from the other medical papyri which only in rare instances discuss diagnosis or symptoms. Of great interest is that the compiler attempted to record and classify systematic observations on the anatomy and physiology of the human body.

forms and equally skilled in silver soldering, yet there is no indication that catheters were ever made or used. Yet, acute retention was known for there are many recommended remedies (in the medical papyri) to help a man to pass water. Even retention of urine after spinal injury is described.

No discussion of Egypt and its contribution to medicine is complete without reference to the important role played by the rite of mummification. This ancient custom contributed much to the ultimate advance of anatomy and physiology.

The earliest definite evidence of mummification is that of a body of the Second Dynasty discovered at Sakkara.[20] By 2700 B.C. at a time of the Fifth Dynasty, mummification reached a high state of perfection. The flexed position in which the predynastic bodies were found was retained in the earliest mummies, but later found in the freely extended attitude. After the application of many layers of fine linen bandage, the mummy* was covered in resin which sets to form a hard carapace. On the outside, the details of the facial features are indicated by paint in the wrappings. The genital organs are modelled with linen and resin. Such procedures were practiced in order that the sex and personal likeness of the dead man might be perpetuated. It is believed that the custom of painting the features on the wrappings of the mummy developed the employment of masks made of cartonage. Subsequent to the masks there developed the use of anthropoid coffins with wooden masks, and still later, in Roman times, by portrait-panels depicting the features of the dead man, with the real face concealed beneath voluminous layers of linen bandages.

The embalmer's art deteriorated during the period of the Middle Kingdom (ca. 2000 B.C.) as evidence by the resultant poorly preserved, fragile mummies of that period. Great progress was subsequently made by the beginning of the Eighteenth Dynasty when new methods were introduced and continued

---

* The word mummy is used exclusively for the embalmed corpses of ancient Egypt. However mummy is not an ancient word. "Uta" and "setekh" are the Egyptian words for embalming, and bandaging was called "ges." The word "Mumia" is actually Persian and in the Arabic tongue, which was the prevalent means of communication among all the Islamic peoples from Persia to Egypt, it means asphalt and other bituminous substances.

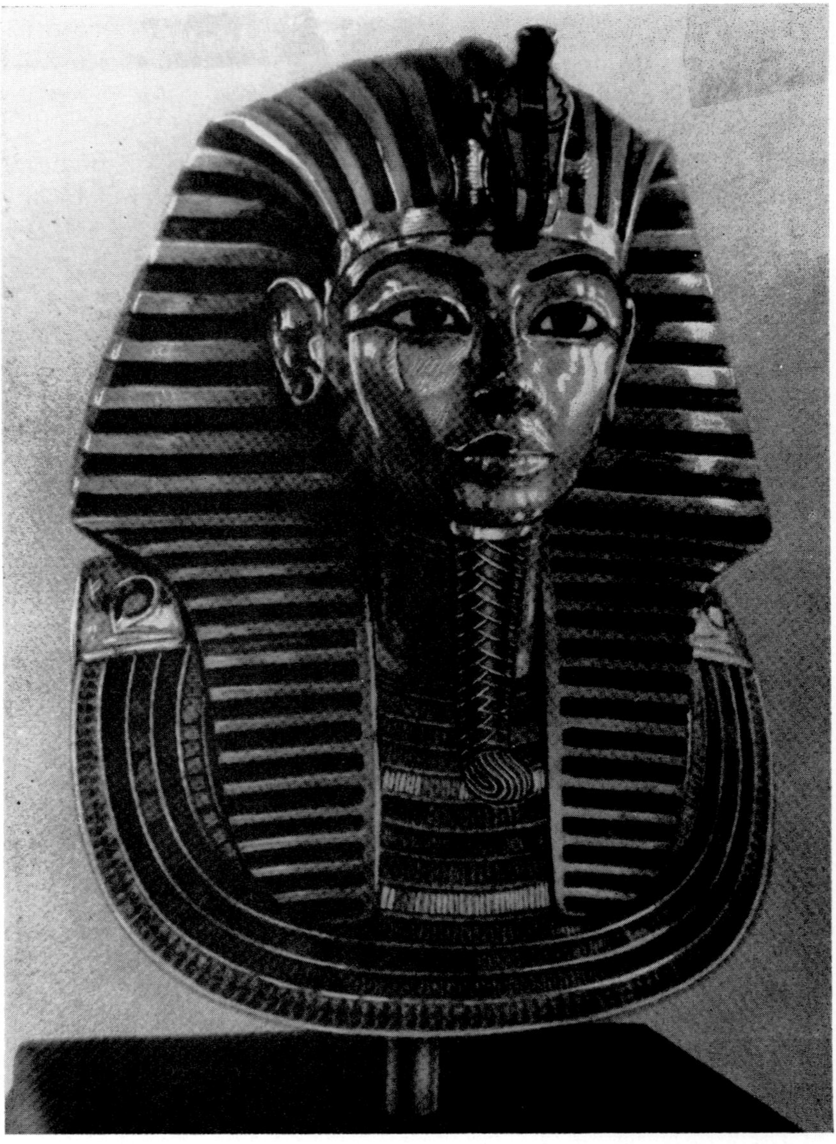

FIGURE 4. Massive gold mask which covered the head of King Tutankhamen's head. The mask is considered an admirable portrait of the king. (Museum—Cairo, Egypt.)

improvements were made from time to time. By the Twenty-first Dynasty, the most amazing methods of mummification were in vogue. By this time, the embalmers succeeded in perfect preservation of the tissues of the body but by an elaborate technique they were able to change the shrunken appearance of the corpse into a fullness of contour similar to that of a living person. They painted the entire body with red ochre and inserted artificial eyes.[21]

The art of mummification underwent a second deterioration.

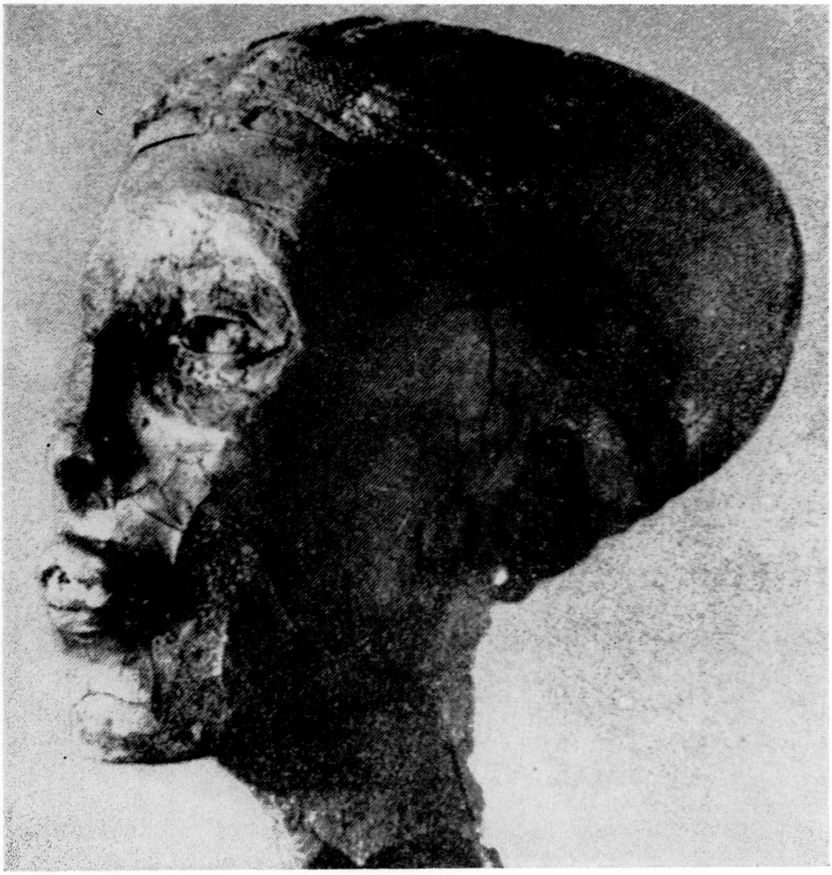

FIGURE 5. The mummified head of King Tutankhamen. Analysis of his mummy reveals that Tutankhamen was between eighteen and twenty years old when he died. (Cairo Museum, Egypt.)

Less was given to the treatment of the body itself—greater attention given to the arrangement of the superficial wrappings. But the basic procedure was maintained and the practice of mummification continued in Egypt for more than thirty centuries and singularly was imitated in many other parts of the world.

Dawson[6] believes that in considering possible origins of the process of mummification one "turns to the belief that death was not the end of life, which has prompted man from the earliest times to bury with the dead, not only amulets for protection, but objects necessary to life: food, pottery, tools, weapons and a host of other articles, which it was believed the dead would still require in a purely physical sense." It therefore soon became evident that the burial of the dead, in a small scooped out grave in the sand could not possibly accommodate the dead person and his needed possessions. This led to the custom of burying the dead in large roomy chambers which unfortunately produced decay of the corpse. This gave rise to the intensive study and ultimate success of embalming or mummification, as it is more commonly known. The modern traveller in Egypt is indeed impressed by the rich historical background and modern evaluation of antiquity when he visits Luxor, the Valley of the Kings, and the Valley of the Queens.

Due to the excellent preservation of certain mummies uncovered in Egyptian excavations, a great deal of interesting urological information has been uncovered. Although it was the custom of the embalmers of ancient Egypt to remove all the internal organs of bodies, including the kidneys, this was not always successfully performed. Since these embalmers worked through set incisions to remove the contents of the cavity of the abdomen, chest and skull, they often over-looked the kidneys. Perhaps due to haste or because of the retroperitonal location, these organs could easily be overlooked.*

* Contrary to this belief is the more scholarly explanation which explains that during the process of mummification the kidneys were left in situ in the abdomen. The Egyptians fully realized the importance of the kidneys and held them as sacred. Thus in the thirteenth chapter of the *Book of the Dead* reference is only made to the heart and kidneys: "May naught be against me in the presence of the great god, the lord of Amentet. Homage to thee, O my heart! Homage to you, O my Reins."

Ruffer* was able to examine the kidneys of three mummies. The first showed congenital atrophy of the left kidney. The second mummy dating from the Eighteenth Dynasty, around 1500 B.C., had bilateral multiple renal abscesses in which masses of bacilli were identified by microscopic examination. The third mummy dating from around 2000 B.C. or about the Twenty-first Dynasty showed ova of Bilhariza, mostly in the right ureter. Ruffer, in the same publication, reported his examination of three renal calculi obtained from the prehistorical excavations of Flinders Petrie, who found them in the debris of a male skeleton dating prior to the First Egyptian Dynasty. The first calculus weighed 30 grams, the second 24 grams. The third weighed 12 grams, and was examined chemically and microscopically. It contained leukocytes and epithelial cells and also an organic mass that could not be identified. The surrounding layers contained a mixture of phosphates and uric acid.

Gray,[22] in discussing *Radiography of Ancient Egyptian Mummies,* decries the lack of use of radiography in the study of paleopathology. He points out that though the gross anatomy of mummies has been well covered by Smith and Wood-Jones[23] and the histologic aspects by Ruffer[24] in 1921 and by Sandison[25] in 1963, they were destructive studies for they entailed the unwrapping and dissection of the specimen.

Shortly after Roentgen's epochal discovery, Petrie recognized the value of radiography.[26] He published unusual radiographs of the legs and the feet of some of his mummies. As empha-

---

* Dr. Marc Armand Ruffer, a French physician, first came to Egypt in 1893, after an extensive career in bacteriology. He was one of the founders of the British Institute for Preventive Medicine (now the Lister Institute). Ruffer journied to Egypt because of illness which he thought would be benefited by the climate in Egypt, which ultimately became his home and destiny. He became intensely interested in Egyptian mummies and actually he is regarded as the founder of "paleopathology." Sir Marc Ruffer (he was knighted for his services to England) was from the very beginning fascinated by the wealth of human remains being discovered in Egypt and published a remarkable series of papers on the subject. From 1909 until his death in 1917, he published many articles which were gathered together and published in book form under the editorship of Roy L. Moodie in 1921. This book has had a great influence on paleopathology and these papers are constantly studied and quoted by workers in this discipline. (Ref., Sandison, A. T.: *Sir Marc Armand Ruffer (1859-1917), Pioneer of Paleopathology. Medical History* 150-155.)

sized by Gray, it was extraordinary that Petrie made no mention of these radiographs in his text. On the other hand, Moodie,[27] in 1931, described his radiographic findings in 17 *Ancient Egyptian Mummies.*

Because radiography has no deleterious effect on a wrapped mummy, and particularly in view of the paucity of reports on the radiologic examination of mummies, Gray obtained permission to radiograph the specimens in the museums of Great Britain and other Eruopean countries. As objectives of the work, he stressed: (1) the presence or absence of human bones; (2) to determine the age and the sex of the person; (3) to correlate the radiographic findings with the various embalming techniques; (4) to demonstrate amulets within the wrappings; and (5) to demonstrate pathologic changes.

Gray's findings are as follows:

(1) ***Determination of Presence or Absence of Human Bones.*** "The large museums of Great Britain and other European countries contain many mummies purchased in Egypt by early nineteenth century explorers and travelers. The native dealers were quick to realize that a good profit could be made from the sale of 'souvenirs' and mummies—and forgeries were by no means uncommon. . . . On many occasions, a traveller had been sold not a mummy but a modern fake. Sometimes, a coffin proved to be empty or perhaps contained only a few bones. In one case, the wrappings of what was purported to be a mummy with a painted vellum mask concealed a concoction of wire and wood. In some instances, there was nothing inside the wrappings; in others, there was a centre core of wood or clay about which the bandages had been wrapped. Some small mummies, ostensibly those of children, were, in fact, the bandaged remains of birds."

(2) ***Determination of Age and Sex.*** "A coffin can usually be dated by its orthography and style, but it cannot be assumed that the coffin contains its original inhabitant. For example, a coffin bearing the names and the titles of a man may contain the mummy of a woman, and vice versa. Furthermore, the period to which the coffin belongs may differ widely from that of its occupant. In one case, a specimen appeared to be the un-

wrapped mummy of a woman 75 years old. Radiography, however, showed it to be that of a girl about 17 years old."

(3) ***Correlation of Radiographic Findings with Known Embalming Techniques.*** "It has been possible to correlate radiographic findings with known embalming techniques, especially in mummies of the Twenty-first Dynasty wherein the salient features are visceral packs within the body cavity, artificial eyes, and subcutaneous plumping of the body. Visceral packs between the legs suggest embalment during the later dynasties. Masses of solidified resin within the body cavity and the skull are characteristic of mummies of the Ptolemaic period."

(4) ***Demonstration of Amulets.*** "For religious reasons, amulets, made either of faience (pottery) or metal, were frequently incorporated in the wrappings. Being radiopaque, the amulets can be detected easily, and when desirable, can be and have been localised with ease and removed through small incisions in the wrappings."

(5) ***To Demonstrate Pathologic Changes.*** Under this heading, Gray lists the conditions encountered such as osteoarthritis, lines of arrested growth, fractures, other bony features, dental conditions and lesions of the soft tissues. The interested reader is referred to Gray's original articles.[28, 29] No evidence of urological disorders are reported in this unusual exploration into diseases of antiquity (evidence of malignant neoplasia, tuberculosis, syphilis, leprosy and rickets were not encountered in this study).

Among the many thousands of mummified remains which have been examined from Egyptian graves, it is remarkable that so few have shown evidence of vesical calculi. Further, the examination of these bodies was carefully performed and it is doubtful that any specimens were overlooked. G. Elliot Smith[30] remarks about this scarcity as follows:

> "The first Egyptian body that I ever saw in situ—at Mr. MacIvers excavations at El Amrah in 1901—was a prehistoric youth with a vesical calculus. Although I have been constantly on the look-out for other examples since then, I have never seen another case, although close upon ten thousand bodies must have been examined either by Dr. Wood Jones or myself

> in Nubia and Egypt. I have seen two cases of renal calculi, both in Ancient Empire graves in Egypt and one case of gall-stones (in a mummy of the New Empire).

Thus, from its rarity one can only conclude that as compared with present day frequency among civilized people, calculi were almost absent among the ancient Egyptians.

Bitschai and Brodny[31] believe that additional information concerning genito-urinary disease is furnished by medical papyri. For example in the Edwin Smith Surgical Papyrus, much space is devoted to wounds, fractures and dislocations. Unfortunately, it confines itself to a description of lesions of the thoracovertebral column and ignores the lower half of the body. There is, however, one case of particular urological interest because it identifies for the first time in history the relationship between the spinal cord and the genito-urinary organs:

> "You may examine a man suffering from a dislocation of a vertebra of his neck, and you observe that because of this he has no sensation in his arms and legs, while his penis is erect and urine escapes without his realizing it. If, however, the middle vertebra of the neck is affected, the result is release of semen . . . there is an emission of semen from the penis; that means that his penis is erect and that there is a discharge from the end of it. You would say that it remains stationary when it can neither fall nor rise. . . . The urine falls by drops and cannot be restrained."

All would agree that this description is that of a paraplegic with a lesion of the spinal cord. It is extraordinarily clear despite the then meagre knowledge of basic physiology.

In the Berlin Papyrus can be found a formula for diagnosing the sex of an unborn child:

> "To know if a woman will give birth or not—every day she puts wheat or spelt, the size of a date and enclosed in two small bags, into her urine. When both sprout it is a boy and if only the spelt sprouts, it is a girl; when they do not grow at all she will not conceive."

Another writing, again more superstitious than many of the accurate facts, handed down by the Egyptian can be found in the Kahuh Papyrus. It is a test to indicate whether a woman is sterile or whether she is pregnant. Strange as it may seem it still exists today in several regions of the world. The patient drinks a watermelon mixed with breast milk from a mother who had borne a male child; if she vomited, she was pregnant, but if she only belched she was sterile.

The Ebers Papyrus is the largest and best preserved of all the Egyptian Papyri. It is a complete document, in 108 hieratic columns. The material in the Papyrus seems to have been brought together from a number of separate sources. It is primarily a collection of prescriptions, without description of diseases, but it also contains some surgical advice and rudimentary anatomy of the vessels. Unfortunately, hundreds of technical terms of this great papyrus, especially names of diseases and drugs, have not as yet been accurately translated. It begins with three general "recitals" and then proceeds with many hundreds of recipes, classified rather loosely in accordance with the diseased states to be treated. However it also contains "cases" in which material is organized by title, examination, diagnosis, prognosis and treatment. In this historical document, the physician was advised to inspect not only the sick man's body but also what came out of it—urine, feces, "what is lifted by cough" or blood which in the case of intestinal hemorrhage is described very grapically as being "like pig's blood after it is fried."

Egyptian physicians were highly respected and in great demand for thousands of years. Homer believed they were the best available. Persian emperors and other Eastern potentates requested their services. Herodotus the Greek historian found the Egyptian doctors grouped into specialties. He wrote, "the practice of medicine is so divided amongst them that each physician is a healer of one disease and no more, some of the eye, some of the teeth, some of what pertains to the belly."

The kings of many nations used all methods to attract Egyptian physicians to their courts. Thus Cyrus sent to Egypt for an oculist, and Dovius obtained an Egyptian specialist to treat his mother's eyes. When the Greeks (sixth century, B.C.) began to take their important place in the medical world, they utilized many of the Egyptian theories particularly the Egyptian materia medica.* Egyptian medicine possessed many valuable vegetable drugs still included in the modern pharmacopeia, materia medica as reflected in the works of Dioscorides and Galen were unquestionably enriched from Egypt as will be seen in our study of Greek medicine.

---

* For example, the use of castor oil in antiquity is well confirmed by the Papyrus Ebers which has a very interesting passage on the ricinus plant which is quite unique in the medical literature of Egypt. Sigerist[12] (p. 340) quotes Dawson's translation as follows:

> "List of the virtues of ricinus: it was found in an ancient book concerning the things beneficial to mankind. If its peel is brayed in water and applied to a head that suffers, it will be cured immediately as though it had never suffered. If a few of its seeds are chewed with beer by a person who is constipated, it will expel the faeces from the body of that person. The hair of a woman will be made to grow by means of its seeds. Bray, mix into one mass, and apply with grease. Let the woman anoint her head with it. Its oil is made from its seeds. For anointing sores with a foul discharge (the trouble will depart as though nothing had occurred. It will disappear by anointing thus for ten days. Anoint very early in the morning in order to expel them (the sores) a true remedy (proved) millions of times."

Chapter IV

The World of Hippocrates

Greece

AS in all peoples of antiquity, the origin of Greek medicine dates back beyond recorded medicine. It is characterized by a peculiar mixture of mythology and rationality. Greek medical practitioners were less handicapped by ritual or religious customs than were medical practitioners in other countries. Between the millennium of 500 B.C. and 500 A.D. the art of medicine in the ancient world developed most remarkably in Greece. Before this unusual millennium, Greek medicine followed the pattern of magico-religious practices. During the creative period (500 B.C. and 500 A.D.) the name of Hippocrates dominated all medical thoughts and medicine became an art, a science and a profession.

It is difficult to assess the development of medicine in Alexandria but there is no question that it attracted the best scientific and medical talent. The young doctor of antiquity wisely planned to study at Alexandria, just as the young doctor of today plans to study in a large medical center. Such training in antiquity, as even today, was essential for recognition and success.

The scholars at Alexandria also gathered together most of the available medical writings. The result of their efforts was the *Hippocratic corpus,* believed by scholars to be the remnants of the medical literature which had circulated anonymously in the fifth and fourth centuries. For philological reasons and also to add authenticity to the writings, they were attributed to Hippocrates.[32]

Sigerist[12] delightfully and brilliantly introduces a reader to Greek* history in the following manner:

"The Fifth Century B.C. was the Golden Age of Greek culture, the time to which Greeks and Romans always looked back as their classical age, the time that formulated ideas and ideals and set the style for centuries to come. In this cultural development, Athens was foremost, a small town with a small hinterland Attica, and a total population which probably never exceeded 300,000 including over one-third slaves and about 40,000 metics or resident aliens. Pericles made the city one of the most beautiful in the world. Architecture, sculpture, and paintings flourished as never before. Even in the present ruined state, the Acropolis of Athens presents an overwhelming sight with its stairway over which the processions marched; the Prophylaea, a monumental gateway; the graceful temple erected to Nike, goddess of victory; the Erechtheum, house of a mythical king of Athens, with its 'Porch of the Maidens,' and the noble structure of the Parthenon, of Pentelic Marble, which today looks and feels like old ivory, built and decorated by the best artists of the time to house the protectoress of Athens, the virgin goddess Athena."

Before we delve into the contributions of Greece to medicine and urology, it is well for the reader to bear in mind that medicine, wherever it originated, whether in archaic times, among the Chinese or the Indians, in the old cultural centers of Mesopotamia, Egypt or in classical Greece, it was always associated with religion. For example, the medicine of ancient Greece is traditionally associated with the name of Aesculapius, an image after the likeness of Imhotep, in Egypt. The only difference is that Imhotep was deified by the decree of a Pharaoh, whereas the more democratic Greeks, justified the deification

---

* Greece was apparently uninhabitated in Paleolithic times, but the remains of Neolithic peoples occur throughout the Aegean area. Their ethnic character remains unknown, though they presumably did not speak an Indo-European tongue and were related among themselves.

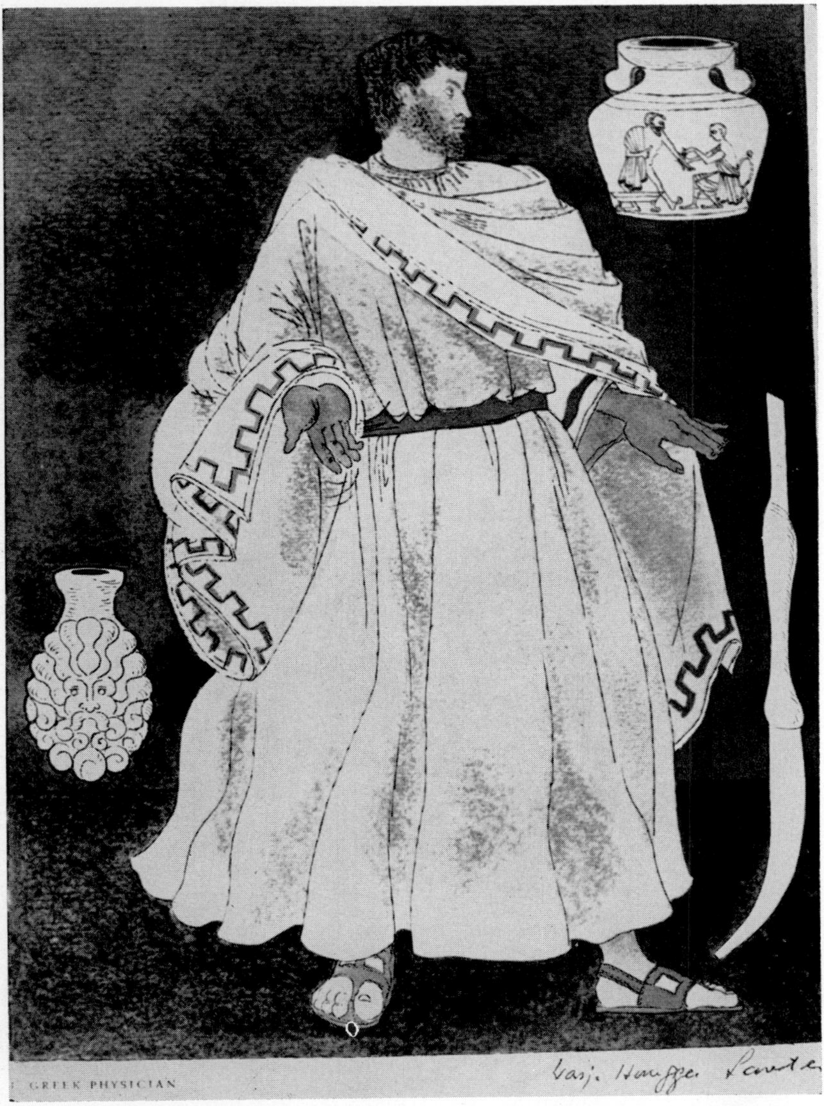

FIGURE 6. Greek Physician. (Courtesy of Abbott Laboratories: Collection of Medical Costumes, portrayed by Warja Honegger—Lavater.)

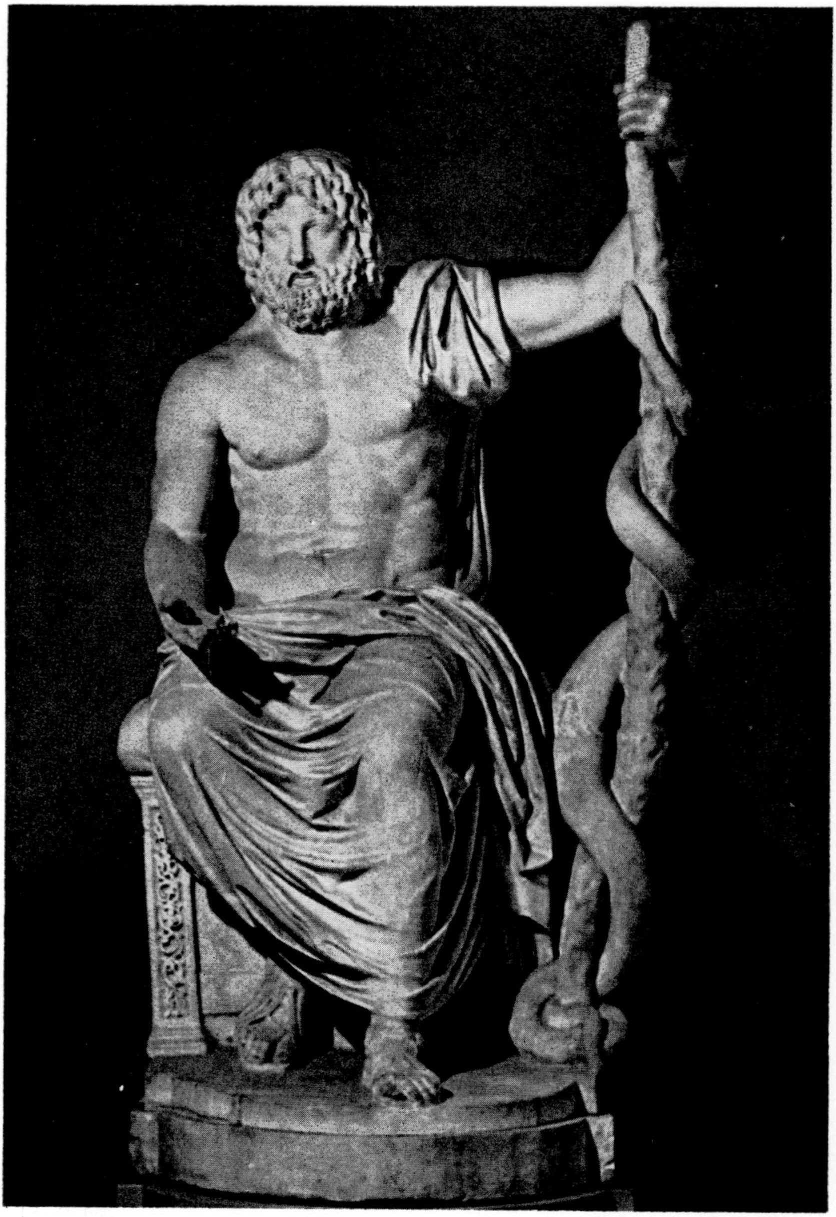

FIGURE 7. The Staff and Serpent, the traditional symbol of medicine, has a long lineage. Ancient Greece and Rome had abundant representations, of which this "Enthroned Aesculapius" is an example, dating back to Rome of the 4th Century. Artist not known. (The Ny Carlsberg Glyptothek, Copenhagen.)

of Aesculapius, by accepting the belief that he, Aesculapius, was the son of Apollo. This was easily accepted by the Greeks, who were familiar with the polygamous habits of their Olympian Gods and their predilection for carnal union with human females.

Greek philosophy and medical thought is the accumulated treasures of two thousand years of Babylonian and Egyptian thought. Credit must therefore be given to Egypt and Babylonia for their basic success in astronomy and mathematics which served as a stimulus to the Greeks. Bettman[33] summarizes the Greek inheritance in the following manner: they sorted it out, tried to discard magic, and merge the remainder into a rational structure. The new edifice took time to build, and it required new methods, careful observation (in place of blind beliefs), plus the certainty that disease was a natural phenomenon, and not a divine infliction. But once the structure was up, it stayed up, and remains, even today, one of the most significant landmarks of Western civilization.

No one will deny that the Greeks invented the science of medicine for it was Hippocrates who separated medicine from philosophy. Classical Greek medicine was an art, not a science and the truly Hippocratic doctor was primarily concerned with the patient, not with the disease. In fact, throughout antiquity, the good physician tried to reject the myth of scientific nomenclature; for him, the symptoms were the disease and he treated the patient and not the organs of the body. When etiological and anatomical thought became predominant it was accepted as signs of decadence rather than progress and accomplishment. The Hippocratic books, generally speaking, consider knowledge of the structure of the human body a help to the physician; the functioning of the organs as such does not explain disease. The work of the founders of human anatomy may have tended to divert the attention of the researcher from the whole to the parts of the body, as Galen subsequently stressed in his writings.

There is no question that Greek medicine followed an entirely different course than that of Babylonian and Egyptian medicine. Many have attributed this deviation to the creative power of individuals living in enlightened Greece. Nevertheless, as so patly stressed by Edelstein[34] in his Garrison Lecture of 1960, other factors must be taken into consideration.

The first is that medicine in Greece remained free from all legislative interference. In Egypt, as Aristotle pointed out, any change in treatment before four days have passed is prescribed by the doctor at his own risk. In our discussion of Babylonian medicine, Chapter II, the code of Hammurabi is quoted that he who is unsuccessful in surgery will have his hands cut off. Such prohibitive regulations make men cling to tradition and stifle the courage to attempt ever new things. Thus Greek inventiveness, unhampered, led to many improvements and changes, in the field of medicine. Despite this freedom, the Greeks and the Romans developed a strong code of medical ethics not found in other parts of the world.

At one time in Greece as well as in Rome, diseases were believed to be sent by the gods. By the fifth century B.C. this view no longer existed and the Hippocratic writings discuss the divine origin of only one disease, epilepsy. All other diseases were the result of natural causes. Paradoxically, it was believed that divine power could heal disease and this was not discouraged.

In the days prior to Hippocrates, Grecian medicine was in the hands of a religious organization, the priests of Aesculapius, the deified Grecian hero of medicine. Haggard[35] describes the setting as follows:

> "The marble temples dedicated to this god were on the country hillsides, overlooking the blue Aegean. Olive groves and columned porticoes made them beautiful sanatoria. Beyond the entry of each was a statue of Aesculapius,* represented as a bearded man of kindly mien holding a staff about

---

* The family of Aesculapius and his descendents devoted themselves to healing, which they considered their special prerogative. They built shrines, and served in the temples of the hero-god. Sacrifices were offered to his wife Epione at Epidauros, while his daughters assisted him in the ritual, and administered to the sick. Hygieia was not a healer, but represented health. She aided in receiving the suppliants and cared for the sacred serpents.[36]

which twined a snake—the caduceus,† the emblem of the physician even to this day. Besides him were representations of his daughters, Hygieia and Paracea . . . the ill applied for admission to these temples. They slept before the statue of the god. In their dreams he and his daughters were supposed to minister with divine healing to the worshippers. The following day the priests would administer such simple medicaments as their knowledge provided, perform crude surgical operations, and prescribe baths and diet. . . . These healing priests assumed no responsibility. The gods, so they said, brought disease; the gods and only the gods could relieve it. The priests could intercede for divine aid, but they had no incentive to seek the cause of disease or to search for means for cure and prevention. Under such a system of medicine no progress could be made; for all its dignified and beautiful surroundings the ancient Grecian medicine was, in principle at least, no better than that of early savage men. The will of deified heroes had come in to replace the malign influences of spirits; but the change indicated progress of religion, not of medicine."

---

† The origin of the caduceus motif is of most ancient vintage. The actual origin of this symbol (caduceus) of the American Medical Association is a fascinating and complex historical problem. The serpent staff dates even further back than the Graeco-Roman era, for example beautifully carved flint knives, dating from the late Gerzean Period of Egypt, circa 3100 B.C., have intertwined snakes incised in gold-foil or ivory handles. These knives are of extraordinary beauty and they may well have been used for ceremonial purposes in cultic rites. "Comparative study," writes Bunn,[37] "of designs on the knife handles with those of Mesopotamian cylinder seals clearly demonstrates that the pattern has a Mesopotamian origin and were borrowed by Nile dwellers." Indeed, certain cylinder seals, circa 3500 to 3000 B.C. are decorated with intertwined serpent-necked lions and intertwined copulating vipers which were prime religious symbols for the gods of fertility.[38]

Of even greater historical interest is the libation cup of King Gudea, which is decorated with a two-snake staff. This cup can now be viewed in the Louvre, recovered during excavations at Tellok, ancient Lagash. This cup dates to circa 2000 B.C. On this cup can be seen intertwined serpents going up from the base on either side of a staff and approach to the rim of the cup.

Budge[39] points out the single-serpent staff motif is also most ancient, and describes an artistic portrayal of a remarkable early Egyptian human of the old Kingdom, circa 2800 to 2250 B.C. depicts the goddesses Nekhebet and Sati presenting to Horus, a son of Osiris, the gifts of life and sovereignty symbolized by a staff about which is entwined a serpent. There is no denial of the ancient connection between the serpent and healing. The ancients strongly believed in the dark enshrouded historical background of the serpent as a factor in death or life.

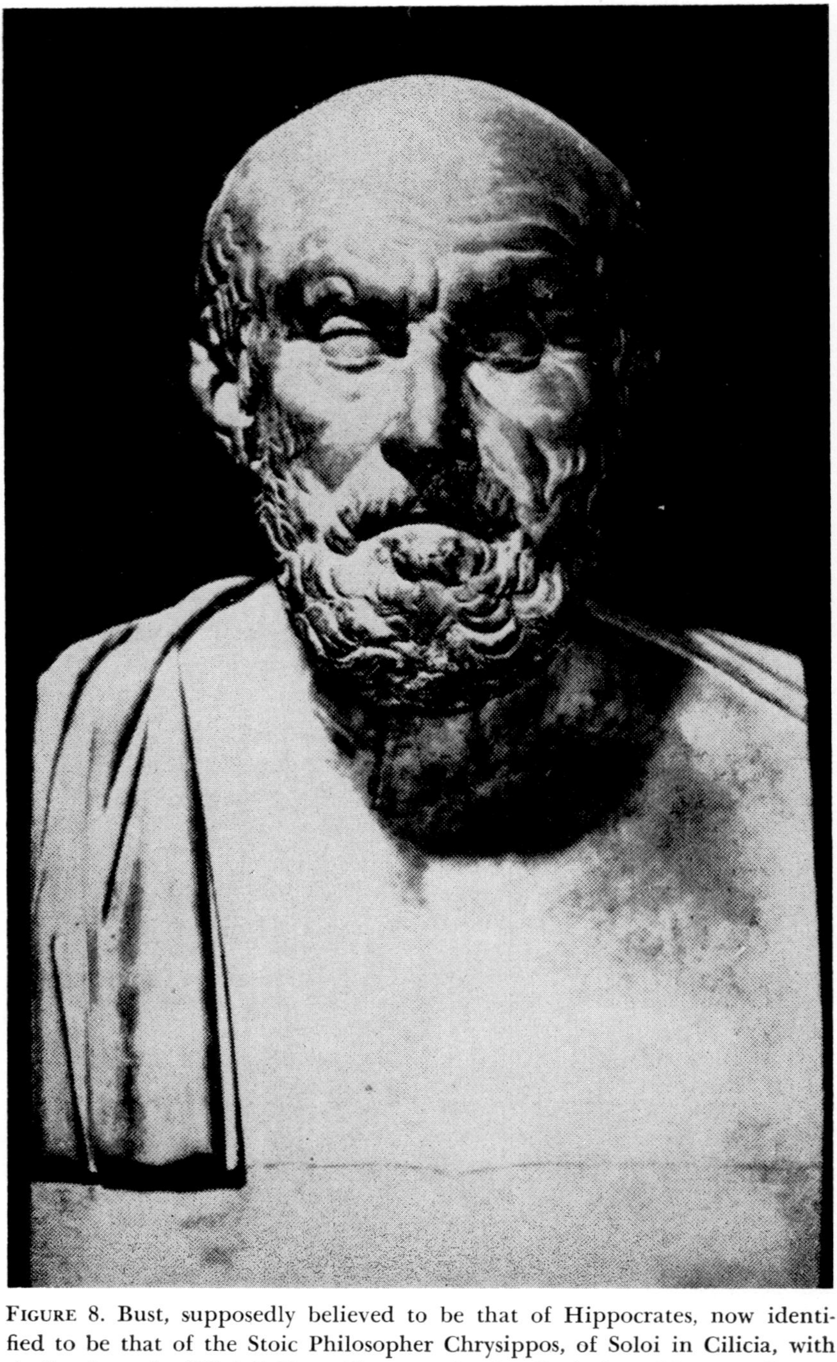

FIGURE 8. Bust, supposedly believed to be that of Hippocrates, now identified to be that of the Stoic Philosopher Chrysippos, of Soloi in Cilicia, with similar busts in Uffizi Gallery, Florence; in the Capitolene Museum, Rome; and in the British Museum.

Now, when we come to the days of Hippocrates* we see a definite change indicative of progress in medicine, at the expense of religion. For it was Hippocrates who separated medicine from religion. He also supplied for the first time a basic philosophy and basic ethics destined to be the great guiding influence of the medicine of tomorrow. It is true that men long before Hippocrates, namely the *Babylonians and Egyptians, had noted certain symptoms* of disease, but Hippocrates took these isolated facts, coordinated them and organized them into a flexible science. In addition, it was Hippocrates who sat beside his patients and was the first to painstakingly uncover symptoms, and record them, which were to him indications of the underlying pathology or the struggle between the patient and the disease. Thus, after much experience, he was able to define and classify disease in a manner which heretofore had never been attempted. Unfortunately, at the very peak of ancient Grecian culture, civilization declined. Within a century after Hippocrates we find this decline quite apparent and medicine haltingly brought to a stop in its progress and emancipation. It now remained for Galen (600 years later), the last of the great physicians of the Roman period, to revive Hippocratic medicine, which we shall see as our story unfolds itself.

---

* According to Garrison and Morton, classical philologists consider that many of the writings attributed to Hippocrates were in fact written by members of the Hippocratic school, of which he was one. Hippocrates himself is, by common consent, the greatest physician of all time, the "Father of Medicine."

Little is known about Hippocrates and many misleading and confusing statements concerning his birth, education and life have been published. For many years, and until about twenty years ago, the accepted portrait of Hippocrates was that of the BUST in the Uffizi Gallery in Florence. This bust is now identified as that of the stoic philosopher CHRYSIPPOS, of SOLOT in Cicilia. Similar heads of the same individual are found in the Capitolene Museum, Rome, and in the British Museum. New evidence unearthed in the ancient and abandoned city of Ostia at the mouth of the River Tiber, revealed the bust of an elderly bearded man, with fragments of the nose and right side of the face, broken off, now accepted as the likeness of Hippocrates. Despite the disfigurement, it is a sensitive and interesting face, quite different from the previously accepted "Hippocrates." A similar head is on a well known coin of the island of Cos. Further confirmation points to the fact that this head is of someone important like Hippocrates. Four other busts have now been identified as the same man. One is in Florence, one in Naples, and one in Copenhagen, and one in the Vatican. These busts had previously been identified with another Hellenistic philosopher named Karneades.[40]

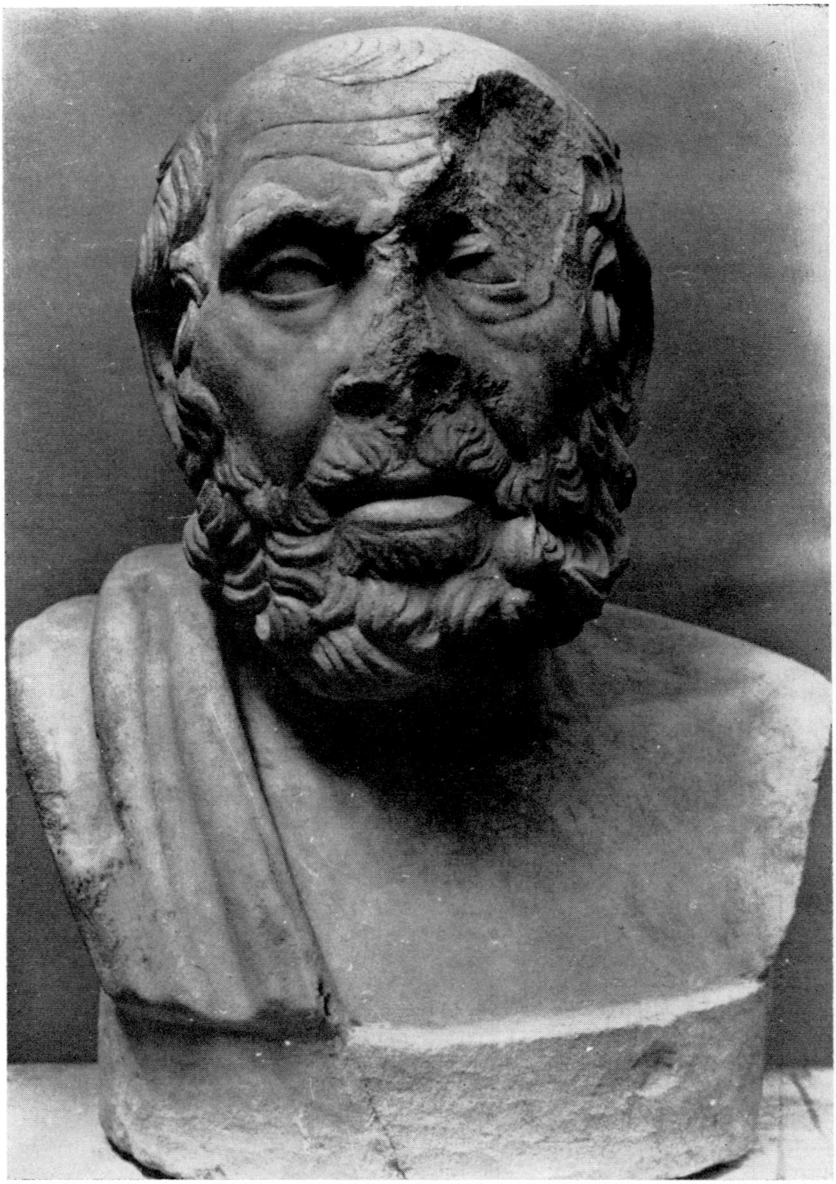

FIGURE 9. This is a photograph of a bust discovered in the abandoned city of Ostia at the mouth of the Tiber River. It is now accepted as the likeness of Hippocrates. Richards believes this head corresponds closely with that on a well known coin of the Island of Cos, of a date of the first century A.D., showing the initials ITT (Hip), and a caduceus. (Photograph courtesy of Dr. Dickinson W. Richards, Jr., and *Journal of the American Medical Association.*)

The Hippocratic physician has been described as a craftsman who had to compete for his existence and for whom prognosis was a means of furthering his reputation rather than a form of scientific interest. These men were the first to insist that a mass of anonymous medical writings of the fourth and fifth centuries were attributed to Hippocrates. It is most likely that this was done to insure authenticity and thus guarantee the adoption of new ideas.

The Hippocratic Oath, so familiar to all physicians, has within recent years also come under close scrutiny by many medical historians. Edelstein, in discussing this ancient document, raises the ambivalent interpretation of the Oath. Thus the physician swears to maintain "purity and holiness" in his life and in his art, yet this cannot be accomplished if the Oath is specifically followed. This can only be explained by assigning the Oath to a particular group of physicians who were followers of the Pythagorean principles. If this be so, the Oath was of a relatively later date and could not possibly have much influence during the centuries preceding the Christian era.

A further explanation of this Oath follows study of the social circumstances of the Hippocratic doctor. This reveals the relatively low social status and the means he used to establish and maintain his reputation. Such an attitude is contrary to the universal belief that the Hippocratic physician was a scientist-philosopher, trying to live up to the lofty principles of the *Hippocratic Oath.*

Edelstein,[34] after eliminating the Aristotelian and Epicurean schools as advocates of *Hippocratic Oath,* attributes the dogma of the Oath to the Pythagoreans. This he did for among all the Greek thinkers, the Pythagoreans alone outlawed suicide. Actually, suicide to the Pythagoreans was a sin against God who had allocated to man his position in life as a post to be held and to be defended. Thus, "Any physician who accepts such a dogma naturally must abstain from assisting in suicide or even from suggesting it. Otherwise, he would be guilty of a crime, he no less than his patient, and in this moral and religious conviction the doctor can well find the courage to remain deaf to his patient's insistence, to his sufferings, and even to the clamor of the world which disagrees almost unanimously with the stand taken by him." Thus, the physician is enjoined in the *Hippocratic Oath,* influenced by Pythagorean doctrines, to refrain from aiding or advising suicides.

Similarly, the Pythagorean influences disapproved of abortion; whereas most of the Greek philosophers commended abortion. Plato recommended abortion, particularly when the parents passed the age advantageous for begetting children. Aristotle believed a well-ordered community could only be maintained by control of the population and acceptance of abortion was a good procedure to accomplish this.

Of interest is that Artistotle advocated abortion to be performed before the foetus had attained animal life, for if performed later, abortion was not compatible with holiness. Here again, the Pythagoreans differed and believed that the embryo was an animate being from the moment of conception, and regardless of when abortion was practiced, it meant destruction of a living being.

The Pythagoreans had marked ascetic rigorism, concerning sexual matters and matrimony in general. They disapproved of extramarital relations and even in matrimony coitus was advocated only to produce children. They considered it a moral obligation to beget children so that adequate worshipers of the gods would exist. Thus, when the physician swears never to give poison or abortive remedies: "In purity and holiness I will guard my life and my art," it actually must be the purity and holiness of the "Pythagorean way of life" to which he dedicates himself.

The ambivalence of the Greek physician is further demonstrated by his negative approach to many diseases. Thus, they seemed to be satisfied with the statement that *such and such a person can be helped no more.* In fact, they advised against treating patients who cannot be cured and believed it essential to know when a case was hopelessly incurable, and in such cases avoid any therapy. No one can deny that this is indeed an inhuman behavior. When the art of the physician is no longer available, the afflicted one resorted to incantations and prayers, for it was the belief that when the physician could not help, the gods would help. In this respect, the Methodists were the first to treat chronic diseases regularly and were the only physicians who objected to the possibility of divine interference. "But in general," writes Edelstein, "religious medicine is, throughout antiquity, a subsidiary of human healing by surgery, diet, drugs, and music."

The urologist of today as well as others who swear by Apollo to the *Oath of Hippocrates* are puzzled by: "I will not use the knife either on sufferers from stone, but *I will give place to such as are craftsmen therein.*" It is puzzling for the treatment of stone by operation is one of the oldest surgical procedures. Many scholars and philologists who question why this operation is forbidden by the *Oath,* believe this is only so to distinguish between the practice of internal medicine and that of surgery. Throughout antiquity, surgery was accepted as beneath the dignity of the physician and was confined to those so-called barber surgeons. Some scholars have even suggested that since impotence frequently followed such a procedure (perineal lithotomy) its practice was not advocated. But if this were so, i.e., the physician for moral reasons refused to do the operation, he morally cannot assign the task *("I will give place to such as are craftsmen therein").*

It is indeed a dilemma. The words must mean what in the opinion of all early interpreters they seemed to mean, namely that lithotomy is here excluded because the performance of operations was held to be incompatible with the physicians craft. The one example given by the *Oath* intends to exclude surgery from the field of the physician. It is possible that originally more operations were named as forbidden but that these references are missing only in the preserved text. Such a hypothesis has not as yet been verified. It is more probable, however, that the statement as it stands is intact but in itself carries broader implications. In short, the *Hippocratic Oath* could not possibly be an expression of the common Greek form of medicine. Instead, it is an ethical code which probably reflects opinions characteristic of a small and isolated group, namely, the Pythagoreans.*

It seems but natural to assume, that as man's basic quasi-scientific knowledge grew, that abnormal changes in the appearance of the urine would be noted and be associated with bodily disease and afflictions. This did not, however, definitely become established until early in the Grecian period, with more definite indications and applications of uroscopy quite devoid of magic and superstition.

Hippocrates devoted a special book to the study of urine

---

* In the study of antiquity we read a great deal about the *Dogmatists* and the *Empiricists* as well as the *Methodists* who were the most important physicians in Imperial times. Statements about *Methodist* doctrines are encountered in the writings of Celsus and Galen. From records now available, it appears that all three groups believed in human individuality and to influences of climate of geographic location. The *Methodists* differing from the *Empiricists* and *Dogmatists,* believed it was unnecessary to know what part of the body is sick or may have caused the illness. The disease alone is the index of what one needs to know and he is therefore advised to observe certain general conditions of the body. For example, he should be aware of the body's dryness, its fluidity, and a mixed condition, as well as variations of this in different parts of the body.

Thus, it follows that such knowledge must affect and influence treatment. Advice is then given to make a dry body moist and a moist body dry. The treatment is aimed at the whole body for it is the whole body that is sick. Even in surgical problems, many *Methodists* believed it possible to practice on nothing more than the three conditions named above, and that only in cases of foreign bodies is the philosophy altered.

Of course, such philosophy was not universal and opponents of the *Methodists* raised violent objections to this thinking. The objectors believed that the omission of observation of season and locality and failure to take into consideration the human constitution meant a narrowing of medicine and placed treatment of human beings in the same category as the treatment of animals.

Of singular interest is that in the first century A.D., *Methodism* was more highly thought of in Rome than were *Dogmatism* and *Empiricism.* Why did the Romans prefer *Methodism?* It is possible that this preference existed because *Methodism* used fewer drugs and also because the routine advised gave greater consideration to usual routine or in many instances left it unchanged. This partiality was significant, for the history of *Methodism* was determined by the master race, whose appreciation of medicine differed greatly from that of the Greeks.

Methodism continued to play a vital role even in the Middle Ages. At the beginning of the Renaissance, little value was given to this philosophy. Yet, it had some influence on the development of medicine even in the 17th and 18th centuries. In the following century, its influence was purely historical.

which was entirely disassociated from magic and superstition. He wrote:

> In fevers the urine is best when the sediment is white, smooth and consistent during the whole time, until the disease comes to a crisis. The most deadly of all kinds of urine are the fetid, watery, black and thick; in adult men and women the black is of all kinds of urine the worst, but in children the watery. If the urine is passed in deficient quantity with a noise, it indicates either that the man stands in need of purging, or that the bladder is diseased. A small quantity of blood passed without fever and pain does not indicate anything bad, but proves a solution to a state of lassitude. If the urine is passed with pain and if pus be passed along with the urine in fever, the physican should announce that the patient will thus be relieved of his complaints. Thick urine having a thin sediment indicates some pain and swelling around the joints.

Hippocrates basically recognized four conditions of the urinary tract. In Greek thought, the number four was somehow of special significance. For example, the so-called primary elements were four in number—earth, air, fire and water; the primary qualities—hot, cold, moist and dry were similarly four; Alcmaeon held to the four regions of the body-causes and as described above Hippocrates held to the four humors which corresponded to the four temperaments. Of course, a single humor could assume many forms, for example nasal mucus could be watery and transparent, or thickened and colored, or dried and hard, all in various degrees.

> "One should consider respecting the kinds of urine which have clouds, whether they tend upwards or downwards with the colors as described are to be reckoned good and commended; but such as are carried upwards with the colors as described are to be held bad and are to be distrusted."

In cases of fever, Hippocrates laid great stress on the examination of the urine: "One may judge from the urine what is to take place, for if it is thicker and more yellowish so much the better, but if it be thinner and blacker so much the worse."

Theophilus, who lived under Heraclius (A.D. 610-641), mentions the application of heat to urine as a diagnostic test referring to the cloudiness caused by heating albuminous urine. He described other pertinent observations of the urine in disease: "The urine of persons leading a sedentary life had more sediment than that of those who followed an active vocation; the urine of women from this cause has generally more sediment than that of men; that of children more than that of adults; and that of persons who live grossly than the urine of temperate persons." Theophilus described the character of oily urine, "when the appearance of the urine resembles oil still more, it indicates an increase of the melting of the fat; and when the urine in consistence and color appears exactly like oil of a dark color, it prognosticates a collapse and death."

Theophilus wrote a confirmation of one of the aphorisms of Hippocrates: When in ardent fevers the urine has an oily sediment it prognosticates death. Tar-like urine, as it is called from the resemblance of the sediment to the color of tar (ervium ervilia) which according to Wellcome might be better called the frumous, since, as Acturaris explains, the deposit bears a close resemblance to clots of blood. Such urine was believed by Theophilus to be indicative of the melting of the flesh. It is of interest to note that the scaly urine derived its name from small substances resembling husks or hulls of grain in the urine, and in febrile diseases was supposed to indicate great disorder of the general system, but otherwise to be connected with an affliction of the bladder.

The word *furfuraceous* is frequently encountered in these writings, and it derives its name from the resemblance of the sediments to bran. It, too, was believed to be symptomatic of a local disease of the bladder, or of a constitutional disorder with fever. The word gritly and its application to urine, was so called because of the resemblance of the substances in the urine to large particles of grown grain, and Hippocrates regarded it to be of very serious significance in fevers.

But what about anaesthesia? Archer[41] writes that Aesculapius, the god of medicine was supposed to have used a potion, nepenthe, to produce insensibility in his patients, before he operated upon them.

The Greeks (later the Romans) used a form of local anaesthesia by placing in the region they desired to be anaesthetized the "stone of Memphis" treated with vinegar. Kleinman[42] believes that the anaesthetic effect produced was the result of a chemical reaction. Since the Memphis stone was composed of carbonates, when exposed to the vinegar, it liberated carbon dioxide which presumably numbed the affected part.

The famous Greek physician of the first century A.D., Dioscorides, utilized the root of the mandragora plant boiled in wine for anaesthesia to his patients before he performed any surgery. This same plant was used for centuries in Asia by the Chinese and the Hebrews in cases of criminologic investigation. The suspected criminal was forced to drink a concoction in a form of infusion with other drugs. A confused mental state took place which often led to a confession of crime. Paradoxically, it was also used to aid in the relief of the sufferings and tortures endured by accused persons, and was then referred to as the "potion of the condemned."

Herodotus tells of the ancient Scythians who breathed fumes produced by a form of hemp *(Cannabis Indica)* and in this way obtained a state of mental excitation followed by sleep. The Arabians as well as the Egyptians used the same plant which they called hashish, from which they also obtained a state of mental excitement. In the third century, Hua T'O, the celebrated Chinese physician, utilized Indian hemp to narcotize his patients.

In the *Antidotarium* of Nicholas of Salerno (about the twelfth century), is a reference to the soporific sponge as follows:

> *Spongia Somnifera*
> Take . . . of opium the baicum, juice of hyoscyamine, unripened berry of the blackberry, lettuce seed, juice of hemlock, poppy, mandragora, ivy . . . put these all together in a vessel and plunge therein a new sea-sponge just as it comes from the sea, taking care that fresh water does not touch it, and put this in the sun during the dog-days until all the liquid is consumed. And when there is need, dip it a little in water not too warm, and apply it to the nostrils of the patient, and he will quickly go to sleep. When, moreover, you want to awaken

> him, apply juice from the root of the fennel and he will soon bestir himself.

Keys[43] writes, "The action of the medicated sponge was uncertain because there could be no standardization for the drugs used, and it therefore fell into disuse. It is probable that anaesthesia in general was slow in developing because drugs could not be standardized. No attempt was made to purify them or to regulate dosage. Often, a drugged sleep resulted in death. This in itself discouraged the more staid physicians from the conquest of pain. Then, too, pain was considered in a holy light; which is to say, something that God deemed good for mankind."

Hippocrates and the great physicians of the Hellenistic world infused new life into the science of medicine. These men of genius, however, did not entirely extinguish the ancient medical lore that had held sway for centuries before their time. Much of it survived and spread far and wide. In fact, the Greeks themselves borrowed not a little from the medicine of Egypt and Mesopotamia.

Chapter V

Ancient Rome—Galenic Urology

NO discussion of Roman medicine is possible without acknowledging the great inheritance bestowed upon the Roman medical profession by the Greek physician.[44] Three hundred years after Hippocrates, Roman armies destroyed Corinth, "the pride and light of Greece," and thus Grecian medicine came into Rome. The Romans were much less interested than the Greeks in theoretical systems; they cared more for practical applicability. It follows, therefore, that the practically thinking Roman would be interested in practical doctrines of medicine, inaugurated by the Greeks, and confirmed by many years of practice.

The first healers or physicians in Rome were slaves whose medical knowledge was limited and primitive. Beginning in the fourth century B.C., Greek physicians began to emigrate to Rome despite the opposition to them by the Romans. Their superiority in medical procedures and surgical problems soon overcame this opposition, and in 46 B.C. Julius Caesar bestowed the right of citizenship upon all free-born Greek physicians on Roman soil. Indeed, more privileges soon followed, such as the exemption of doctors from taxation, military service, and the duties of taking lodgers and accepting offices.

Since there were no licensing boards, medical schools or restrictions, it now became necessary to determine who was to be a physician and by what rights he could assume this social position, which gradually was becoming more enviable than ever before. During the time of Antoninus Pius, certain rules were introduced, under which only five to seven or perhaps ten doctors could be identified as such in any Roman city, depending upon its size. Such men were called the *valde docti*, and were required to prove that they possessed medical knowledge. Thus a form of license was originated, and served to protect the physician and the patient.

Medicine among the Romans only reached a high level in the century before and after the beginning of the Christian era. This was made possible by the writings of such men as Celsus,* Dioscorides,† Aretaeus,‡ and Galen (Claudius Galenus).

The most versatile and perhaps the most successful Roman physician of later antiquity was Galen§ (130-200 A.D.). He strongly

* *Celsus,* although not a physician, was a prolific writer and a wealthy patron of science and literature. In scholarly manner, he compiled in an encyclopedic form the medical knowledge of his time. Many centuries later, during the Renaissance, his volumes were among the first medical books to be published, mainly because of the elegant literary style in which they were written.

† *Dioscorides* was a Greek surgeon under Emperor Nero. He has been recorded in history, for he was the originator of the *materia medica.* While a surgeon in the army, he studied all of the medicinal herbs of each country that he visited, and was able to accumulate data about 600 plants and plant substances. Of these, some 90 are still in use today. The work of Dioscorides remained as the official *materia medica* until the 17th century. His work was first printed in Greek by Aldus Manutius in 1499; the first Latin translation was published in 1478.

‡ *Aretaeus* was a famous Roman physician. In many ways, he resembled Hippocrates for his keen clinical methods of observation. His descriptions of pneumonia, tetanus, emphysema, the aura of epilepsy, and mental disorders still remain as great classics. He first diagnosed epilepsy resulting from a depressed fracture of the skull. Aretaeus advised bleeding to relieve the liver in melancholia, purging with aloes, and natural hot baths during convalescence. He also wrote on diabetes, to which he gave its present name. He emphasized the part which thirst plays in the symptomatology. Aretaeus' description of ulcerations about the tonsils, according to Garrison, clearly resembles diphtheria, and is unquestionably the first description of this disease.

§ According to Garrison and Morton, Galen, the founder of experimental physiology, stands second only to Hippocrates in importance during the period of Roman medicine. He was the most prolific of the ancient writers and his writings dominated medicine until the time of Vesalius. His anatomical writings are a repository of all contemporary knowledge, together with some of his own views and discoveries. He had a good knowledge of osteology and myology, some knowledge of angiology and less of zoology. Although not to be regarded as the founder of the science of anatomy, he is nevertheless the first important figure. Until Harvey, Galen was the most important figure in experimental physiology. His system of physiology was accepted until the middle ages.

Galen devoted six books to pathology. His ideas on inflammation and tumors led him to make many valuable deductions. He was familiar with cholera, hydrophobia, malaria and the relations of urinary calculi to the kidney, ureter and believed in and practiced the manifold therapeutic armamentarium of the disciples of Hippocrates. He united the principle of supporting the healing powers by solicitous symptomatic treatment with a scientifically founded, careful administration of medication.

Galen followed largely the teaching of Hippocrates, and in his *Commentary* praises him for the acuteness of his prognosis of the urine. Like other physicians of antiquity, Galen paid great attention to the characters of urine in disease, and his knowledge of the subject was remarkable considering the state of learning at the time.

For one thousand years after the death of Christ, Galen was the unquestioned authority on matters pertaining to medicine and physiology. Indeed, his reputation was so great that few of his hypotheses were seriously challenged for ten centuries. He was especially interested in the secretion of urine and the function of the kidneys, ureters and bladder. His writings are accepted as among the earliest accurate concepts of urologic physiology.[47]

Six hundred years separated Hippocrates from Galen and in this interval tremendous changes took place in material civilization, social behavior, and cultural environment. Just what were these changes and influences? The great age of Pericles was drawing to a close; Greek philosophy reached its final peak; the Macedonian empire rose and fell; the face of the western world was being altered by Rome's successful wars. Rome was the center of a great empire, yet ultimately it, too, was to fall.

In Green's translation of Galen's *Hygiene De Sanitate Tuenda,*[48] Sigerist writes an introduction of great simplicity and accuracy. This is a "must" for all who are interested in the story of Galen. In his scholastic introduction, Sigerist says:

---

bladder, and he was able to recognize pyuria. Galen's classification of tumors persisted for more than 1000 years. He considered neoplasms to be due to an excess of black bile which solidified in certain sites. He recommended purges to dissolve the black bile and, if these were unsuccessful, the knife. He was not familiar with internal tumors and employed the term "sarcoma" for any fleshy-like superficial swelling. Galen is also credited with establishing a system of medicine in the minutiae of pulse variations, which persisted into the 18th century. (Herophilus of Chalcedon is said to have counted the pulse with a water clock.)

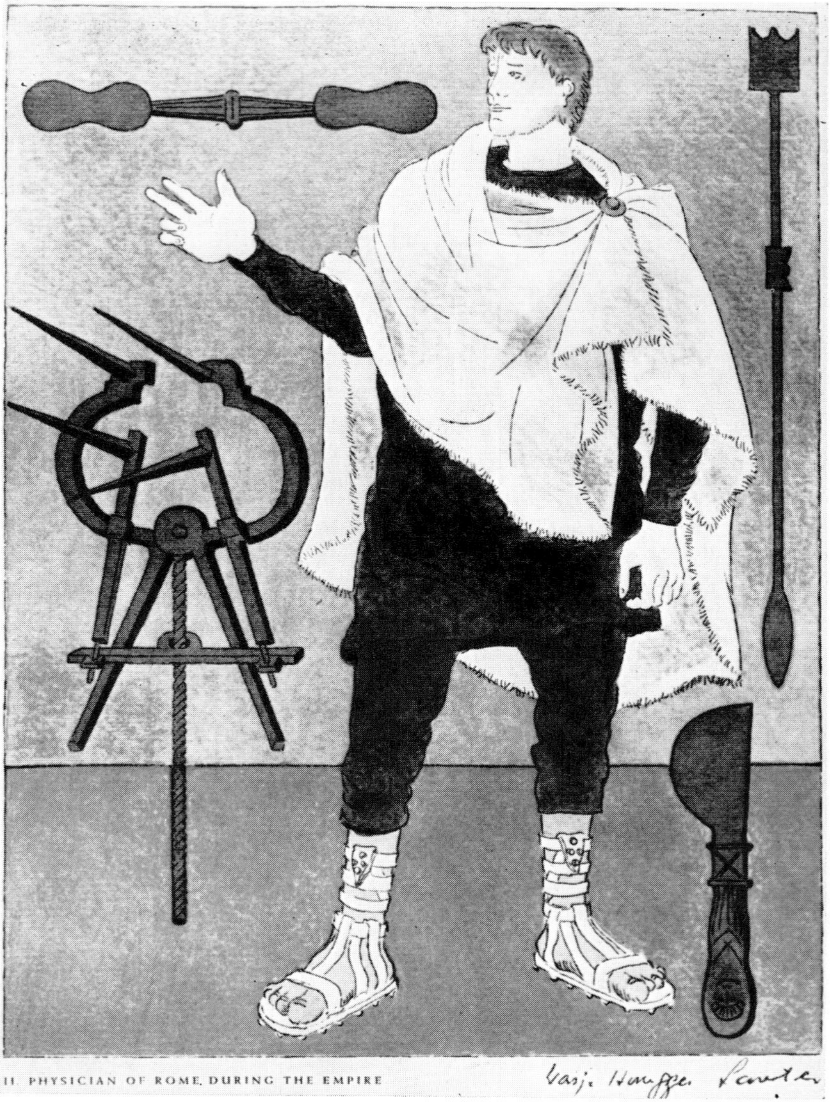

FIGURE 10. Physician of Rome during the Empire. (Courtesy of Abbott Laboratories: Collection of Medical Costumes, portrayed by Warja Honegger—Lavater.)

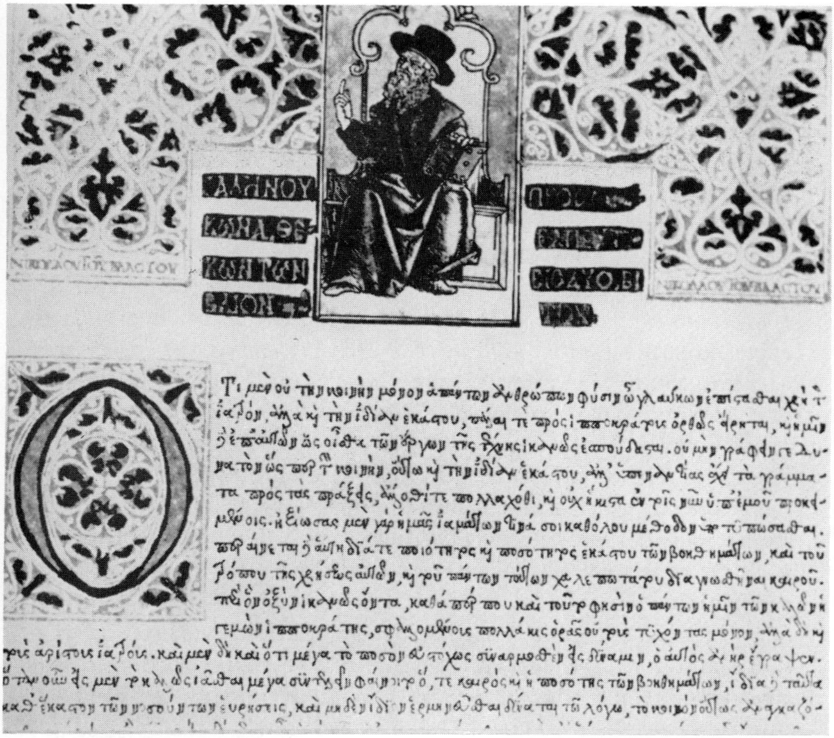

FIGURE 11. Decorative border and miniature of Galen teaching. (Therapeutica, Venice 1500. From the copy in the Wellcome Historical Medical Museum and Library. By courtesy of "The Wellcome Trustees.")

"The reader who having studied a Hippocratic treatise and turns to Galen, Hippocrates' greatest admirer and follower, feels rather bewildered. He misses the clarity and simplicity of the Hippocratic writer, his straightforward way of putting things, and finds Galen verbose, quibbling, hair-splitting at times. However, he should not let himself be discouraged, should keep reading and he will soon discover that Galen was a very great physician who has a great deal to say. Times have changed since the days of Hippocrates; almost six centuries had elapsed, generations of sophists had systematized knowledge and taught the art of disputation, and gone were the days of the democratic city states of ancient Greece. Galen wrote most of his books in imperial Rome, in the whirl of a metropolis that was the capital of the entire world."

Sigerist continues:

> "Galen's works are of capital importance for one more reason. The collection of Hippocratic writings, which includes books of different authors from various schools, gives us a splendid cross-section through the medical literature of the fourth and fifth centuries B.C. And then, for a period covering hundreds of years, we have not a single medical book preserved. The Alexandrian school flourished. Herophilus and Erasistratus attracted students from all over the Mediterranean world. Numerous and important books were written on every conceivable subject of medicine and all of them perished. If we are not totally ignorant of the theories and achievements of the Alexandrian physicians, this is merely due to the fact that they were frequently quoted by later writers. Foremost among them was Galen, who knew the books of his predecessors very well indeed, quoted them and frequently attacked them when he happened to disagree with their views. Thus his works are a huge repertory of ancient medical literature reflecting the medical lore of several centuries. The study of Galen's writings is a task equally fascinating for philologists and physicians and the first step obviously must be to prepare editions and translations which then will make it possible to analyze and evaluate the content of Galen's teachings."

Green[48] describes Galen as one of the most remarkable figures in medical history. Although we have since the days of Galen acquired much knowledge that makes us realize the inadequacy of his writings, we cannot deny that his thinking was fundamentally sound. Some of his beliefs were modern in theory. "Actually," writes Green, "Galen was a thousand years ahead of his time and it took mankind over 10 centuries to catch up with him. For nearly 1500 years, he ruled the medical world, and many of his works, thoughts, and phrases are not only embedded in our medical canon, but current in our daily speech."

Galen lived in the second century A.D., during a time characterized by stoic philosophy, early Christianity, high culture and much sophistication, accompanied by great material achievement and considerable unrest. He was born in Pergamon, in Asia Minor, probably in A.D. 130. His father (Nicon) was an architect, cultured and well educated, who directed young Galen in receiving a fine liberal education, and ultimately in the study of medicine. He studied at Pergamon, which was the site of a very famous Aesculapian temple, but furthered his medical education in Smyrna, Corinth, and finally in Alexandria, where he studied for several years and there cultivated the tenets of the School of Alexandria.

At the age of twenty-eight, he returned to Pergamon, where he was assigned as physician to the gladiators. This gave him a great deal of experience, but he shortly left for Rome, where he established a fine reputation as practitioner as well as anatomist. For some reason, probably political, he left Rome and returned to Pergamon, but was ordered by the emperor to join the army at Aguileia (close to where Venice now stands). After serving in the army, the emperor again sent him back to Rome, as medical attendant to the prince Commodus. He continued to live in Rome until about A.D. 192, and returned again to Pergamon, where he died in 200.

Galen enriched anatomical knowledge of the kidneys, bladder and sexual organs, but his real contribution was his concept of renal physiology based on animal experimentation. His writing is best exemplified in the following extract from an essay on the *Failure of Asclepiadus* to Understand the Functions of the Kidneys and Ureters:*

> "The extent of exactitude and truth in the doctrines of Hippocrates may be gauged, not merely from the way in which his opponents are at variance with obvious facts, but also from the various subjects of natural research themselves—the functions of animals and the rest. For those people who do not believe that there exists in any part of the animal a faculty for attracting its own special quality, are compelled repeatedly to deny obvious facts. For instance, Asclepiadus, the physician, did this in the case of the kidneys. That these are organs for secreting the urine was the belief not only of Hippocrates,

* Asclepiadus of Bithynia in Asia Minor (born 124 B.C.) was the first Greek doctor to introduce the Hellenic medicine in Rome. He is the teacher of Themison of Laodicea, the founder of the Methodist School.

Diocles, Erasistratos, Praxagoras, and all other physicians of eminence, but practically every butcher is aware of this, from the fact that he daily observes both the position of the kidneys and the duct, or ureter, which runs from each kidney into the bladder, and from this arrangement he infers their characteristic use and faculty. But, even leaving the butcher aside, all people who suffer either frequent dysuria, or from retention of the urine, call themselves 'nephritics' when they feel pain in the loins and pass sandy matter in their water.

"I do not suppose that Asclepiadus ever saw a stone which had been passed by one of these sufferers, or observed that this was preceded by a sharp pain in the region between kidneys and bladder, as the stone traversed the ureter, or that when the stone was passed, both the pain and the retention at once ceased. It is worthwhile, then, learning how this theory accounts for the presence of urine in the bladder, and one is forced to marvel at the ingenuity of a man who puts aside these broad, clearly visible routes, and postulates others, which are narrow, invisible, indeed entirely imperceptible. His view, in fact, is that the fluid which we drink passes into the bladder by being resolved into vapors and that, when again these have been condensed, it thus regains its previous form, and turns from vapor into fluid. He simply looks upon the bladder as a sponge, or a piece of wood, and not as the perfectly compact and impervious body that it is, with two very strong coats. For, if we say that the vapors pass through these coats, why should they not pass through the peritoneum and the diaphragm, thus filling the whole abdominal cavity and thorax with water? But, says he, of course the peritoneal coat is more impervious than the bladder, and this is why it keeps out the vapors, while the bladder admits them. Yet, if he had ever practiced anatomy, he might have known that the outer coat of the bladder springs from the peritoneum (I think here he refers to the endopelvic fascia) and is essentially the same as it, and that the inner coat, which is peculiar to the bladder, is more than twice as thick as the former."

The essay continues: "Perhaps it is not the thickness or thinness of the coats, but the situation of the bladder, which is the reason for the vapors being carried with it? On the contrary, even if it were probable for every other reason that the vapors accumulated there, yet the situation of the bladder is situated below, whereas vapors have a tendency to rise upwards; thus they would fill all the regions of the thorax and lungs before they reached the bladder.

"But why do I mention the situation of the bladder, peritoneum, and thorax? For surely, when the vapors have passed through the coats of the stomach and intestines, it is in the space between these and the peritoneum that they will collect and become liquified, as in dropsical subjects it is here that most of the vapors must necessarily pass straightforward through everything which in any way comes in contact with them, and will never come to a standstill. But if this be assumed, then they will traverse not merely the peritoneum but also the episgastrum, and will become dispersed into the surrounding air; otherwise they will certainly collect under the skin.

"Even these considerations, however, our present day Asclepiadeans attempt to answer, despite the fact that they always get soundly laughed at by all who happen to be present at their lectures on these subjects—so difficult an evil to get rid of is this sectarian partisanship, so excessively resistant to all cleansing processes, harder to heal than any itch.

The competence of the vesicoureteral junction is vividly described by Galen:

"Thus, one of our Sophists who is a thoroughly hardened disputer and as skillful a master of language as there ever was, once got into a discussion with me on this subject; so far from being put out of countenance by any of the above-mentioned considerations, he even expressed his surprise that I should try to overturn obvious facts by ridiculous arguments! 'For,' said he, 'one may clearly observe any day in the case of any bladder that, if one fills it with water or air and then ties up its neck and squeezes it all around, it does not let anything out at any point, but accurately retains all its contents. And surely if there were any large and perceptible channels coming into it from the kidneys the liquid would run out through these when the bladder was squeezed, in the same way that it entered.' Having abruptly made these and similar remarks in precise and clear tones, he concluded by jumping up and departing, leaving me as though I was quite incapable of finding any plausible answer!"

The reader will now enjoy Galen's rebuttal, which entirely depended upon his observations made in animal experimentation:

"The fact is that those who are enslaved to their sects are not merely devoid of all sound knowledge, but they will not even stop to learn! Instead of listening, as they ought to, to the reason why liquid can enter the bladder through the ureters, but is unable to go back again the same way—instead of admiring nature's artistic skill, they refuse to learn; they even go so far as to scoff, and maintain that the kidneys, as well as many other things, have been made by nature for no purpose! And some of them who had allowed themselves to be shown the ureters coming from the kidneys and becoming implanted into the bladder, even had the audacity to say that these also existed for no purpose; and others said they were spermatic ducts, and that this was why they were inserted into the neck of the bladder and not into its cavity. When, therefore, we had demonstrated to them the real spermatic ducts entering the neck of the bladder lower down than the ureters, we supposed that, if we had not done so before, we would now at least draw them away from their false assumptions, and convert them forthwith to the opposite view. But even this they presumed to dispute, and said that it was not to be wondered at that the semen should remain longer in these latter ducts, these being more constricted, and that it should flow quickly down the ducts which came from the kidneys, seeing that these were well dilated. We were, therefore, further compelled to show them in a still living animal the urine plainly run out through the ureters into the bladder; even thus we hardly hoped to check their nonsensical talk.

"Now the method of demonstration is as follows: One has to divide the peritoneum in front of the ureters, then secure these with ligatures, and next, having bandaged up the animal let him go (for he will not continue to urinate). After this, one loosens the external bandages and shows the bladder empty, and the ureters quite full and distended—in fact almost on the point of rupturing; on removing the ligatures from them, one then plainly sees the bladder becoming filled with urine.

"When this has been made quite clear, then, before the animal urinates, one has to tie a ligature around his penis and then to squeeze the bladder all over; still nothing goes back through the ureters to the kidneys. Here, then, it becomes obvious that not only in a dead animal, but in one which is still living, the ureters are prevented from receiving back the urine from the bladder. These observations having been made, one now loosens the ligature from the animal's penis and allows him to urinate, then again ligatures one of the ureters and leaves the other to discharge into the bladder. Allowing, then, some time to elapse, one now demonstrates that the ureter which was ligatured is obviously full and distended on the side next to the kidneys, while the other—that from which the ligature has been taken—is itself flaccid but has filled the bladder with urine. Then again, one must divide the full ureter and demonstrate how the urine spurts out of it, like blood in the operation of venesection; and after this one cuts through the other also, and both being thus divided, one bandages up the animal externally. Then when enough time seems to have elapsed, one takes off the bandages; the bladder will now be found empty; and the whole region between the intestines and the peritoneum full of urine, as if the animal was suffering from dropsy. Now if anyone will but test this for himself on an animal, I think he will strongly condemn the rashness of Asclepiadus, and if he also learns the reason why nothing regurgitates from the bladder into the ureter, I think he will be persuaded by this also if the forethought and art shown by nature in relation to animals."

It is indeed stimulating to read of such keenness at a time when so little was known about the circulation of the blood and human physiology. Let us now read further in Galen's *On Natural Faculties,* particularly in his concept of renal perfusion and renal secretion:

"Since, then, we have talked sufficient nonsense—not willingly, but because we were forced, as the proverb says, 'to behave madly among madmen'—let us return again to the subject of urinary secretion. Here let us forget the absurdities of Asclepiadus, and in company with those who are persuaded that the urine does pass through the kidneys, let us consider what is the character of this function. For, most assuredly, either the urine is conveyed by its own motion to the kidneys considering this is the better course (as we do when we go off to market) or, if this be impossible, then some other reason for its conveyance must be found. What, then, is this? If we are not going to grant the kidneys a faculty for attracting this peculiar quality as Hippocrates held, we shall discover no other reason. For, surely everyone sees that either the kidneys must attract the urine, or did the veins exert a propulsive action when they contract, they would squeeze out into the kidneys not merely the urine, but along with it the whole of the blood which they contain. And if this is impossible, as we shall show, the remaining explanation is that the kidneys do exert traction.

"And how is propulsion by the veins impossible? The situation of the kidneys is against it. They do not occupy a position beneath the hollow vein (vena cava), as does the sieve-like (ethmoid) passage in the nose and palate in relation to the surplus matter from the brain; they are situated on both sides of it. Besides, if the kidneys are like sieves, and readily let the thinner serous (whey-like) portion through, and keep out the thicker portion, then the whole of the blood contained in the vena cava must go to them, just as the whole of the urine is thrown into the filters. Further, the example of milk being made into cheese will show clearly what I mean. For this, too, although it is all thrown into the wicher strainers, does not all percolate through; such part of it as is too fine in proportion to the width of the meshes passes downwards, and this is called whey (serium); the remaining thick portion which is destined to become cheese cannot get down, since the pores of the strainers will not admit it. Thus it is that, if the blood-serium has similarly to percolate through the kidneys, the whole of the blood must come to them, and not merely one part of it."

Galen continues in his essay, and one is amazed at the clarity and keenness of observation in his clinical approach and philosophy concerning urine formation:

"Concerning the secretion of urine, however, he (Hippocrates) writes that this occurs through the kidneys, but does not add in what way it occurs. I do not think he could say that this was from the tendency of matter to fill a vacuum, for, if this were so, nobody would have ever died of retention of urine, since no more can flow into a vacuum than has run out. For, if no other factor comes into operation save only this tendency by which a vacuum becomes refilled, nor more could ever flow in than has been evacuated. Nor could he suggest any other plausible cause, such, for example, as the expression of nutriment by the stomach which occurs in the process of anadosis; this had been entirely disproved in the case of blood in the vena cava; it is excluded, not merely owing to the long distance, but also from the fact that the overlying heart, at each diastole, robs the vena cava by violence of a considerable quantity of blood.

"In relation to the lower part of the vena cava there would still remain, solitary and abandoned, the spacious theory concerning the filling of a vacuum. This, however, is deprived of plausibility by the fact that people die of retention of urine, and also, no less by the situation of the kidneys. For, if the whole of the blood was carried to the kidneys one might properly maintain that it all undergoes purification there.

But, as a matter of fact, the whole of it does not go to them, but only so much as can be contained in the veins going to the kidneys; this portion, only, therefore will be purified. Further, the thin serous part of this will pass through the kidneys as if through a sieve, while the thick sanguineous portion remaining in the veins will obstruct the blood flowing in from behind; this will first, therefore, have to run back to the vena cava, and so to empty the veins going to the kidneys; these veins will no longer be able to conduct a second quantity of unpurified blood to the kidneys—occupied as they are by the blood which had preceded, there is no passage left. What power have we, then, which will draw back the purified blood from the kidneys? And what power, in the next place, will bid this blood retire to the lower part of the vena cava, and will enjoin on another quantity coming from above not to proceed downwards before turning off into the kidneys?

"Now those near the times of Erasistratus maintain that the

parts above the kidneys receive pure blood, whilst the water residue, being heavy, tends to run downwards; that this, after percolating through the kidneys themselves, is thus rendered serviceable, and is sent, as blood, to all parts of the kidneys.

"For a certain period at least this view also found favor and flourished, and was held to be true; after a time, however, it became suspect to the Erasistratians themselves, and at last they abandoned it. For apparently the following two points were assumed, neither of which conceded by anyone, nor is even capable of being proved. The first if the heaviness of the serous fluid, which was said to be produced in the vena cava, and which did not exist, apparently, at the beginning, when this fluid was being carried up from the stomach to the liver. Why, then, did it not at once run downwards when it was in these situations? And if the watery fluid is so heavy, what plausibility can anyone find in the statement that it assists in the process of anadosis?

"In the second place there is this absurdity, that even if it be agreed that all the watery fluid does fall downward, and only when it is in the vena cava, still it is difficult, or, rather impossible, to say through what means it is going to fall into the kidneys, seeing that these are not situated below, but on either side of the vena cava, and that the vena cava is not inserted into them, but merely sends a branch into each of them, as it also does into all the other parts.

"What doctrine, then took the place of this one when it was condemned? One which to me seems far more foolish than the first, although it also flourished at one time. For they say, that if oil be mixed with water and poured upon the ground each will take a different route, the one flowing this way, and the other that way, and that, thereafter it is not surprising that the watery fluid runs into the kidneys, while the blood falls downwards along the vena cava. Now this doctrine also stands already condemned. For why, of the countless veins which spring from the vena cava, should blood flow into all the others, and the serous fluid be diverted to those going to the kidneys? They have not answered the question which was asked; they merely state what happens and imagine they have thereby assigned the region."

Polk[47] in his *Notes on Galenic Urology* writes, "Handicapped by his own misconceptions about the flow of blood, nonetheless

Galen's contribution to existent knowledge of the secretion and evacuation of urine remains an outstanding exhibition of clinical, investigative and persuasive talent."

A good insight into the basic principles of Galenic physiology is given by Singer and Rabin,[49] as these authors discuss Galen's physiology as it probably influenced Vesalius in his pioneer thoughts. Thus wrote these authors: "Standing behind all anatomical teaching before the seventeenth century is Galen's physiological system. It is set forth or implied in the various texts that were printed in the early collected editions of Galen's works. Until the boyhood of Vesalius, however, Galenic teaching reached the student of medicine mainly through Avicenna. By the time Vesalius began to study at Paris (1533), the anatomical works of Galen had been translated into Latin by Guenther and others . . . the basic principle of life in the Galenic physiology is a *spirit, amina* or *pneuma* drawn from the general world-soul in the act of respiration. This pagan stoic principal is, strictly interpreted, inconsistent with Christian, Moslem or Jewish doctrine, an awkward fact omitted or slurred or misrepresented or misunderstood in medieval writings. Thus, the medieval physiological system is basically unintelligible. . . . Food traversing the alimentary tract is absorbed as 'chyle' from the intestine, collected by mesentric veins into the portal vessel by it, and conveyed to the liver. That organ has power to elaborate the chyle into venous blood and to imbue it with a spirit of pneuma which is innate in all living substances, the natural spirit *(spiritus naturalis)* of the medievals and is ultimately derived from the world spirit, charged with natural spirit, but also with the nutritive material derived from the food, venous blood is distributed to the body by the liver, through the vena cava, which runs the length of the body. This vena cava arises from the liver much as the aorta arises from the heart, that is to say from the left ventricle.

"This highly ingenious physiology," continues Singer and Rabin,[49] "is not derived from an investigation of human anatomy. It is fanciful and, insofar as it is related to actual structures, they are those of animals and not of men. He (Galen) specifically states that he did not dissect human bodies, either of enemies killed in war or of exposed children, but he does not say that he never dissected a foetus. His anatomy is derived mostly from apes, supplemented for special purposes from cattle and swine."

Not only was Galen an expert at writing clearly and emphatically, but he was also a clever politician. When the court physician Demetrius died, Marcus Aurelius, then fighting on the Danube, appointed Galen as court physician. When the emperor returned to Rome at the end of 176 A.D., he became ill with an acute stomach upset. The attending doctors diagnosed the trouble as a feverish paroxysm, and treated it with purgatives. No improvement following, Galen was called in. The following is Galen's account of what then happened:

> "Hereupon I was summoned to spend the night in the Palace, a messenger coming to fetch me, by order of the Emperor, just as the lamps were being lighted. Three physicians had seen him in the morning and at the eighth hour, and two had felt his pulse (no mention is made of uroscopy) whilst to all did appear the beginning of an attack. I, however, remained silent; then the Emperor perceiving me, asked why I had not, like the others felt his pulse. I replied: 'Two doctors have already done that and from their experiences on the journey with you they are better able to judge of your present condition.' As I said this he called on me to feel him, and as the pulse, taking into consideration his age, circumstances, and constitutional aspects, seemed to me inconsistent with an attack of fever, I declared that none was to be feared; but that the stomach was overloaded with nourishment which had been coated with phlegm. This diagnosis called forth his praise, and he thrice repeated: 'Yes, that is it; it is exactly as you say; I feel that cold food is disagreeing with me.'
>
> "He then asked me what was to be done. I answered him frankly that if another than he had been the patient, I should have, following my custom, given him wine with pepper.
>
> "With sovereigns like yourself, however, doctors are in the habit of employing the least drastic remedies, therefore it must suffice to apply upon the abdomen wool with warm spikenard.
>
> "The Emperor replied that warm ointment on purple wool was his usual remedy for pain in the stomach, and called Dr. Peitholaos to apply it and let me go. This being done,

and his feet warmed by rubbing with heated hands, he demanded Sabine wine, threw pepper into it and drank, after which he said to Dr. Peitholaos that now, at last, he had a physician and a courageous one, repeating that I was the first of physicians and the only philosopher; he had tried many, not only the covetous, but those greedy of fame and honor and those filled with envy and malice. I am of the opinion that in this case my diagnosis was remarkably correct."

Galen habitually castigated all charlatans, berated all physicians who attempted to rival him. He delivered his theories as infallible dogma, and declared: "Whoever seeks fame need only become familiar with all that I have achieved."

Galen was a great experimenter and researcher, and since Roman law prevented the use of human cadavers, he confined himself to a criminal's skeleton picked clean by vultures and the remains of a corpse washed out of a cemetery in a flood. His anatomic studies were amazingly correct. He delved into physiology with experiments on dogs, swine, horses, birds, fish and once an elephant. He created cerebral and spinal lesions so he could trace the nerve pathways, and he is credited with finding the link between the brain and the larynx. He described in detail and with amazing accuracy the two eyelids, and six eyeball muscles and the maxillary group of muscles, as well as many muscles of the head, neck, trunk and extremities. His extensive *materia medica* included 540 vegetables and 180 animal and 100 mineral substances, all of which formed the basis of what ultimately became known as the famous herbal "galenicals."

Even though Galen's theories ultimately disappeared from the lecture halls as a guide to medical students, his life was a fruitful one for the world. He uplifted medicine in the Roman Empire to a high status and greatly advanced medicine, surgery, and hygiene. He gave all contemporary and future doctors much to think about. Indeed, few men in any age have ever done so much.

Chapter VI

Islamic Medicine with Facets of Urology: Rhazes, Avicenna, and Maimonides

ARABIC medicine played a definite role in the development of medical science. At the end of the 7th century, the Arabs had already swept from Arabia, through the Eastern Roman Empire, and over Egypt, North Africa, and Spain. Indeed, the very fate of Western Europe was undetermined until the Arabs were finally defeated in the Battle of Tours in 732.

These conquerors now repulsed in further advance, settled in their newly occupied lands and built up a civilization, unique in its great interest in cultural pursuits and a most particular interest in science. They translated* the Greek and Roman manuscripts into Arabic, and we are forever indebted to them.

* Meyerhof[50] believes that the first Arab physicians who turned to account the translations of the most important medical works of antiquity, and who arranged their practices accordingly were obviously the translators of these important manuscripts, consequently, almost throughout the entire 9th century medical practice in Bagdad was in the hands of Christians. A passage in one of the texts of the brilliant Moslem theologian and writer al-Jahiz tells of a physician of Bagdad who was living in miserable circumstances and when he was asked why he had so few patients replied, "In the first place I am a Moslem, and even before I studied medicine, people were of the opinion that Moslem doctors were good for nothing. Furthermore my name is Asad, when it should be Saliba, Juh anna, or Bira and I should have the surname Abu Isa, Abu Zakariza, or Abu Ibrahim, instead of my surname Abu 'l-Harith. I wear a white cotton garment, but it should be black silk; and my tongue is Arabic, when it should be that of the people from Gondeshapur (Syriac or Persian)."

The Nestorians† were the founders of the medical schools of Edessa and Nisibis, which reached its height of importance toward the end of the fifth century. These Christians of the Orient who had been expelled from home by religious persecution brought the Greek civilization with them into exile, translated the Greek texts into Syriac, and spread knowledge of them through the Orient from Syria to Mesopotamia. When the Arabs in their religious fanaticism to expand had conquered Syria and Persia, they came in contact with these ancient schools of which they had some knowledge before. The great power of Islam now expanded further and new schools were founded. At Cordova, a library of over 300,000 volumes existed. Of even greater significance is that in this period of Arabian domination art and poetry had their maximum development yet medicine was considered as the most precious of all forms of education.

Although Hippocrates and his *Amphorisms* were greatly admired, Islamic science seemed to favor Galen more emphatically. Haggard[35] gives the following reasons why these peoples were more inclined to accept Galen's theories over those of Hippocrates: The theorizing of Galen, his subtle, showy expla-

---

† The principal translators of Greek medicine were the Nestorians, who were mainly responsible for preserving the ancient Greek classics into Arabic. The Nestorians were adherents of an heretical Christian sect who followed the teachings of Bishop Nestorius, a monk from Euprepius and a pupil of Diodorus of Tarsus and Theodore of Mopsuestia. Nestorius' theology established a schism in the church, and because of this Nestorius was ultimately banished and died an outcast in 449 in Africa.

According to Brody,[51] the Nestorians were chiefly in Asia Minor and Syria, with Edessa and Nisibis as their chief cities and great centers of learning in schools which had been in existence since the fourth century. Here, the Greek classics were translated by the Nestorians into Syriac, a language derived from the ancient Aramaic. The school in Edessa was referred to as the Athens of the Aramaic world and it became the cradle of Syriac literature.

In 451 and 489, the councils of Chalcedon, ordered that the Nestorians be expelled from Syria, causing most of them to settle in Persia. In 489, the Emperor Zeno closed the university at Edessa. Nevertheless, many remained in Syria and Egypt, where they maintained their churches in the sixth and seventh centuries, while occupying themselves mainly as merchants delving in eastern trade. Some historians believe that the Nestorians (perhaps numbering approximately 100,000) represent the oldest Schismatic church in the world.[52]

nations, appealed to the Arabs; the rugged principles of Hippocrates did not. They adopted Galen's theories, his dogmas and his poly-pharmacy to an Arabic form. Soon, at their hands, Galen's theories became dogmas; his beliefs took on the forms of axioms as irreputable as the basic axioms of geometry.

It is believed by many that the adoption of Galen by the Arabs may account for the subsequent readoption of Galen and his theories by the West rather than the adoption of Hippocratic theories. Galenic philosophy thus reached Western Europe, flavored by and through Arabic culture.

These Arabic precursors of European medicine were headed by great physicians. Such a leader was Abu Bakr Mohammed ibn Zakarija al-Razi, better known by the latinized name Rhazes (865-925). He was the first Moslem to utilize the translated literature and greatly enriched the art of medicine. Rhazes was born in Raij in Northern Persia and some have claimed he was a pupil of the famous 'Ali ibn Rabban, which chronologically is impossible. At one time, he was physician and teacher at the hospital founded by the caliph al-Muqtadir at Bagdad in 918. His description of smallpox and measles is a classic and he was accepted as a clever clinician and brilliant diagnostician.

Rhazes was a prolific writer and his many volumes were zealously copied by authors who followed him. His large encyclopedia, especially the famous Kitab-al, Mansuri and the twenty-four volume Kitab al-Hawi fi l'tibb contains many medical theories, which he gathered from the translated literature. It is of particular interest in that one finds in the fourth volume (extant in the Egyptian National Library at Cairo) quotations from Hippocrates, Galen, Rufus, Philagrius, Alexander of Tralles, Oribasius, Paul the Byzantine and many others unknown.

Although Rhazes was a great admirer of Galen and accepted many of his theories, in practice he inclined toward Hippocrates and thus became known as the "Arabian Hippocrates." Like Hippocrates, he based his diagnosis on observation of the course of the disease and paid particular attention to dietetics and hygienic measure plus the use of simple drugs. Thus he wrote, "at the commencement of an illness, choose measures whereby strength may not be lessened; where thou canst cure by diet, use no drugs, and where simple means suffice use no complex ones."

Rhazes warned physicians not to rely too much on uroscopy as a means of making a diagnosis. Uroscopy was extremely popular at this time but unfortunately was utilized by many "quacks" other than the earnest, conscientious physician. This popularity probably can be traced to the story prevalent as early as 760, a century before Rhazes' birth, when Abu Koreish Isa's skill in diagnosing the sex of an unborn child by uroscopy. He predicted the birth of a son to the Caliph's pregnant wife and claimed that he did so by means of uroscopy.

In his treatise, *Upon the Circumstances Which Turn the Head of Most Men from the Reputable Physician,* Rhazes gives us a clear picture of the physician as well as the character of the patients of his day. His advice to physicians as to how to retain the respect and confidence of their patients is just as applicable today. He stresses how easily it may be for people to turn away from intelligent and learned physicians and place their trust in impostors and "quacks." He stressed the fallacy of the layman who expects the physician to know everything:

> "If he inspects the urine or feels the pulse he is supposed to know what the patient has eaten and what he has been doing. This is lying and deception and is only brought about by trickery, by artful questions of speech through which the senses of the public are deceived. Many hire men or women to find out all the circumstances of the patient, and to report what is told by neighbors and by servants."

There were many illustrious doctors in the golden age of Arabian medicine. The reader must bear in mind that when we say "Arabian Medicine," we mean the medicine of the Islamic culture area of the middle ages, whose works were written for the most part in Arabic, while their authors belonged to the diverse peoples of the Near East and North Africa. For clarification of this particular culture, let us delve into that culture that reached its zenith in the 9th and 10th centuries.

At one time, Persia contributed little to the advancement of medicine, but produced great rulers, great soldiers and above all a prophet and poet who taught a pure and highly ethical religion. The *Videvdad* was a code book which is important for it gives valuable information about many hygienic views, and information about the training and practice of physicians. This code book was probably written between 250 B.C. and A.D. 224. It is a law book which states what is allowed and what is forbidden and in many ways reminds one of the Code of Hammurabi. Girls were to be married after their fifteenth year. Women were highly respected and marriage with relatives was recommended rather than condemned. Indeed, it appeared to be the custom, as it was in Egypt and still is in Arab countries. Of singular interest is that abortion was considered a great crime, equal to manslaughter. Thus if a girl was made pregnant and went to an abortionist woman, she, the woman, and the man were all considered equally responsible. Sodomy was rated one of the greatest crimes. The passive and unconsenting victim was whipped to death; but for the active and consenting pederast there was no way of atoning—"he was a daeva and worshiper of daeva forever."

Many pages are devoted to purity regulations. "Fire, water, earth and vegetation were not to be defiled, prescriptions similar to those we found in Hesoid's *Works and Days*. Man became unclean as a result of physiological processes such as menstruation, childbirth, ejaculation of sperm, and death. Whoever touched a corpse, whether of man or dog, became unclean and had to purify himself through elaborate rites."

As formerly emphasized, physicians in antiquity did not require a license to practice. Anyone could claim to be expert in problems of health and disease, and treat sick people for a fee. Despite the low ebb of medicine in ancient Persia, there was some kind of licensing of surgeons. The Persian document dealing with the admission of physicians to the practice of surgery is the earliest preserved regulation of its kind:[54]

> "The Muhtasib was an official appointed by the Caliph to superintend public morality and to insure that the interests of the people were protected. He demanded physicians to

abide by the Hippocratic Oath, making them swear never to administer a noxious medicament or to compound a poison for anyone or to prescribe a drug to bring about abortion or to prevent conception. Doctors had to turn their eyes away from the women's quarters when visiting a patient. They must never reveal a confidence, must never tear aside a veil or venture upon any course forbidden to them. Since there was no definite medical school curriculum or official system of granting degrees after examination there could be no conditions imposed upon the doctor before he started to practice; except apprenticeship to someone who was practicing medicine. Levy tells of the story of a blind doctor in Baghdad who employed a man to lead him about, inspect urine glasses and generally assist in the practice. Unfortunately, the doctor died two months after engaging this assistant, who thereupon immediately opened an office for the treatment of the sick on his own account.

"The Muhtasib authorized a book with instructions concerning the practice of medicine. This manual was also utilized by the doctor upon visiting the sick. Thus he was instructed to first inquire of the patient what it was that brought on the illness, and the nature of any pain he was suffering. In accordance with the answer he received he had to write a prescription, giving a copy to the relatives. On the following day he was expected to pay a second visit, in order to learn how the illness was progressing, *to examine the urine,* and question the patient with the object of discovering if he was better or worse. He now prescribed again, giving a copy of the new prescription to the relatives. This process continued until the patient recovered, or else died. If he recovered, the physician received his fee and an honorarium. If the patient died, the relatives were instructed to present themselves before the Chief Physician, officially appointed in each city, and give him the prescriptions which had been written for the patient. If the Chief Physician believed the treatment prescribed was in accordance with the requirements of science and the art of medicine, with no signs of fault or negligence on the doctor's part, it was his duty to declare that the man's life ended by the termination of his alloted time. If he was of a different opinion he had to say: 'exact the blood-money for your kinsman from this doctor.

> He slew him through negligence and lack of skill.' In this manner excellent precautions were taken so that no one should practice medicine being unqualified and that no qualified doctor should be negligent."

Perhaps the most famous of all Arabic physicians and philosophers is Avicenna the Persian physician (980-1037). His influence extended throughout the Islamic world and Europe. His writings continue to this day to be an inspiration to scholars.

For more than eight hundred years the leaders of European medical thought have paid homage to this Persian scientist and philosopher. He was accepted by St. Thomas Aquinas, and although in Western eyes he was considered an infidel and pagan, Danté nevertheless gave him a place in *Paradise*. For centuries, all important medical schools conscientiously read and re-read his *Canon* of Medicine more accurately called *Al-Qanún*, which has been described by many as the most influential text ever written. It contains more than a million words, both wise and foolish, yet it exerted a tremendous influence on medical thinking. Osler[55] described Avicenna as the author of the most famous medical text-book ever written, and said that it had been "a medical bible for a longer period than any other work."

Tradition has it that on St. Johannestag in 1527 in the market place of Basel, Paracelsus publicly burned the works of Galen and of Avicenna, so that "all this misery may go in the air with smoke." Karl Sudhoff protests. It was not the *Canon Medicinae des Avicenna* that Paracelsus cast into the fires but rather the *Summum der Bücher,* a compendium which had been but recently published in Lyon.

"It is of little consequence," writes Galdston,[56] "at this moment whether truth lies with tradition or with Sudhoff: though parenthetically I would rather gamble on tradition—its version is more in keeping with the Paracelsian temperament. Curiously, the far more pertinent inquiry is: Who was this Avicenna, so intimately coupled with Galen? Should we in the pursuit of this curiousity turn to the medical historians, we'd discover motley divergence of notices and judgment." "Thus" continues

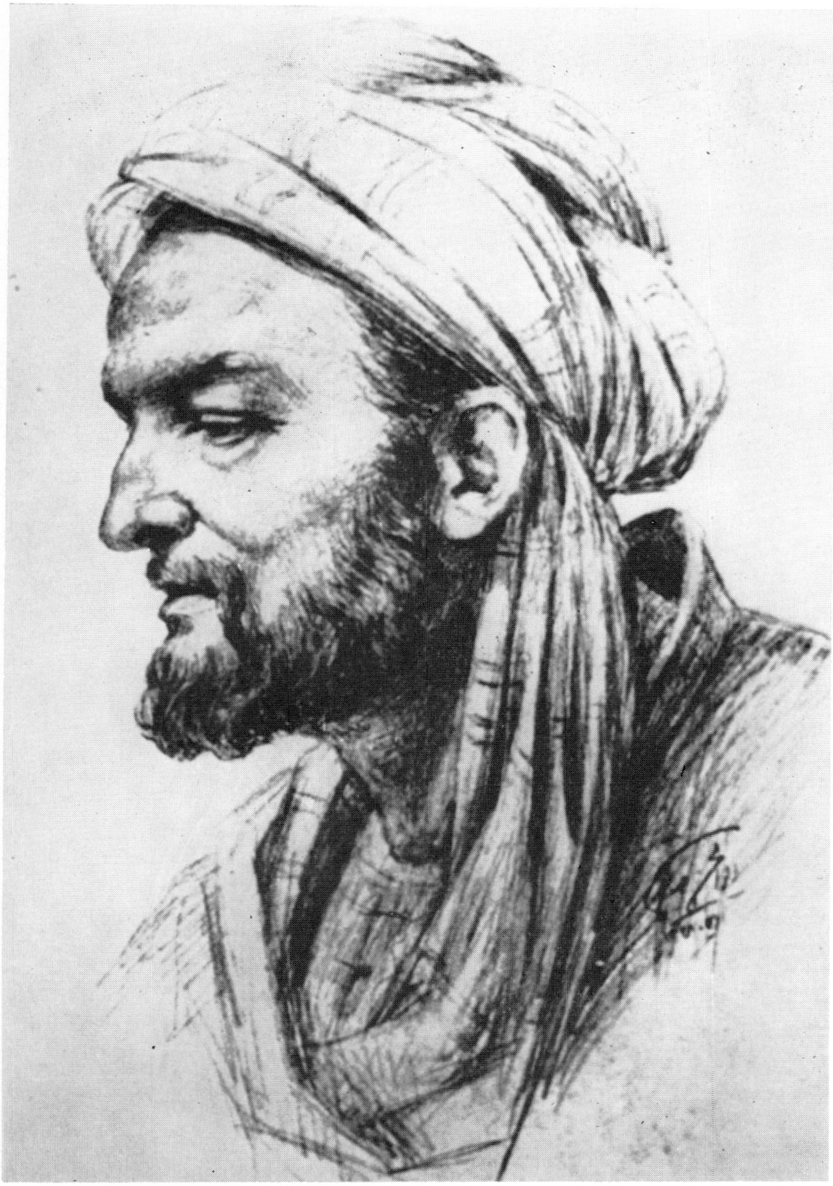

FIGURE 12. Painting of Avicenna. Source unknown.

Galdston,[56] "Garrison devotes a page and a half to Avicenna, and characterizes him as a corvival Omarian spirit . . . one who trod the primrose path at ease and died in the prime of life from the effects of its pleasures." It is a bit difficult to reconcile this portrait of Avicenna as one who trod the primrose path of ease with the more than 200 separate compositions definitely attributed to him. Let us therefore read of the life of Avicenna, physician, scientist and philosopher.

Galdston, a strong admirer and advocate of Avicenna, repeatedly emphasizes his virtues, rather than attacking his character. Thus he quotes Arturo Castiglioni[57] as exhibiting a more sensitive appreciation of Avicenna, and who also did not ascribe Avicenna's early death to dissipation but rather to "a stormy life which led him through many transitions and great suffering." He quotes Castiglioni's comment on Avicenna's *Canon:* "The clarity of the clinical histories, the accuracy of the therapeutic indications, constructed logically and without dangerous exaggerations, and the eloquence of his forcible style were sufficient to confer on this book up to the end of the seventeenth century an almost indisputable authority in the minds of the physicians of all countries."

Not content with finding an ally in Castiglioni with reference to Avicenna, Galdston quotes Kurt Sprengel in his *Versuch einer pragmatischen Geschichte der Arzneykunde,* "No other man in the realm of science, save Aristotle or Galen, has exercised so great and powerful a despotism as Scheikh Reyes (or the Prince of the physicians)—Al-Hussein Abu-Ali Ben Abdallah, *Ebn Sina,* usually called Avicenna. His system predominated for almost six hundred years. The history of this literary despot deserves closer investigation." And in this vein Galdston, as Chairman, on May 20, 1954, opened the meeting, commemorating the Thousandth Anniversary of Avicenna, held at the New York Academy of Medicine, in conjunction with the Asia Institute Association.*

---

* For the reader interested in Avicenna, the papers read at this historic meeting and subsequently published, are available in the *Bulletin of the New York Academy of Medicine,* April 1955, Vol. 31, #4, pp. 300-332.

The elder of two sons born in August, 980 to Abd-Allah, the local governor of Kharmaithan of Ismaili origin and his wife, Sittare, from Afshewa, of Persian descent, was Abu Ali Al-Hussein Ibn Abu-Allah ibn Hasan ibn' Ali ibn Sina, who through the Europeanized Hebrew transliteration of his name has become known to us as Avicenna.

As a child, he was precocious and extremely anxious to learn. By the age of ten, he had memorized the *Quran,* as well as other philosophical writings. Because of this remarkable aptitude he was placed under tutelage to learn Indian arithmetic as well as studying Muslim jurisprudence at the same time. At about the age of sixteen, Avicenna showed an interest in medicine and thereafter read every available book on the subject, with ease and great understanding.

> "Medicine (he comments) is not a difficult subject and in a short space of time, of course, I excelled in it, so that the master of physic came to read with me, and I began to visit the sick. Consequently, there were opened to me the doors to various kinds of treatment which I learnt by experience (or experiment). I was then about sixteen years of age. During the period of hard practice and study which then ensued, I never once slept the whole night through. If a problem was too difficult for me, I repaired to the mosque and prayed, involving the Creator of all things, until the gate that had been closed to me was opened and what had been complex became simple. Always, as night fell, I returned to my house, set the lamp before me and busied myself with reading and writing. If sleep overcame me or I felt the flesh growing weak, I had recourse to a beaker of wine, so that my energies were restored."

"Everything he did" wrote Pope,[54] "bore the marks of his remarkable memory, his fantastic versatility, his long sustained and concentrated labor, together with an insatiable passion for thoroughness and a real dedication to truth." In addition to his medical and philosophical studies, his work in physics, astronomy and mathematics, in geology, and mineralogy, and with such minor accomplishments as the invention of the Vernier instrument, five centuries before Vernier, was indeed evidence of an exceptionally gifted and productive life. In addition to all of these accomplishments he was a serious musician, wrote verse, published over a hundred books, was a politician, translated *Euclid* on the side and accomplished all this by his fifty-sixth year when he died.

Avicenna was once subjected to a test, in the spirit of al-Rhazes little book, *Cure Within the Hour* to cure on the instant a girl serving in the royal apartments, who had bent over and could not straighten up again.

"Take off her veil," ordered Avicenna. This was done, putting the girl in an anguish of embarrassment, yet her body was still locked, immobile.

"Off with her skirt" ordered Avicenna; the girl, in a spasm of emotional shock, straightened up and disappeared. He thus won the challenge and also undoubtedly recorded one of the earliest triumphs for psychotherapy.

It is certain that Avicenna's fame rests as much upon his medical writings as upon his metaphysical compositions which out-numbered his scientific endeavors. He is credited with approximately one hundred works in Arabic and Persian and of singular interest is that the most important ones are still extant. As a matter of fact, we happen to know more about Avicenna than about most of the pioneers of medicine, only because he dictated a record of the first twenty-one years of his life to his friend and pupil Juzjani. This source of autobiography ceased at the time of his father's death, which seems to have brought about a change in his habits and mode of living.

A discussion of Avicenna's works are beyond the scope of this thesis yet one cannot avoid some comment of his writings, with particular emphasis on his use of the *mot juste,* and for his constant usage for succinct classification.

Although *Al Qanum* is by far Avicenna's major contribution to medicine, he is also known in the medical world for his infinitesimally smaller work *Al-Arjuzat fit-tibb* (the *Poem on Medicine*). This has enjoyed great popularity both in the East and in the West. We are greatly indebted to Dr. Krueger[58] for the first English translation of the *Cantica (Al-Arjuzat fit-tibb)* and the reader is strongly recommended to read this first English version based primarily on a French version with frequent reference to German and Latin sources. In fact, Dr. Krueger found it necessary at times to undertake the study of elementary Arabic* so that some of the original words could be expressed more aptly in the English version.

The *Poem on Medicine* was known in Western cultures during the Middle Ages. The first extant evidence of a translation of this work into European language was that done by Gerardo of Cremona who lived between 1114 and 1178, thus placing the translation sometime in the middle of the twelfth century. About one hundred years later, Armengaud de Blaise of Montpellier included a Latin translation of the *Poem*. In 1522, the *Poem* was published in Lyon, by Pierre Antoine Rusticus dofe Plaisance, who omitted the comments but corrected the style and errors and included an index of useful Arabic terms. Space does not permit further review of this extraordinary man. Since our essay is basically concerned with urine, it behooves us to herewith include Avicenna's opinion concerning this substance.

Thus he wrote:

About the Color

"White urine witnesses the quantity of ingested food and drink; it is a sign of bad digestion, phlegm, cold restlessness of hepatic obstruction. Somewhat yellow, it indicates the presence of a certain quantity of bile, the color of fire, that means the presence of a great deal of yellow bile. Very yellow and tinted with red, it proves a super abundance of yellow bile. Dark red

---

* Avicenna, as all the learned men of his age, used principally Arabic as the instrument for his thoughts. Arabic at that time played in the Orient a role analogous to that of Latin in the Occident. It was the *"Langue par excellence"* of art, science, religion and literature. Arabic was used by Avicenna, too, although he was never considered as a literary man with a masterly command of a foreign language, and his Arabic poems were not taken as first rate. He also wrote in his mother tongue, Persian. According to Ardalan, some of his treatises written in Persian are pure, eloquent and clear. His famous work in Persian is called *Danishnama,* and was dedicatel to his great patron, Ala'an-Dowla. In this short work, he summarized in a succinct manner all his philosophical system with a view to making it comprehensive to the Persian Emir, rendering all the philosophic terms into appropriate Persian equivalents.

urine of the one who has not ingested saffron and who has had neither fever nor colic contains blood. When found black after having been dark, it signified that the patient has suffered a great chill. Black after having been very red indicates a poor combustion of humours. Judge the illness according to the odor of urine on the condition that the patient has not ingested a coloring food, certain vegetables, cassia fistula and that which may tint like murri."

On the Density of Urine

"The tenuity of the urine indicates inadequacy of digestion. Sometimes it is fluid after indigestion or obstruction of the liver or because of a tumor. The thickness of the urine indicates good digestion or the abundance of phlegm in the body."

On the Sediment in Urine

"The white sediment indicates recovery; yellow, it marks acuteness of the bile; if it is red like the blood wort, it is a question of disease of the blood. If a similar sediment continues without modification, that indicates an abscess of the liver. Black after having been dark red and that after loss of strength, going to the bottom after having floated, that means the soul is about to escape; the patient can no longer benefit from the prayers of a sorcerer; death is at hand through the excess of humoral combustion. If the sediment appears black after having been dark and it does not occur in the course of an acute illness, especially if this appearance coincides with a favorable sign, and if the origin of the illness is in black bile, it indicates the end of the illness."

On the Location of the Sediment

"If a cloud appears floating in the upper portion of the vial (I presume this refers to the urine container), it indicates crudeness of the illness. If a certain maturity exists in the urine, wind is causing the sediment to reascend to the surface. If the sediment is half-way up, be aware that the wind is in a small quantity. If it is white, after having been yellow, coherent without being thick, falls to the bottom, appears with a changeable color, it marks the maturity of the illness."

On the Consistency of the Sediment

"An ephemeral sediment indicates the weakness of the patient. If there are elements similar to barley meal in the urine, one is dealing with scrapings of the vessels. If the sediment looks like bran and has a bad color, it indicates ulceration within the ducts; like metal filings, it proves the elimination of portions of organs. If pus appears in the vial, it marks the opening of a collection. If the sediment has decomposed blood, there is a phlegmonous tumor. If it goes to the bottom, resembles sperm, it comes from an immature lymph swelling. If one sees sand in it, be aware that there is a calculus."

On the Odor of Urine

"If the urine has no odor, it is that the food has not been digested or has been digested raw. The degree of decomposition agrees with the intensity of the odor of the urine. If this odor is dreadful, be aware that the illness is in the bladder.

"Thus, I have reported on the different kinds of urine; guide yourself by what I have stated about their composition."

In the second part of the *Poem on Medicine,* Avicenna advises as to the *Conservation of Health* through diets and drugs and his section *On the Beverage* is of extreme interest. Thus he writes: if you wish to avoid illness, divide your nourishment into three parts: a third for respiration, a third for food and the rest for water. A little cold water quenches thirst, better than far too much warm water. Too much ice in the beverage is harmful to the nerves; allow it only for the obese and sanguine man with strong tissues. It is not necessary to drink at the table except with the threat of choking, and never after the meal, nor after a warm bath, nor after a violent exercise, nor after sexual intercourse—that can be dangerous. If it is necessary and you can control yourself, drink moderately. When digestion is completed in the lower part of the stomach, then have the amount of water which quenches your thirst with water and wine, if you are thirsty again, drink no more—the thirst is false.

With regard to drinking wine he wrote:

> "As regards drinking, do not misuse wine. Be content with a small amount and, then not every day, nor with fasting, nor after light or acid food. Do not get intoxicated incessantly. If that happens to you, let it be only once a month. Wine taken in small amounts is dangerous. Warm intoxicates the one who stuns easily; give him aromatics and let him eat sour pomegranates, quince, cucumbers at the same time; dilute his wine with water. Give it straight to the one in whom it provokes flatus. The best wine is the strong yellow kind, it is proper to drink it with salty meats. During the summer, it is better to drink a light and thin wine; mix it with water, eat acid meats and, then eat astringent meats."

The death of Avicenna is described by Abu-al-Guzgani, a student of the famous physician, first translated by Paul Krans[59] in 1932. The report in addition to its historical interest also reveals some light on the medicaments employed by Avicenna in his last illness.

> "The master relied upon his powerful constitution until he was overcome by an attack of colic during a campaign. Worried because he feared that his sickness would prevent him from fleeing after the defeat which appeared imminent, he wanted to regain his health without loss of time, and was given eight enemas in a single day. As a result his intestines became inflamed, and he was attacked by dysentery. He was forced to flee and while in flight was overcome by a fainting spell such as usually accompanies colic. Nevertheless, he continued to treat himself with clysters. One day he ordered that two grains of parsley seeds be used for a clyster, so that he would be able to break wind. The acrid parsley seeds only made the dysentery worse. For the attacks of syncope, he took mithridaticum, but one of his slaves put too much opium in it. In this condition he was brought to Ispahan. He was so weak that he was unable to stand on his feet, but treated himself until he was again able to walk. Although he had not yet completely recovered from his sickness, he did not spare himself nor did he give up his dissolute life. He had frequent re-

> lapses from which he repeatedly recovered. However, when the disease again attacked him on one of his journeys, he knew that his constitution was broken and that he could not resist. Thereupon he gave up trying to cure himself. He said: "The physician who treated my body was not adequate to his task. Now all attempts to cure are useless." He remained in this condition for several days, when the Lord took him. He was fifty-seven years of age."

Avicenna was without doubt one of the greatest physicians and philosophers of Islam who attempted to build a complete and logical, and well-rounded system of medicine. Although basically it was to a large extent Greek, he added the experience of several centuries of Arabic medicine and much personal experience. Avicenna thus brought about a system that was no longer Greek but was a powerful expression of Muslim philosophy. This expression was so forceful and persuasive that it dominated medicine in the East and in the West for 600 years.

We have discussed Rhazes and Avicenna, but attention should be given to the accepted fact, that most of the Western Arabians who reached any degree of eminence, date long after Rhazes and Avicenna. One of the foremost of such leaders who in addition to being a physician was a philosopher, poet, astrologer, mathematician and theologian. I refer to Moses Maimonides, through whose writings Greek medicine was preserved and transmitted to Western Europe by way of the Moorish invasion of Sicily and Spain.[60]

One can hardly think of this era, particularly of the Arabo-Spanish Period, without mention of this most learned physician, namely Abu Imran Musa ben Maimuni ibn Abd Allah, known to the Continent as Maimonides, and among Jews as "Rambam" (a contraction of Rabbi Moses ben Maimuni). We include him in this "Galaxy of Ancients" because of his many contributions to medicine and urology. Many historians classify him as only second to Rhazes in Medical knowledge.

Although Maimonides has never been accepted as an authority on medical practice, his criticism of Galen's medical assertions cannot be overlooked. Despite the fact that the authority of Galen was so great that medieval medical writers would not challenge him, Maimonides recognized a number of contradictions and discrepancies in Galen's work. Maimonides emphasized the value of logic and observation. Thus he wrote: "Know, my masters, that no man should believe anything that is not attested by one of these three sanctions: rational proof as in the mathematical science, the perception of the senses, or traditions from the prophets and learned men."

Equally daring and progressive in thought was Maimonides complete rejection of astrology. "Considering how long astrology in the sense of the doctrine of the stars influencing human health and destinies, had dominated men's minds, and how universal was the acceptance of it, Maimonides' strong expressions show how much genius lifts itself above the popular persuasions of its time, even among the educated, and how much it anticipates subsequent knowledge."[61]

Gordon[62] describes Maimonides as one of the most colorful personalities of the twelfth century. "He was an outstanding physician, equally eminent as a commentator, codifer and philosopher. He was born in Cordova, Spain, in 1135. The city at that time had a population of half a million, and an extremely large Jewish population. At the age of thirteen, Maimonides had to leave his birth place and wander from place to place as a religious refugee. Finally, in 1160, he settled in Fez, Morocco where he studied medicine under such famous physicians as Ibn Zuhr (son of the famous Ibn Zuhr-Avenzvar) and Abu Yusuf.

When 30 years of age, he migrated to Egypt where he soon became famous for his medical and literary contributions. In 1193, the English King, Richard the Lion-Hearted, offered him the position of court physician in England. This he refused but continued to work hard and composed the following ten medical works, all written in Arabic. These essays on medical problems are one of the best and most important medical works which antiquity has left us: *The Preservation of Youth; The Extracts (Gleanings from Galen); Commentary on the Aphorisms of Hippocrates; Medical Aphorisms, On Hemorrhoids; On Sexual Intercourse; Discourse on Asthma; On Poisons and the Protection Against Deadly Remedies; Discourse on the Explanation of Fits; Glossary of Drug Names.*

These ten medical treatises were all written in Arabic, probably in Cairo, during the last quarter of the twelfth century. They were immediately translated in Hebrew, and within recent years are appearing in English translations. We are greatly indebted to Gordon for his translation of *The Preservation of Youth,* and highly recommend this source for the interested reader.

It is extremely significant that in his essay *The Care of Patients in the Absence of a Physician or in the Presence of a Physician Who Is Not Adequate and Not Experienced in This Science,* he displayed in his diagnosis and therapeutics the Hippocratic spirit of *"vis medicatrix naturae."* Thus he wrote: "Galen has already explained to us that the ancient Greeks, when in doubt as to what to do in a certain disease, did nothing but left the patient to nature, which they considered sufficient to cure all illnesses. And, Hippocrates sang the praises of nature in many places at great length, considering nature to be wise, clever and capable of doing what is necessary for the sick without resorting to medication. And it is true that the physician should keep nature, support it and do nothing else but follow it."

Maimonides also refers to Razi (Rhazes) and writes: "And Razi said in one of his well-known chapters: If a disease is stronger than the patient, there is no hope that he will survive and the physician will help him; if the strength of the patient is greater than the strength of the disease, he will not need a physician, because nature will cure him; but if the strength of the patient and that of the disease are equal, then one needs a physician to increase the patient's strength. This can be done only by the perfect physician, who knows how to strengthen the patient and take care of him, so that he may overcome the hurdles of nature. However, most physicians commit many errors and, while they think they increase the patient's strength, they really weaken him and interfere with his progress."

Apparently, Maimonides looked further for confirmation and

quotes Aristotle as follows: "And about this, Aristotle said, in his book *De Sensu et sensibili,* that many died from medication because of the ignorance of physicians in understanding nature. When the physicians say 'nature' they mean the power that rules all living creatures, whose presence and true function has been explained in the books of the ancient sages." Of singular interest long before our present knowledge of sulfa, antibiotics, and hormones, Sir William Osler became a "therapeutic nihilist" for the same reasons quoted above. The doctrine of self-limited disease was revived by Jacob Bigelow[63] of Boston, who was the first to effectively protest in America against ill-chosen drugs and large doses and against excessive blood-letting. Dr. Oliver Wendell Holmes believed that Bigelow's stand exerted more influence upon medical practice in America than any work that had ever been published in the United States. Similarly, Osler gave much credit to the homeopaths who avoided drastic drugs, cupping and venesection.

Maimonides' primary position is in theology, where he encompassed the whole of Hebrew law, both canonical and civil, as reflected in his authoritative *Code,* along with ethics and religious guidance, as exemplified by the letter addressed to the Jews of Yemen.[64] In addition, he was an accomplished astronomer and in his letter to the Rabbis of Marseilles he condemned astrology, labelling it as superstitious. All are agreed that he was the foremost Jewish philosopher, who strongly influenced Albert the Great and St. Thomas Aquinas. Maimonides magnum opus was his *Guide of the Perplexed,* translated in 1204 into Hebrew and later into Latin.

All who diligently read Maimonides are greatly impressed by the emphasis that this ancient places on hygienic living. He stressed the need of dealing not only with disease but with Health and Disease, with great emphasis on the former. As stated above he relied greatly on diet, hygienic care, sanitation, and in his essay on the *Preservation of Youth,* recommends special diets and exercise. Indeed, he specifically advises against any excessive movement after eating and recommends the avoidance of activity including sex and bathing after eating: "Because they are very damaging, especially great is the harm to those whose blood vessels are narrow and thin by nature. Yet it is desirable that one should exercise a little the length of his house, so that his food may descend to the lower part of the stomach."

His comments on intercourse are exceedingly interesting: "The interest of most men in intercourse is well known. Not one of them has in mind the care of his health or the prolongation of the human race, but a craving for lust. They have no other intention but the satisfaction of their desire every time and at every opportune moment. And the informed already know that intercourse hurts most people, except the few whose temperament shows that a small amount of it will not hurt them. But the difference among men is only in the amount of harm; some will suffer in many ways and some only partially. Its harm to young men whose bodies are moist is little, and in the case of old people or convalescents or those of a dry constitution, the impairment of health is extensive. . . . And it is not proper for a man to have intercourse before the food is digested in the stomach, and not when he is hungry or thirsty or drunk or has just finished his bath or exercises or had a phlebotomy performed a day before or a day after. Whoever wishes to remain healthy should chase the idea of intercourse from his mind as much as he can."

In Maimonides, we find a man with a rare universal mind which could embrace the whole of the science and philosophy of his period. In his intellect, there was complete harmony of philosophy and religion, of science and ethics and medicine.

Chapter VII

Ars Medica and Uroscopy

AMONG the ancients, disease was believed to be caused by supernatural forces or demons, and that diseases could only be cured through magical rites performed by witch doctors. As man began to observe nature around him he began to acquire some knowledge as to how to cope with disease, and when successful results were thus obtained, the supernatural origin of disease was discarded in favor of a more rational and pseudo-scientific concept. The first rational approach to disease, the basic assumption of cause and effect of disease, was first inaugurated by uroscopy. In the next chapter (Chapter VIII), we will discuss the evolution of uroscopy, but will now confine our discussion of the role *ars medica* played in uroscopy.

For most of us living in the last third of the twentieth century, the historical role of the artist in depicting medicine does not mean very much. Yet, such a role was significant and the artist and his work often proved to be the most authentic source of information concerning certain customs and practices of long ago. These resources actually served as a pictorial narration of the mores of peoples at a specific time.

Melicow[65] believes that there are probably no two professions which on the surface are so unlike as Medicine and Art, but which on closer examination reveal many similarities and interrelationships, which give them both a common origin and heritage. In ancient society the physician and the artist were parts of a trinity consisting of medicine, art and religion. This relationship continued through the dark ages and medicine and art continued to be a part of and to serve religion. With the

Renaissance, a step toward a more scientific treatment of medicine was inaugurated. Art contributed to this as exemplified by the sketches of human bodies made by Leonardo da Vinci. Another example of this unity between artist and physician is well demonstrated by the great teacher of anatomy, Andreas Vesalius, who did not hesitate to utilize an artist of great skill to demonstrate accurately the skeletal system, muscular system and important viscera of the human body. With such a combination, an artist and anatomist, certain anatomical structures were described and accurately depicted for the first time.

By means of an art in the form of paintings, sculpture, wood-blocks, prints and lithographs the essential aspects of medical iconography is reflected throughout the ages. Fortunately for students of medical history, literary sources have often been supplemented with pictorial sources. Since the days of Aristotle, biological and medical books as well as ecclesiastical tomes were illustrated by colorful paintings and sketches.

Paintings give to the student of medical history a definite visual impression of his source of study which must contribute great inspiration to his labors. The historical study of urology would indeed appear dull, inadequate and at times misleading were it not for the numerous paintings depicting the urinal with its contents enthusiastically recommended as a fertilizer, as a skin lotion or taken as an internal or external medication. Actually, interest in urine stimulated the alchemist in his search for the golden elixir, followed by the chemist and finally by the scientist and the establishment of modern urine analysis.

The doctor in the act of "water gazing" is depicted in many manuscripts, dating as far back as the early fourteenth century. It becomes even more common among the wood-cuts of the fifteenth and sixteenth centuries. Scenes representing the physician, the apothecary and even the charlatan in the act of diagnosing the disease of a patient from his urine glass are innumerable. All are of great help to the medical historian.

Works of art undoubtedly contribute a great deal of our knowledge of the history of disease. Of course, they are of particular value for periods for which we have scanty literary material. Although we have many well preserved manuscripts relative to uroscopy, paintings depicting such scenes are of great additional value to the medical historian interested in the study of urine. We are greatly indebted to the artists of the sixteenth and seventeenth centuries for it was during this period, that outstanding artists, particularly of the Dutch School utilized the uroscopist as an interesting subject.*

Wellcome[66] has given us an excellent summation of the role of art in uroscopy. The summation and distinctive description recording of unusual wood-cuts and paintings are indeed of singular historical significance. In describing one of these sources of historical information, Wellcome writes:

"Probably nowhere in medieval art is the uroscopist more characteristically represented than in the frieze in Majolica by the famous master Della Robbia (1400-1482) which adorns the ancient hospital at Pistoja. On a pallet bed in the hospital lies a patient, with face drawn and wasted by disease. By the side stands a monk physician, his finger on the patient's pulse. At the foot of the bed another physician stands, with urine glass in one hand, while in the other he holds a bleeding staff. The whole bas-relief is modelled with great fidelity and characteristic skill, and gives a faithful and touching picture of the hospital practice in the fifteenth century."

A wood-cut of the sixteenth century is described as follows: "The physician is seen dressed in his doctor's robe and cap; in one hand he holds the urine glass, from which he is about to form his diagnosis, and near him stands the patient, awaiting with anxiety the result of the examination. In his hand he carries an osier basket, of cylindrical shape, with a cover, which

---

* Although it is generally agreed that uroscopy was practiced in early Japanese medicine, it is a singular fact that nowhere in Japanese medical art is there any representation of the Japanese physician as a uroscopist. This is in striking contrast to the prevalence of such representation in the Middle East and Western civilizations as is well documented in this chapter. Mestler[67] in his interesting galaxy of old Japanese medical books states that the earliest Japanese work on urology appears to have been composed by Yoshio (1724-1800), a famous physician and interpreter for the Dutch at Nagasaki, with the title Inek Hatsubi, published posthumously in 1815.

was used for carrying the urine glass to and from the physician's house. A basket of this kind was very necessary, as the urinal, being made with a spherical base, could not stand alone."

The basket also served as a safe carrier for the urine glass. The reader must recall that "scientific" uroscopy was derived predominantly from the early Greeks. At the suggestion of Isaac Judaeus,* the urinal was made to partially resemble a bladder and made from transparent glass to allow adequate inspection. In many of the paintings and wood-cuts the physician is depicted holding the urinal up against the light. Indeed it was advised by many that the urinal be held with the left hand and if the sun be intense, the right hand could shield the urinal from the direct rays of the sun so as to avoid faulty examination.

Holbein's famous painting the *Dance of Death,* shows death holding up a urinal before the physician. A well known Dutch engraving of the sixteenth century, depicts Christ, as a physician, inspecting a urinal. A wood-cut (from Brunschwig, H., Cyrurgia, Strassburg, 1497) shows two medieval physicians at a patient's bedside. The physician on the patient's left side feels his pulse, while the one on his right holds up a urinal.

Teniers the elder, of the Dutch School, has been credited with painting more canvases depicting the uroscopist than any other painter of his time. In his paintings, the doctor is shown as a man of grave demeanor, generally old and venerable with gray or white hair and usually with a beard. On his head, he wore a cap or bonnet trimmed with fur, sometimes in a gown and sometimes in the ordinary costume worn by the middle classes of the period.

In the interiors painted by Teniers, there is little variation in the background. As a rule the walls are bare, only furnished with a few shelves on which stand some bottles, and pots of ointment; occasionally some books and a few surgical instruments; a stuffed crocodile or curious stuffed fish hanging from

---

* Isaac Judaeus, an early Jewish physician, taught in Salerno, and was an ardent water-caster (uroscopist). He wrote copiously about urine. He gave the most minute directions for examining color, density, quality and sediment of the urine.

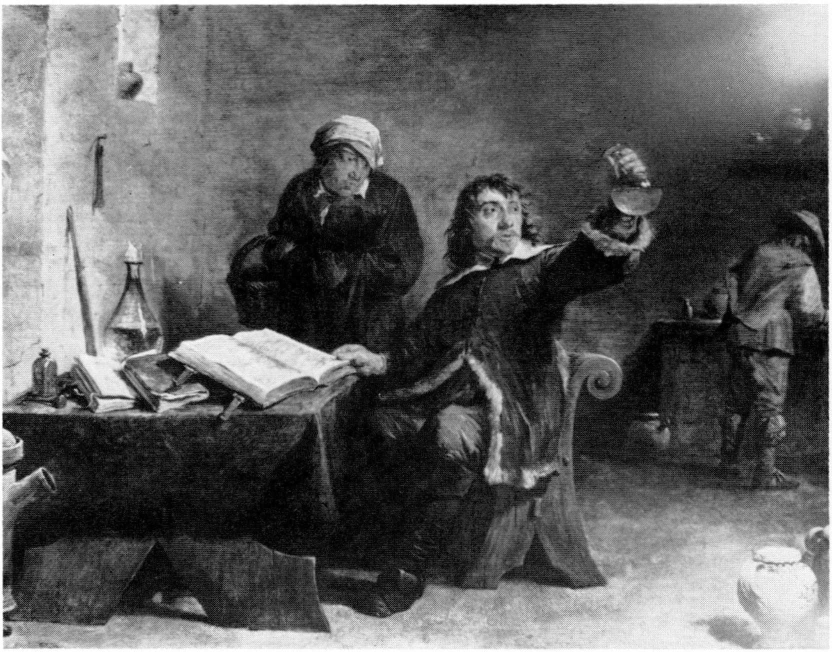

FIGURE 13. The Village Doctor, painted by David Teniers the Younger (1610-1690) Museum of Brussels, gives us a fine opportunity to view this phase of uroscopy. Note the serious attitude of the doctor and the apprehension of the patient. (Photograph by courtesy of Photographie Giraudon, Paris, France.)

the ceiling. At other times he would include some animal skulls and packages of herbs as part of the interior accessories. There is no doubt that Teniers was a believer in uroscopy for he treated the subject with great seriousness.

Ostade (1610-1685), a native of the Dutch city Haarlem, similarly showed great enthusiasm in depicting the uroscopist and characteristic interiors representing common scenes in the domestic life of the country he was so familiar with. In addition to the physician, he included the surgeon and the chiropodist as subjects for his canvases. One of the best known of his paintings show a physician, as a man of about middle age, wearing a velvet bonnet bordered with white, and garbed in a dressing gown. He is alone in his private sanctum and he is carefully examining the urinal glass, which he holds in his right hand,* while he leans his left on the table. Paper, pen, a large botannical book, opened at a page on which illustrations of some plants can be detected, and a pharmacy vase in blue and white delft, bearing the inscription "Ad Scabiam" can be seen on the table. To the left can be seen the doctor's library, divided from the study by a curtain, and at the back a door, half-opened which clearly demonstrates a room lighted by a stained glass window. Thus, the viewer of this painting is given the opportunity of studying the environment of the scientific practitioner of his time, who was a great reader, profound thinker and master of his craft. This was prior to the time when uroscopy fell into the hands of uromantics (uromancy) who were truly charlatans. Such fakers travelled around the country dressed in elaborate gowns and head-dress with solemn mien, and a mysterious urine-glass serving only to hood-wink the illiterate for a fee.

Gerad Dow† (1613-1685), one of the finest painters of the Dutch School, was equally partial in his selection of the physician with the urine glass as a model for his paintings. His most famous picture called *The Doctor,* the original of which hangs in the Imperial Collection in Vienna, is well known because of the many reproductions made from it. In this painting, the physician is represented as a young man with fair curly hair, wearing a velvet cap and dressed in a long brown robe, belted around the waist. He stands in the full light of an arched window, holding the urinal upraised in his *left hand,* while he makes an explanatory gesture with the right. Behind him can be seen an old woman, apparently in trouble for she is weeping and drying her eyes. Of singular interest is that on the

---

* Ismail, a Persian physician, who practiced toward the eleventh century advised that urine should be examined in daylight, but that the bottle be shaded from the sun. He also wrote that the physician is too sacred to hold a bottle containing urine with his own hands. The attendant should take the bottle in his left hand and show it to the physician. He also warned about keeping the urinal away from one's shadow and dress, as images are liable to give erroneous ideas and make the color look different. It is unfortunate that this early Persian idea is not recorded on paintings in any great number.

† May also be spelled Gerrit, Dow, or Douw.

window-ledge a richly colored cloth falls on a bas-relief representing the passions, and on it rests a barber's dish of copper, an ornamental bottle, an open book bearing an anatomical drawing and the name of Andre Vesale.

Gerad Dow is noted for another fine painting *The Water Doctor.**

Perhaps one of the greatest of paintings by Gerad Dow, and which now hangs in the Louvre is, *La Femme Hydrophique.* In addition, to being of medical interest it is a work of great skill and is much admired by artists for its tone, perspective and general execution. The painting depicts a fine apartment, furnished with great luxury and undoubtedly the home of a wealthy burger. A woman of middle age reclines in a chair and the artist clearly demonstrates her puffed eyelids, distended stomach and swollen feet. Kneeling by her side is a young girl, sobbing and looking up with great anxiety into the face of the patient, who in all probability is her mother. Behind the patient and leaning over her shoulder is an elderly woman, the servant or nurse, who is administering stimulant from a spoon.

"It is difficult to describe the piteous expression on the face of the patient other than to say it arouses great sympathy—sadness and silent suffering is clearly depicted in this scene

---

* According to Smith[9] the uroscopist was at first referred to as water doctor and in later years when his reputation was dwindling as water-caster, water juggler, water judge and even later as piss-prophet. "This last expression as one might guess," writes Smith, "was used ironically, and first appears in a volume by J. Hart. The editor of the *Journal of the American Medical Association* requested that the full title of Hart's work he included in the original publication of this essay and I let him have it: 'The anatomic of Urines: Containing the conviction and condemnation of them; or the second part of our discourse of urines; detecting and unfolding the manifold falsehoods and abuses committed by the vulgar sort of practitioners, in the judgement of diseases by the urines only; together with a narrow survey of their substances, chiefe colours, and manifold contents, joyning with all the right profitable and detectable histories concerning this subject; collected as well out of the ancient Greeke, Latine and Arabian authors, as out of our famous physicians of severall nations; their authoritie; quoted and translated out of the original tongues, together with some of the authors owne observations.' London, RoMylbourne, 1625, p. 32. "Now would I willing demand of the most cunning Pisse-prophet, what could he have found out by either of these urines." Smith concludes in his usual satirical and humorous vein, "And modern editors complain about the length of titles of scientific papers!"

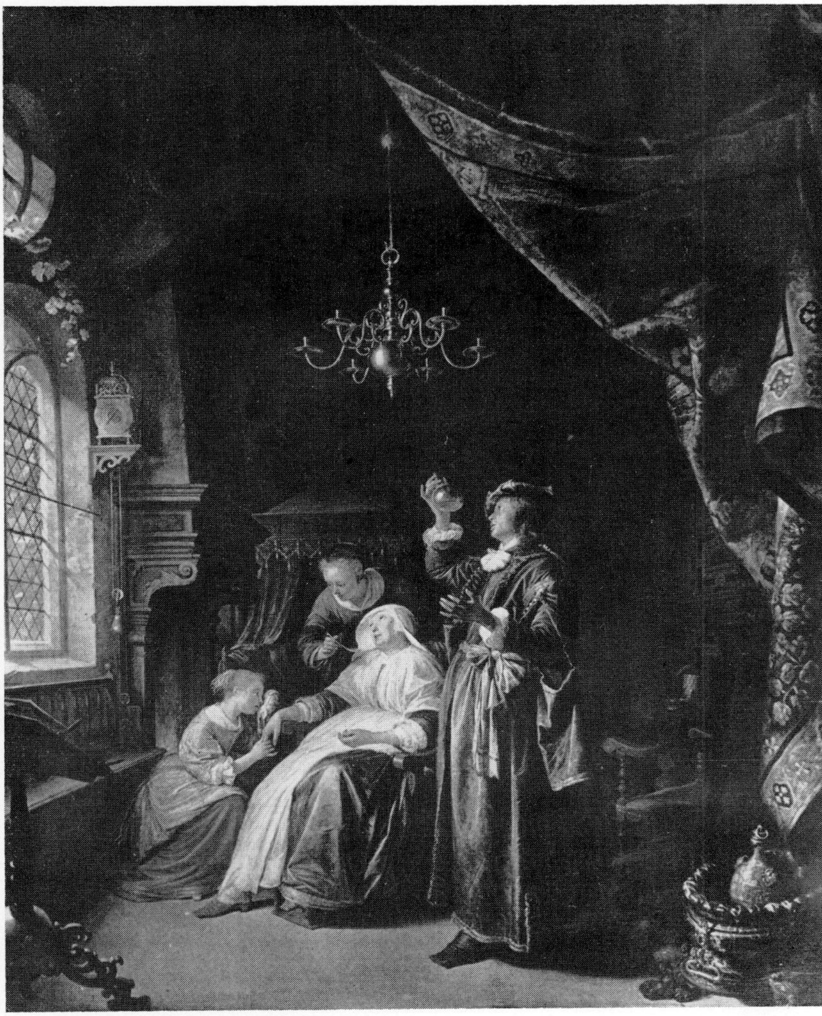

FIGURE 14. Gerad Dow (1613-1675). A realistic view of the Doctor, "Analyzing Urine—Uroscopy." Louvre, Paris. (Photograph by courtesy of Photographie Giraudon, Paris, France.)

which is strikingly contrasted by the bright sunlight which shines through the window, and "even the green leaves of a spray of creeper have crept through into the room, giving a subtle effect as a Nature's smile."

The figure of the physician has been remarkably portrayed by the artist, as he stands out almost in relief in the foreground. He is tall and dignified, graciously posed, and wearing a rich and sumptuous robe. In his right hand (should correctly be in the left hand) he holds the urine glass between the light and his eye, while with serious expression he examines the color of its contents. The remainder of the painting is completed by a rich oriental curtain which is draped back to the right side, on which the light falls and all are agreed that the entire work is a masterpiece of composition and technical execution.

The Dutch School often resorted to paintings representing languorous young women, with sunken eyes and waxen complexions, who appear extremely melancholic. Such a patient has been cleverly depicted by Gerad Dow, in the painting *Mal d'Amour*. In this painting, the doctor appears grave and dignified, fashionably dressed in a long robe and velvet bonnet trimmed with fur. In his right hand (Dow favors the right hand in all his paintings), he holds the urine glass to the light. The fingers of his left hand rest on the pulse of the fair patient, whose pale face and languorous look betray the symptoms of her distress.

Wellcome[66] describes a painting by Metzu which depicts a uroscopist as a young and fashionable doctor; attractive in face, and handsomely dressed in black velvet trimmed with fine lace, who handles the urine glass with an air of grace. He appears to be mingling compliments with the scientific phrases in which he is describing the complaint to his pretty client, while she, in an audacious negligee, abandons herself to the listless reverie which was a characteristic feature of *Mal d'Amour*. In the background are a young man and an old woman, who are evidently exchanging confidential opinions on the case, and who could no doubt afford more truthful evidence of its cause than the liquid which the physician is so carefully examining in the glass.

The physician and the medical profession have come in for

their share of caricaturing throughout history. "The positive role which the physician plays in the lives of his patients, in health and sickness, in sadness and despair, and in birth and death the physician's humanness and vulnerability, his ineptness and fallacies, and his apparent preoccupation with financial gain are most forcefully and revealingly expressed. But it has remained for the caricaturist and for many who are not preeminently caricaturists but artists to highlight the physician and the medical profession in all their defect—real and imagined."[68]

Such an artist was Jan Steen* of the Dutch School. This artist differed in his handling of the uroscopist by generally treating him in a humorous fashion. At times, he ridiculed the patient and at other times the physician. He rarely depicted the physician as giving serious attention to the urine glass. Instead, he usually portrayed him as if employing this method of diagnosis more as a matter of form than as a necessity. However, in his famous painting *A Judgement from Urine* he reverts to the traditional execution of a scene with a uroscopist. In this scene the physician is depicted as a man of bulky proportions, examining a specimen of urine with due gravity. The patient, evidently ill, appears emaciated and pale, is seated awaiting the doctor's verdict. Directly behind the doctor and the patient is an elderly woman crying as she pitifully gazes at the invalid, who undoubtedly is her husband. On a table near the physician is another urinal glass and a basket: the latter undoubtedly for carrying the urinal glass.

Ryckaert (1612-1661) painted several pictures with the uroscopist as his model. In one painting, Ryckaert shows original detail in the accessories of the scene. The physician is depicted by the artist as an old man with a long beard. He is dressed in a fur-trimmed robe, and is seated at a table, on which lie many books and papers. On the table can also be seen an inkstand, a

---

* Jan Steen (1626-1679) of Leyden was one of the leading Dutch painters of his day. His work consisted mainly of scenes of town life interpreted in a humorous, moralizing manner epitomized in his famous painting *The Lean Kitchen.* The modern physician scrutinizing this painting would be interested in analyzine the nutritional status of Steen's subjects.

vase, and a skull and the entire scene is lighted by a smoking candle. Here the physician holds the urine glass in his left hand and in the liquid can be seen floating a little figure of a foetus, at which the urologist is gazing with astonishment. Behind the physician sits an old woman, who undoubtedly brought the specimen. She is patiently awaiting the verdict with her hands clasped. Unfortunately, the charlatan of this era claimed to be able to determine pregnancy by uroscopic examination.

MacKinney*[69] discusses Byzantine Uroscopy utilizing a manuscript from fifteenth century Byzantium; Bologna, University, MS 3632, folio 51. Theophilus Protospatharius, On Urines, in Greek:

The picture portrays uroscopy in a Greek setting. Seated at top left is a famous seventh century Greek expert on urology, Theophilus, whose treatise *On Urines* was much used in the Greek East and in the Latin West (in translation). Handing Theophilus a urine flask that has been taken from a carrier-basket is his assistant, Posos (according to the Greek caption above him). Both men are clad in long robes and curious bonnet-like caps distinctly Eastern in style. Below, are rows of uroscopy flasks, twenty-one in number. Over each flask is a caption indicating the type of urine therein (the text of the treatise describes in detail the various textures and colors of urines, and their significance). Noteworthy in our illustration, states MacKinney, "is the shape of the flasks, very different from those depicted in Western Manuscripts, which are round-bottomed and large necked." The reader is here reminded of the description of flasks depicted in scenic illustrations of uroscopy by painters of the Dutch School.

---

* Loren C. MacKinney (1891-1964), an outstanding scholar in medieval history, devoted much of his career to medieval medicine. We are greatly indebted to him for his untiring researches into manuscript sources where he gave undivided attention to miniatures and illuminations that illustrated particular facets of medical practice such as uroscopy. Thus, many medieval manuscripts gave unequivocal evidence of the need and methods of proper diagnosis. Since uroscopy was deemed especially important as a diagnostic procedure and since there were many procedures in the examination of the urine, much data has been accumulated from a study of such manuscripts with miniatures and illuminations so brilliantly described by MacKinney.

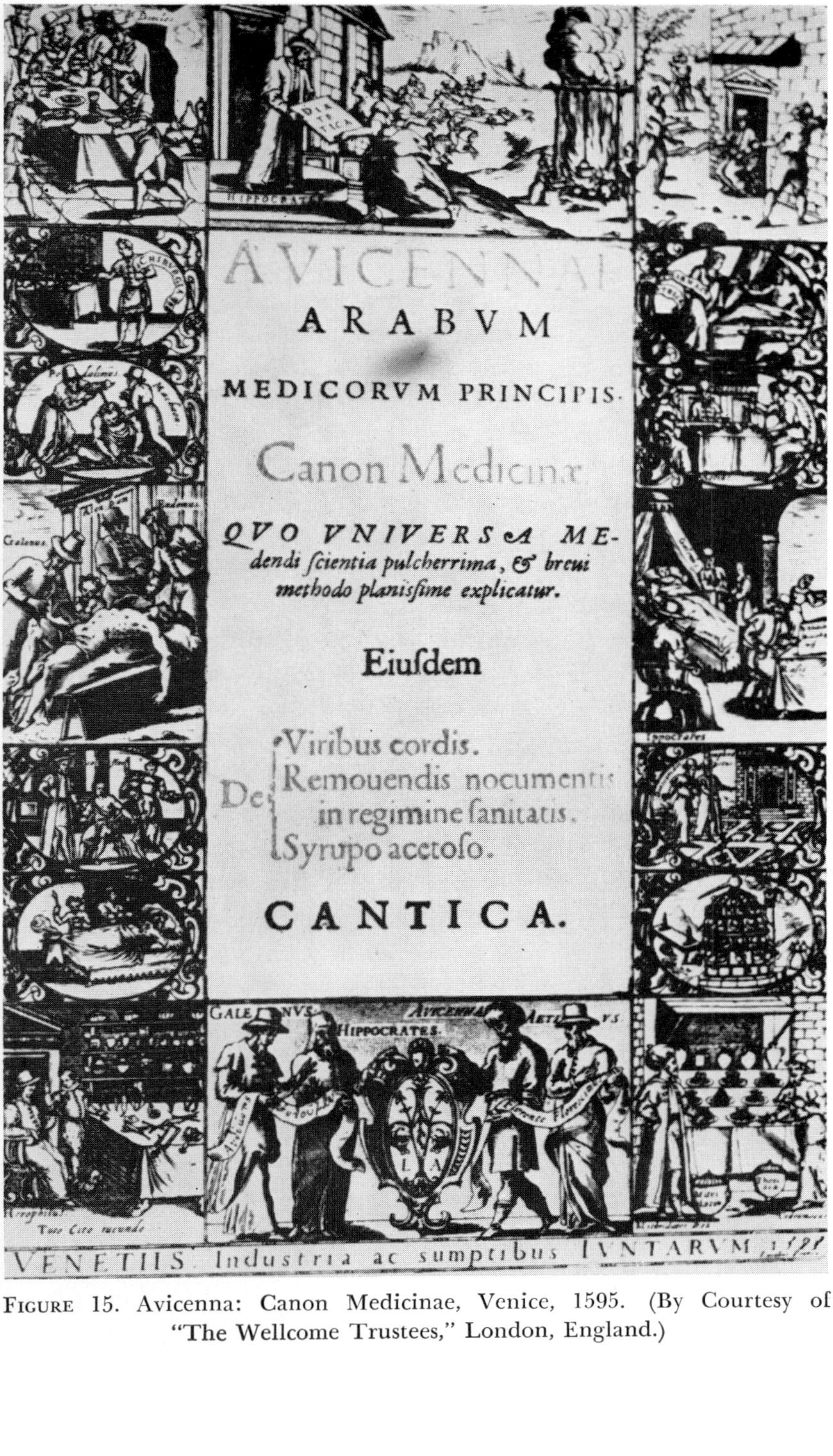

FIGURE 15. Avicenna: Canon Medicinae, Venice, 1595. (By Courtesy of "The Wellcome Trustees," London, England.)

In a manuscript from fifteenth century Flanders (Glasgow, Hunter, MS 9, folio 84 Avicenna, *Cannon*, I ch. 2), can be seen a manuscript miniature, depicting delivery of a urine flask at a diagnostic clinic. Many of the manuscript miniatures of uroscopy picture the delivery of the patient's urine sample to the physician in the characteristic flask, usually carried in a basket container. Here is a colourful representation of such a scene. At left is a woman (perhaps pregnant) who, after handing the flask to one of the four physicians, makes an explanation concerning it. In her hand she holds the flask-carrier (which, incidentally, seems too small for the somewhat oversized uroscopy flask). The flask is about to take its place on the shelf along with five others. One of the physicians (all of whom are clad in ermine-trimmed robes and academic birettas) points to a flask on the shelf, making comments to one of his colleagues. The picture illustrates a section in Avicenna's *Cannon* concerning the "significance of the colour of urine." (See Avicenna.)

A word about Constantinus Africanus, also known as Constantine the African (c. 1020-c. 1087), translator of Arabic works into Latin.[70] He was probably born at Carthage, lived for a time at Salerno, and finally retired to the Benedictine monastery at Monte Cassino. His translations had an important influence on European medicine from the twelfth to the seventeenth century. His fame has been compared to Galen's in Rome, Theophilus's in Byzantium and Avicenna's in Islam. In a manuscript from the fifteenth century (Oxford, Bodley, MS Rawl. c. 328, folio 3), are twelve anonymous illustrations of uroscopy and cautery: the text above the picture reflects the exaggerated merits attributed to him (Constantinus Africanus). It reads as follows: "This is Constantinus, Monk of Monte Cassino, who is as it were the fount of that science of long standing concerning the diagnosis of urines (indicilis urinarum) and all ailements. In this book and many others, he has set forth the true cure. To him come women with urine, so that he may tell the ailement in the case."

The illustrator skillfully depicted the famous monk, seated with what doubtless was intended to represent one of his books, which he explains to the patients approaching with their urine-filled flasks. First comes a woman, presenting her flask with a hopeful expression on her face. She is followed by a man with his flask and by one other person.

In a Paduan manuscript of the year 1434 (Munich, folio Bartholomaeus de Montagnano) appears a medieval scene of uroscopy. The physician is portrayed holding the flask of urine to the light to evaluate it as to colour and texture. "In this picture, Bartholomaeus de Montagnano, a prominent Paduan physician carefully inspects a flask of urine. Before him on the lectern and shelf are two open books. They may be Theophilus *On Urines,* or the section of Isaac Judaeus or of Avicenna's works which treat of urines in detail. On such books Westerners relied heavily. . . . At times, however," comments MacKinney, "they tested their physician's efficiency by playing tricks, such as the following: 'A famous monastic physician of St. Gall during the tenth century . . . was about to examine (the urine of) the Duke of Bavaria. As a trick to test Notker, the Duke substituted for his own urine that of a woman who was pregnant. But Notker, after having made his examination, without any apparent sign of suspicion made the solemn announcement that: God is about to bring to pass an unheard of event; within thirty days the Duke will give birth to a child. Whereupon the Duke was said to have blushed.' "

One of the most dramatic of the numerous medieval miniatures portraying uroscopy and clinical patients is seen in a French Manuscript from fifteenth century France (Cambridge, Fitzwilliam Museum, Bartholomaeus Anglicus, De proprietatibus, rerium, V, 1. in French). Clad in the usual splendid robes of a physician, and wearing a skull cap, he explains the uroscopy diagnosis apparently for the patient on the floor, who is afflicted with dropsy. . . . The text above the miniature explains that, "properties in general, and then in particular" will be considered next; the text below explains that "according to Avicenna the members (of the body) are organs composed of the primary combination of humours." The French version, done in 1372 by Jean Corbechon for King Charles V, is only one of several translations; e.g., into Provencial (before 1391), into Spanish (fifteenth century) and into English (1397-1398).

Although we are primarily interested in the history of uroscopy we cannot omit some mention of pulse taking, which in conjunction with uroscopy actually made up the physicians' entire armementarium at this time.

Some medieval writers believed that pulse taking was more important than uroscopy. Thus in the introduction to a pulse treatise by an anonymous writer in a fourteenth century manuscript, the writer explained that urine indicated the status of the heart; therefore it seemed reasonable to assume that since the heart was more important than the liver, pulse reading was more important than uroscopy. It is probable that such logic was influenced by the practical factor of the simplicity of taking the pulse. But there was a definite intelligent and professional approach to the art of pulse taking. In this then considered complicated procedure, certain factors were to be considered, such as the seasons, the patient's sex, age, emotional condition and patient's case history including habits of eating, drinking, sleeping, exercise, bathing and the like.

In a manuscript from fifteenth century Flanders (Glasgow, Hunter, MS 9, folio 76 Avicenna, *Cannon,* I) is a fine miniature depicting the physician taking the pulse of a bed-patient: Here we see an emaciated patient anxiously watching the physician's fingers on his wrist. Noteworthy is the clear portrayal of the physician's four fingers on the inner side of the wrist, a method still taught medical students. However, the artist misrepresented, or the physician failed to use, the best ancient and medieval technique; viz, to grasp with his *right* hand the *right* hand of the patient thus bringing the tips of the four fingers to bear on the radial artery where the beat is strongest (an ancient Hindu treatise advised taking men's pulse on the right hand, women's on the left). Ancient and medieval writers . . . advised the physician to take a position at the foot of the bed, but under no circumstances should he sit on the bed itself. Celsus, Galen, and others give detailed advice on these matters.

Thus, as early as the ninth century, young physicians were reading instructions in the technique of pulse-taking such as: "Learn how to take the pulse so that you can do it standing or seated. . . . If you are holding the right hand with your right hand, let the fingers be uppermost. Let two fingers, the index and middle fingers, be placed together inside on the upper part of the artery. Hold the pulse for a long time so that you can detect the up and down beat."

A double action manuscript miniature depicting the two principal types of diagnosis is seen in a manuscript from the fifteenth century Flanders (Dresden, MS pp. 92-93, folio 293V, De pulsibus et urinis 2). Here, the physician in the person of Galen, clad in splendid ermine trimmed robes and ermine head-dress, holds a uroscopy flask in one hand, while with the other he takes a lady's pulse.

MacKinney tells us that this illustration is one of several hundred done expertly in colour with elaborate decorations in a manuscript of various Galenic works. "Partly water-damaged during World War II, fortunately it survived. A photo facsimile, with several folios in colour, was published by E. G. Van Leirsum and W. Martin, *Codices Graeci et Latini . . .* (Leiden, 1910). From this our reproductions were made, inasmuch as it was impossible to obtain colour microfilms at Dresden in 1960."

Nathan *et al.*[68] emphasize the role played in medical history by portraits of physicians. The first medical portrait is that of Imhotep, circa 3000 B.C., who was physician to Pharoah Zoser, great architect (pyramid of Sakkara), priest, statesman and demi god in Egyptian mythology. Contemporary portraits of the great philosopher-physician of the Greek period are hardly known. Thus no portraits of Hippocrates, Herophilus or of Diocles are known, nor is it known whether any ever existed. Many sculptures believed to be those of Hippocrates have never been positively identified as such. Indeed, many historians often question the actual existence of Hippocrates.

Great strides in art continued and from the fifteenth to the eighteenth century we see portrait paintings of outstanding physicians replacing the historical paintings of former centuries. Of interest is that the artist now did not resort to props to identify the subject or scene. Many of the portrait painters became famous as a result of their contribution to the painting of famous doctors of the time. Andreas Vesalius was painted by Jan Stephen van Calcar (1500-1546). Calcar went to Venice where he became a pupil of Titian. Francesco claims that not infrequently Calcar's paintings were believed by great artists to have been painted by the master himself. Calcar was a friend of Vesalius and illustrated his work, the famous *Fabrica* with wood cuts. He painted Vesalius in Italy, and in the style of the country. (See Chapter 000—Vesalius.)

One can hardly speak of the School of Titian without mentioning Tintoretto. In Tintoretto's portraits, "as in his other paintings there appears for the first time a hint of Baroque art. While Titian intensifies and emphasizes the beauty, splendor and power of the people whom he portrays, Tintoretto represents them as integral embodiments of the offices that they occupy. An engraving after Tintoretto shows Michele Mercati, papal physician and an outstanding mineralogist. He regards us with eyes as clear as water, and not the slightest sign in his face indicates what sort of a person Michele Mercati actually was."

In Francesco's essay,[71] he selects as a representative picture of a doctor from among the master portraits of the seventeenth century, a portrait of Lazarus Maharkijzus, a physician of Antwerp, painted by Anthony Van Dyck. The painting dates from the years 1627-1632. "When Van Dyck returned to his native city from Genoa" writes Francesco, "he was overshadowed by the fame of Rubens and spent a few unhappy years. Not long after, it became fashionable in high society to be painted by Van Dyck, and as the prices asked by the painter were very high, this fashion remained restricted to the very wealthy.

MacKinney[69] clearly differentiates between ancient and medieval illustrations. Thus, from about 500 A.D. onward, the manuscript became important, and manuscript illustrations were used to elucidate medical texts. "Byzantine manuscripts from these centuries picture in graphic, though sometimes crude, detail the time-honored medical practices: uroscopy, the taking of the pulse, the reduction of a dislocated jaw, shoulder or vertebra, the bandaging of a head, chest or arm, the gathering of medicinal herbs, and the writing of prescriptions. . . . From the eleventh century onward, there is an increasing number of miniatures and an occasional full-page illustration. Practically

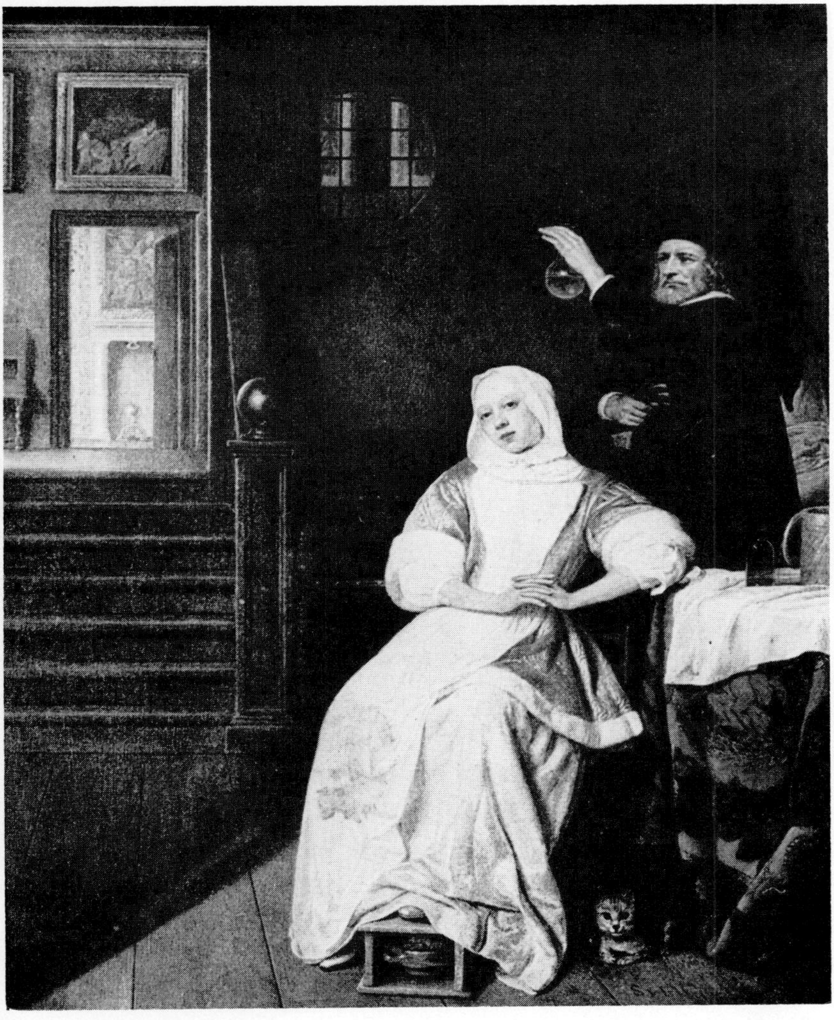

FIGURE 16. This painting of "The Sick Lady" by Samuel Van Hoogstraten (1627-1678) reveals the perplexity of the physician who is confused by the pallor of the patient and the gross dark appearance of the urine which could represent gross hematuria in a woman with glomerulonephritis.

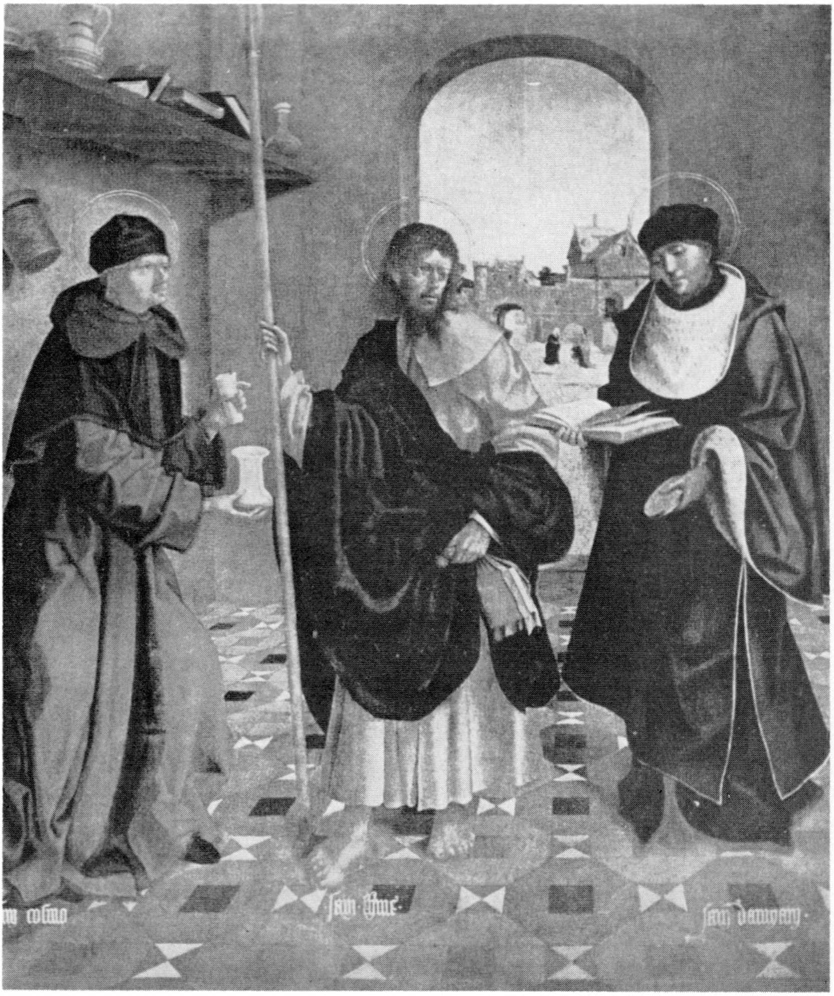

FIGURE 17. In the above painting (The Museu Nacional de Arte, Antiga, Lisbon) of Cosmas and Damian, the Saints flank St. Thomas. The painter is not accurately known but he is believed to be a Portuguese Master who lived about 400 years ago. St. Cosmas and St. Damian are traditionally accepted as the patron saints of the physician and apothecary. The two brothers were Syrian Christians, and believed to have effected many miraculous cures before they suffered martyrdom in the reign of the Emperor Diocletian (A.D. 303). They have been pictured many times in paintings, miniatures and prints, and usually represented with the attributes of their profession, namely, the urine flask and the cordial-beaker and spoon.

all of the pictures seem to have been deliberate efforts at elucidating some part of a medical text. Thus their purpose is fundamentally didactic or illustrative, rather than artistic."

As the Middle Ages waned, it remained for the Renaissance to establish medical historiography and to provide it with a basic idea that has remained present until today. Obviously, the interest of Renaissance writers confined mainly to the biographies and writings of famous physicians and made more vivid by accompanying illustrations. This had already made its appearance in the thirteenth century, manifesting itself in biographies of saints and of famous lay contemporaries.

In the many paintings of saints, few are as illustrative and of medical historical value as those of St. Cosmas and St. Damian. Figure 17 (a reproduction of painting in the Museu Nacional de Arte, Antiga, Lisbon) is a portrayal of Cosmas and Damian and shows the saints flanking St. Thomas. The object held by St. Cosmas appears to be a urine flask.

St. Cosmas and St. Damian are traditionally accepted as the patron saints of the physician and apothecary. The two brothers were Syrian Christians, and were believed to have produced many miraculous cures before they suffered martyrdom in the reign of the Emperor Diocletian (A.D. 303). Their bodies subsequently taken first to Cyrus in Syria, then to Asia, and finally brought to Europe. In 963, the Archbishop Adaldag, in a solemn ceremony, buried them in the Cathedral of Bremen. In 1400, a golden reliquary shrine was prepared for them and in 1648 it was taken to the Jesuit Church at Munich.

Proof of the popularity of the brothers, according to Gerlitt,[72] is confirmed by the fact that in antiquity many Christian physicians assumed the names of Cosmas or Damian. At the time of the Crusades, a knightly Cosmas and Damian Order existed for some time whose purpose it was to care for sick pilgrims and to exchange prisoners. In addition, many cities chose Cosmas and Damian as their patron saints. In 1226, the Surgeon's Guild of Paris chose Cosmas and Damian as its patrons. Since the Guild met in the Church of St. Come, this first special school for surgeons received the name "College St. Come" which existed until taken over by the Academie de Chirurgie. (See p. 199 in Chapter on Ambroise Paré.)

The urine flask in the Middle Ages and even later as described and illustrated in manuscripts practically became the symbol of the medical profession. Its progress formulated a strong *Ars Medica* which ultimately was to be supplemented by photography and reduplicating machines, not to overlook the role of television as an aid in medical education.

Chapter VIII

Uroscopy: From Antiquity to the Sixteenth Century

IN the beginning (see Chapter I) it is probable that ancient man was awed by the status and meaning of the urine. Indeed long before the true significance of this waste product of the body was properly assayed and evaluated it played an important role in the evolution of medicine. This was first based on pure superstition, later by folk-lore, still later by charlatans and finally truly evaluated by the transition of alchemy to chemistry.

Although the real significance of urine was poorly understood, it was soon suspected of being an important index to an individual's state of health. Thus abnormal changes in the appearance of the urine ultimately attracted the attention of man and eventually he associated it with bodily disease. If the ancients were aware of changes signifying disease no evidence of this knowledge appears until the early Grecian period; when one finds *uroscopy* established as a diagnostic means of detecting disease. Hippocrates devoted a special book to the study of the urine and recognized at least four conditions of the urinary tract that could be evaluated by the nature and appearance of the urinary outflow, namely colic due to stone, suppuration, hematuria and probably tuberculosis or malignant disease.

Galen subsequently adopted the Hippocratic belief that the appearance of the urine was an aid in diagnosis. Indeed, Galen went even further in an attempt to explain the physiology of the kidneys and formation of the urine (see P. 63 *et seq.*).

The empiric contemplation of the urine flask lasted down to

the sixteenth century when it reached its zenith in popularity. It was the principal if not the chief diagnostic method available to the orthodox physician who supplemented it with pulse taking, and at times study of the facies, the appearance of the tongue and excrements.

After the fall of Rome, anatomical and physiological inquiry seemed to come to a complete halt. There now was ushered into history "A Thousand Years of Darkness." Although many scientific theories formulated prior to this period were bizarre and mainly philosophical, they at least represented progress toward additional knowledge of the human body and its functions.

An excellent example of continued tolerance of ambiguous pursuit in medicine during this era was the great popularity of uroscopy, both in the East and in the West. Uroscopy* also spoken of as water casting† was originally advocated in a serious and quasi-scientific manner. Unfortunately, it fell into the hands of quacks and charlatans whose unscrupulous practices ultimately labelled the procedure as uromancy.

In the eleventh century, the art of uroscopy was quite extensively used, particularly by disciples in the School of Salerno.† Thus a Salernan physician on visiting a patient, after paying the

---

* Homer Smith[73] defined uroscopy as "the art (if we may call it such) of making a diagnosis and prescribing therapy solely on the evidences afforded by looking at the urine, for which purpose the urine was studied carefully in a specially shaped flask by an almost ritualistic procedure."

† Shakespeare in *Two Gentlemen of Verona* (Act II, Scene I) refers to water casting when he makes Speed say: "These follies are within you and shine through you like the water in a urinal, that not an eye that sees you but is a physician to comment on your malady."

Again in *Twelfth Night,* Shakespeare alludes to the practice of water casting when Fabian speaks of "carrying his water to the wise woman," and again in King Henry IV when the doughty Sir John Falstaff asks, "Sirrah, you giant, what says the doctor to my water?" His page replies: "He said sir, the water itself was a good healthy water; but for the party that owned it he might have more diseases than he knows for."

† The School of Medicine at Salerno dispelled the stagnation of medicine which had persisted throughout the Dark Ages. Its professors were the first medieval physicians to cultivate medicine as an independent science. Many of the documents of the school have been found in the Breslan Codex of the mid-twelfth century discovered in 1837. The School at Salerno was eclipsed by the rise of Montpellier and Bologna to the front rank; it was suppressed by Napoleon in 1811.

formal salutation and compliments, would probably proceed to a careful examination of the pulse. Since he had no stethoscope and was not particularly versed in other modes of examination, he would then ask for an inspection of the urine. In an era when all clinical methods and scientific investigations were unknown, it was but natural for the physicians to resort to an inspection of the urine. On inspection he would note the color, the consistency, the quantity and any sediment that had deposited. He was keen in his evaluation and also knew that the quantity of urine voided should be in proportion to the amount of fluid taken in.

Chemical tests of urine were not employed for they were unknown. The only chemistry employed was in reality alchemy. As time went on, the inspection of the urine (uroscopy) became more popular. It appealed from a spectacular point of view, as strongly to the patient as to the physician.

A great deal of our present knowledge concerning uroscopy comes from literary sources and significantly interesting is supplemented by pictorial sources. For thousands of years, because of no definite universally accepted nomenclature identifying plants, herbals were frequently illustrated in texts. Similarly, what the uroscopist saw while scrutinizing the urine has been illustrated in many ancient manuscripts. Despite the abundance of such material (see chapter Ars Medica), the written word was the main source of information (except for a dearth of such information in Egypt, where uroscopy was never popularized).

Constantinus Africanus* (1015-1087), one of the founders[74]

* It is believed by some that many of the writings of Constantinus Africanus were merely translations into Latin from Greek, Arabic and Jewish writers. His importance stems from the fact that by such latinizing he placed Muslim thought and culture at the disposal of European medicine from the 12th to the 17th centuries. From his earliest youth, Constantinus devoted himself to the study of medicine and supposedly made long journeys to Syria, India, Ethiopia, and Egypt. After remaining at Salerno during its "Golden Period," he became a Benedictine monk of the monastery of Monte Casino. He devoted the remainder of his life to intensive study and writing and died at Monte Casino in 1087. The first edition of the works of Constantine appeared in 1537 in Basel, in seven volumes. Practically all of the text of this and later editions are translations from the Arabic. He even translated from the Arabic the *Aphorisma* of Hippocrates as well as Galen's commentaries on the *Aphorisms*.

of the School of Medicine in Salerno in his work, *De Instructione Medici,* wrote that "urine is better than the pulse to discover the disease from which the patient suffers." The doctrine taught at the School of Salerno, and which was accepted by other medieval medical schools, was that the indications drawn from the urine, although relating to the whole of the body, referred more especially to the liver and the urinary ducts."

Gilles de Corbeil,* who lived during the twelfth and thirteenth centuries,[75] a graduate of Salerno, and first physician to Philip Augustus, wrote an elaborate poem on the urine, entitled *Liber de Urinis* and several treatises on urinary disturbances which were considered very favorably throughout Europe for about four centuries. His work served to popularize the practice of uroscopy and for several centuries this practice came close to excluding all other types of medical observation.

Corbeil begins in his writing to first study the etymology of the word urine, and then referring to the composition of this excretion, wrote that, "urine is composed of the residue left in the blood and other humors in the kidneys." (This is extremely prophetic for it was not until the advance of scientific urine analysis more than six hundred years later, that the attention of the chemist and clinician turned to the study of blood.) Next, Corbeil proceeds to lay down in detail rules for its examination, placing for the guidance of the uroscopist, special emphasis on the aspect, the consistence, the quantity, the nature and the things contained therein. He also advised the physician to take into consideration the circumstances of place, the number, the time, the age, the sex, the exercises indulged in, as well as the temperament and diet of his patient.

This author distinguished no less than twenty different colors in the urine from which he drew his conclusions. He gave

* Pierre Gilles de Corbeil (c. 1200) was a celebrated French physician who attended the School of Salerno and Montpellier and then went to Paris, where he was archiater to Philip Augustus, and probably taught at the University. He was the author of a didascalic poem, which described the different kinds of pulse, methods of examining the patient, of studying the urine, advice about the behaviour of the physician, and inectives against the pharmacists, presented in facile and elegant form. The book on the urine, which is the first in the poem, was regarded up to the end of the sixteenth century as the classical text on uroscopy.

specific instructions as to the kind of urine glass to be used, stating that it is to be of "glass, transparent, and to be in the form of a bladder. The place for examination must neither be exposed to the sun nor in the darkness, and if it be necessary to make an inspection in the sunlight, the hand should be interposed so that the various colors of the residue may be seen more distinctly. If made by candlelight care is to be taken that the rays do not fall directly on the glass."

Bernard de Gordon,[53] of Montpellier (1285-1318), who also studied at Salerno, and was the author of *The Lily of Medicine* wrote that the examination of urine for the purpose of diagnosis is without rival, and recommends it to the physician as the first proceeding. He further declared that the "science of judging the urine is so easy that all can learn what they wish to know."

In many of the medieval transcripts, pertaining to uroscopy the physician is advised to take certain precautions in dealing with patients of various classes and their relatives. Apparently many patients tried to deceive the uroscopist when they sent their urine for examination. It is quite likely this was done to test the doctor's knowledge and skill. It follows that some steps were necessary to guard against such trickery.

Henry Sigerist[75] has given the following fine translation of *Arnaldi de Villa Nova de Cautelis Medicorum* attributed to Arnold of Villanova. This treatise is divided into three parts but part I is most applicable to our dissertation and is therefore herewith reproduced:

On the Precautions that Physicians Must Observe

"We must consider the precautions with regard to urines, by which we can protect ourselves against people who wish to deceive us. The very first shall consist in finding out whether the urine be of man or of another animal or another fluid; and if it is human urine it is diagnosed in four ways.

"The second precaution is with regard to the individual who brings the urine. You must look at him sharply and keep your eyes straight on him or on his face; and if he wishes to deceive you he will start laughing or the color of his face will change, and then you must curse him forever and in all eternity.

"The third precaution is also with regard to the individual who brings the urine, whether man or woman, for you must see whether he or she is pale, and after you have ascertained that this is the individual's urine, say to him: 'Verily, this urine resembles you' and talk about the pallor, because immediately you will hear all about his illness. It commonly happens with poor people and those of moderate means that they go to the doctor when they are afflicted very seriously.

"The fourth precaution is with regard to sex. An old woman wants to have your opinion. You inquire whose urine it is, and the old woman will say to you: 'Don't you know it?' Then look at her in a certain way from the corner of your eye, and ask: 'What relation is it of yours?' And if she is not too crooked, she will say that the patient is a male or female relation, or something from which you can distinguish the sex. Should she say: 'We are not related' then ask what the patient used to do when he was in good health, and from the patient's doing you can recognize or deduce the sex.

"The fifth precaution is that you must ask if the patient is old. If the messenger says yes, you must say that he greatly suffers from the stomach, and that he spits a lot, and in the morning more than at any other time, for old people have by nature a cold stomach.

"The sixth precaution: whether this illness has lasted for a long time or not. If the messenger says that it has, you must say that the patient is altogether irritable and that one can help him, or some such talk. If he says no, you must say that the patient is altogether oppressed because in the beginnings of diseases there is much matter that oppresses the organ.

"There is a seventh precaution, and it is a very general one; you may not find out anything about the case, then say that he has an obstruction in the liver. He may say: 'No, sir, on the contrary he has pains in the head, or in the legs or in other organs.' You must say that this comes from the liver or from the stomach; and particularly use the word, obstruction, because they do not understand what it means, and it helps greatly that a term is not understood by the people.

"The eighth precaution is with regard to conception. An old woman consults you because the patient cannot become pregnant. Perhaps you do not know the cause but say that she cannot hold her husband's sperm which she could have done very well if she has been well disposed.

"The ninth precaution is with regard to a woman, whether she is old or young; and this you shall find out from what is told you. Should she be very old, say that she has all the evils that old women have, and also that she has many superfluities in the womb. Should she, however, be young say that she suffers from the stomach, and whenever she has a pain further down, say that it comes from the womb or the kidneys; and whenever she has it in the anterior part of the head, then it comes from the stomach; and whenever on the left side, then it comes from the spleen; whenever to the right, then it comes from the liver; and when it is worse and almost impedes her eyesight, say that she has pains or feels a heaviness in the legs, particularly when she exerts herself.

"The tenth precaution: you must keep yourself very busy spitting or blowing your nose and if the old woman pesters you with the urine say casually: 'What concern is this of yours?' or 'Why do you pester me so much?' If she says: 'Yes, it concerns me' then you shall know the sex. If she says, no, ask as has been explained under the fourth precaution.

"The eleventh precaution is taken with regard to white or yellow wine. If you have any doubts in this respect, be cautious and put the lid on the urinal down and pour out a little of the content in such a way that the wine in being poured out touches your finger. Then you must give her the urinal and act as if you were going to blow your nose whereby you put the finger that has been dipped in, on or next to your nose; then you will smell the odor of wine, whereupon you must take the urinal again and say to her: 'Get away and be ashamed of yourself!'

"The twelfth precaution is taken with respect to fluid made from figs and also nettles. Although you could recognize this under the first precaution, yet you will clearly see that the residue extends in the form of a circle touching the urinal and does not make a rotundity or pine cone like a true sediment.

"The thirteenth precaution: whenever the old woman asks what diseases the patient has, you must say: 'You would not understand me if I told you, and it would be better for you to ask what he should do.' And then she will see that you have judgement in the matter and will keep quiet. But perhaps she will say: 'Sir, he is very hot; therefore he seems to have a fever.'—'Thus it seems to you and other lay people who do not know how to distinguish between fever and other diseases.'

"The fourteenth precaution: When you have been called to a patient, feel the pulse before you examine the urine and make them talk so that the condition of the animal virtue becomes apparent to you. After having recognized these factors you will be able to evaluate the urine better and with more certainty and you may proceed thus.

"The fifteenth precaution is: should the patient be in a bad condition so that you think that he may die the following day, do not go to him but send your servant to bring you the urine, or tell them to bring it tomorrow in the early morning because you wish that they prepare for the meal and that after you have seen the urine you will tell what they shall administer. And so from the report of the person who brings the urine you will be able to form an opinion about the patient, whether he is in good or bad condition.

"The sixteenth precaution is that when you come to a patient you should always do something new lest they say that you cannot do anything without the books.

"The seventeenth precaution is that if by hard luck you come to the home of the patient and find him dead and somebody perhaps says: 'Sir, what have you come for?' You shall say that you have not come for that, and say that you well knew that he was going to die that night but that you wanted to know at what hour he had died.

"The eighteenth precaution is that if you have a competitor whom you believe to be a shameless crook, be careful when you go to the house of the patient; perhaps he will stir up to urine for you and you will not be able to form a certain judgement from it.

"The nineteenth precaution is the following: If two urines of the same patient are presented to you and you wish to know which was the first, ask at what time of the night he got up, for if he did at dawn or after digestion had taken place that urine which is more digested and red will be first, if it has sediment. If, however, he got up before midnight or around that time, you may judge that the less digested and less red urine is the first.

"No other deception can occur outside of these, but these points must be kept in mind, and you must be cautious because the physician is greatly honored if he knows how to be cautious, for he is asked questions many times."

A remarkable fable written in the thirteenth century, called *Roman du Renart* is the first strong evidence that uroscopy was being questioned.[76] The poem is an extremely entertaining satire on the medical practice of the time particularly with regard to uroscopy. In this poem, the sick lion calls for the fox (the physician) to attend him.

"Come soon to my rescue," said the lion to the fox;
"I abandon myself entirely to you,
And thou, fox, think of me,
Lest thou shoudst take hasty care.
What thou wouldst have done, shall be done.
Nor will I speak more or less
I am entirely in your hands."

"In my head I feel a great pain,
Such as it seems to me (so God love me)
That it is being broken to pieces.
And my sight is troubled,
That I often see nothing,
My mouth is so bitter
That nothing for me has a taste.
I feel much pain all over the body,
The worst is that only with great pain
Can I draw my breath.
I can tell you but half the ills,
On account of the pains which make me shiver."

Fox, the physician, then proceeds:

"So," said Fox, "you shall be cured,
When the third day has passed
Bring me a urinal,
And we shall see therein the ill."

Fox now claims that if he be allowed to examine the urine, he will then be able to discover the cause of the disease. To this the lion yields graciously.

The urinal was brought.
Noble is sitting upright,

and urined more than half.
And Fox said, "just so,"
Took it and went into the sunlight;
Lifted high the urinal,
Looked at it externally,
Turns it over and over again
To see whether it will alter."

. . . .

"Sire, he says, by God's help
I see you have ague
Yet I have the potion which kills it.
Sir King, I shall have to administer it to you."

The Fox now continues his examination, feels the pulse, touches the sides, the chest, the hips, and raises the head.

"A little longer and I should have been too late.
The sickness of your body I will cure.
The quartanc fever will go off,
Which takes away your breath so much."

All were not entirely blindfolded. A charming and highly suggestive reaction to the uroscopist appears in the works of Von Hutten,[77] a German knight of the fifteenth century. He writes a supposed dialogue between himself and a being whom he personifies as "Fever." Fever has attacked his body, and persists in staying in his body. Von Hutten then threatens to summon his physician, Dr. Stroemer "whom," he says "will check you, for in him I have faith." "Yes," replies Fever sarcastically, "the physician. Quite so, call Stroemer; as if I knew not your ways. You would prefer being ill for a whole year than partake even of two scruples of rhubarb, helleware or any other purgative. You had better call against me the physician who saw an oatgrain in a urinal and stated that the patient had eaten a horse."

Montagnana, the famous Italian physician, published (1487) a treatise on the signs furnished by the urine. He designed a chart by means of which the physician might compare the deductions to be drawn from the various colors as observed by him. In the chart, he shows twenty-one urine glasses, partly filled with a liquid colored in various shades, from bright yellow to brown, pink and red, and from blue to black.

The earliest book published in the English language on examination of the urine is entitled, *The Judycyall of Uryns,** and is believed to have been printed by Wynken de Worde in 1512. Bale believes this work is a translation of a manuscript written by Henry Daniel, a monk, in 1379. The title page bears a wood-cut of the physician holding a urine glass, and the text according to Wellcome, is mainly a repetition of that found in earlier works giving the signs which may be judged from the various colors of the urine.

Johannes Actuarius wrote an elaborate treatise on uroscopy: De urinus libri VII, apud A Cratandrum (1529). He was the first to use a graduated glass for the examination of urine.

Wellcome[76] writes of another work on the subject which was printed about 1540, and reads:

> *Here begyn/neth the seynge of urynes/*
> *Of all the colors that/urynes be of*
> *with the me/dycines annexed to every/*
> *uryne/every ury/ne his urynal*
> *michne/profitable for every/*
> *man to knowe.*

The work is undoubtedly an epitome of *The Judycyall of Uryns.* Each paragraph is preceded by a crude wood-cut of a urine glass, and the colophon advises that the work was "Emprynted at London in Foster Lane by John Waley."

In 1548, Robert Recorde published his *Urinal of Physick.* It gives elaborate particulars for *Making the judgement* as follows: "The urine should be kept to see which is first made after mid-night, and should be made in the urinal in which it is to be examined." He is also demanding as to the requirements of the urinal: "It should be of clear glass, not thyck nor greene in color, without blottes or spottes in it, or flat in the bottom, nor too wyde in the neck, but widest in the myddell and narrow styll toward bothe the endes, lyke the facyon commenly of an egg, or of a very bladder beyng measurably blowen (for the urinal should represent the bladder of a man) and so shall every thying be sene in his dew place and coloure.

"Besydes this also must ye mark the tyme dew to behold

---

* In the catalogue of the John A. Benjamin Collection of Medical History now at the University of California Library, Los Angeles, 1964, this book is listed (#368) as *Judycyall of Uryns.* London, P. Treveris, C. 1527. STC 14836.

urines. Fyrst, when the urine is made, whyle it yet is somewhat hotte. You shall consyder the coloure of it and lykewayes the thyckness of the substance of it. All other thynges, as the bubles and the contentes shall be judged somewhat after when the urine is somewhat cooled, and they be duly settled in their proper places."

In 1541, Fletcher, in his published work, *The Differences, Causes and Judgements of Urine,* writes: "Almost all signs of sickness or health, whereby the skillful physician is led into the knowledge of the states of the body, two are of most general and certain signification which are taken from the pulse and urine, without which all knowledge of physicke besides is obscure, doubtful and uncertain."[76]

Of interest is Fletcher's standards of a urinal: "A perfite forme of the urinal, wherein the urine according to its height is divided into three regions for the distinction of the three contents mentioned. 1, 2, 3, 4, the lowest region for the sediment; 5, 6, 7, 8, the middle region for the maze; 9, 10, 11, 12, the uppermost region for the cloud.

Fletcher further directs: "The physician should not view the urine in a place either too light or too darke, or by candle light, for so the colour will appear altered. Or else too light, or the sunne beams make the colour more remisse. Therefore put your hand or a blacke cloth betwixt the light and the urinal on the opposite part of the urinal that the colour and the contents be better discerned and your eyes be not dazzled with the light."

Thus, uroscopy, an art up to the sixteenth century; practiced for more than four hundred years, made little scientific progress. Contrary to the early advocates who were sincere in their belief; the "art" unfortunately fell into the hands of charlatans and quacks who travelled around the country side and took advantage of the credulity of the ignorant and misinformed.[71]

Chapter IX

Primitive Science—Ancient Chemists—Alchemy—Chemistry and Urine Analysis

UROLOGY, as we think of it today, first entered the scientific domain, when it passed from empiric contemplation of the urine glass and man began to investigate the chemical nature of urine. This took many centuries to accomplish and our story must now again revert to the time of the Babylonians, Egyptians, and Chinese.

The first discovery that permitted primitive man to carry on chemical reactions on any extensive scale was fire. Through the millennia, as primitive man slowly developed his cultural patterns, fire gradually made possible an increasing number of weapons and implements with which new advances could be made. The ancient craftsman did not think of the act of smelting a metal as a chemical operation nor did he distinguish it from any other act of his life. "Yet, as discoveries were made, they were incorporated in the technical processes of the culture and, in time, some were fitted into the cosmological patterns from which ancient science finally evolved."[78]

A good illustration of this is found in the history of iron. Analytical data indicates that the first iron used in both Mesopotamia and Egypt was probably of meteoric origin. This metal, called by the Egyptians iron of heaven, gave rise perhaps to the idea, that the source from which the iron came was composed of an iron plate.

Archaeological discoveries reveal that the earliest metals used by man were those that occur in native form. Copper and gold are found in the most ancient graves located in Egypt and Mesopotamia. It is quite probable that following the utilization of native metals, man attempted to extract metals from their ores.[79] Thus smelting of copper was probably discovered very early by the Sumerians in their prehistoric home in Southern Iran.[80]

In Egypt, bronze has been found as early as Dynasties III or IV (about 2500 B.C.) and at Ur and Eridu in Mesopotamia bronzes were known in the most ancient period, 3500-3000 B.C. It is of interest to note that copper continued to be used even after bronze was known, and remains found at sites on the Sinai peninsula where it was mined by the Egyptians show that the chief ore, malachite, was reduced by wood or perhaps charcoal.*

Lead, tin and iron were used in the ancient civilizations at later periods than copper, bronze and gold. After their introduction, the metal workers and smiths became a recognized class of artisans. They occupied a special place in all early cultures. Most of the metallurgical work was done in compounds attached to the temples, and though the priests themselves probably did not do the actual work the association of metals with the gods clearly and firmly became established.[79]

Besides the metals, the ancients had a great number of other chemical substances. Thus glazes were made at a very early period in history and later developed into true glass. Lapis lazuli, believed to have originated in Babylon, was valued and imported into Egypt, where it was classed with the metals. Artificial lapis lazuli was made in Babylon. "Egyptian Blue," a complex silicate of calcium and copper, was extensively used throughout the ancient world. Indeed it was used in the Roman era, when the architect Vitruvius described its preparation.[82]

---

* An interesting art that was long ascribed to the ancient Egyptians was the supposed power of transforming base metals into silver or gold. The ascription is undoubtedly wrong. There is abundant evidence that the art which later acquired the name of alchemy made its first occidental appearance in Greek-speaking Egypt, a little before or after 100 A.D. For such a date the most important and decisive testimony is that of Pliny the Elder (23-79 A.D.) whose *Natural History* covers every existing field of investigation and shows special interest in metallurgy, medicine and magic. It forms in fact the finest single source for the historical background of alchemy, but does not reflect a single idea that can be properly called alchemical. His book reveals a medley of aspirations, beliefs and superstitions, amongst which the idea of the transmutation of metals was apparently ready to burst into bloom, but the bud had not yet opened."[81]

From increased knowledge in metallurgy came a great interest in the stars and heavens, only to give birth to astrology, and from this to alchemistry. It seemed only logical to assume that the great and mighty powers in the heavens, correspond to lesser subjects on earth which they controlled. A change in one, meant a change in the other. Thus, they called the great world the macrocosm; the lesser world, the microcosm, and both were inseparable.

The streams of cosmological philosophy and crude science of the two great ancient civilizations (Babylon and Egypt) mingled with one another for a period of two thousand years, and eventually focused upon Greece, whose intellectual curiosity, fed by older concepts furthered a later science of pure Grecian origin.

The science of chemistry represents a gradual development from the much older alchemy* which had its incipiency from

* A word about the etymology of the word "Alchemy." Many early scholars originally believed the word "alchemy" to be of earlier Egyptian origin. Even after the general idea was abandoned, it was still the fashion among reputable scholars to try to derive the word "alchemy" from the ancient Egyptian language. In its present form, it comes from the Arabic, which passed it on into Latin and thence into the modern languages. The syllable *al* is the Arabic definite article, seen in such words as alcohol, algebra and alhambra. The main root comes from the Greek *chemia,* which also went over directly into Latin, and so gives us the modern word "chemistry," more readily recognizable in the French or German "chemie."

Wilson[83] believes that the etymology of so important a word is a matter of no small interest. "Whenever we use such terms as chemical and chemist, we are really employing an Egyptian root. The Greek lexicon of Suidas, compiled in the 9th or 10th century A.D., defines *chemia* as 'the preparation of silver and gold.' But it does not sound like a native Greek word, nor can it be traced back into the classical period. The Egyptians on the other hand, had a word *chem* or *gem,* meaning 'black' for which the original pictograph is thought by some to have represented a pile of charcoal. A derivative *chemi* was one name for Egypt itself, apparently meaning literally the 'black earth,' i.e., the fertile soil of the Nile Valley, as contrasted with the 'red earth' of the surrounding desert. Plutarch, writing in Greek about 80 A.D., once used *Chemia* as a proper name for Egypt. This is evidently a direct transliteration from the Egyptian."

The word *chemica* is not derived from Egyptian, and is also not to be found in early Greek.[84] Wilson believes the solution is probably a matter of orthography, since from Hellenistic times the Greek spelling was a flexible and uncertain affair. The consonants were fairly stable, but the vowel system of the classical Greek period broke down almost completely, ai, ē, e, ei, oi and y (sometimes transliterated also as u) being all pronounced as i. It is, therefore, not surprising to find the word often spelled chymeia, and this is accepted by most authorities as the original Greek form.[85, 86]

the first to the third centuries A.D. and gradually progressed on through to the fifteenth century, at that time taking on the influence of the Spagyrists. The latter, after developing for a century and a half, gave birth to the period of chemical analysis. Chemistry owes the discovery of many processes to the alchemists. Much of the apparatus used by chemists were devised by alchemists. "Therefore to the spagyrists, particularly, the chemistry of urine is greatly indebted."[87]

Alchemy was chemistry in the service of the ancient belief that gold and silver could be made from basic metals by artificial means. The idea had its origin in Egypt, was believed by Plato and Aristotle, and was actively promulgated by the Hellenistic School in Alexandria. It spread to Europe during the Middle Ages because of the Byzantine Empire and the Arabic conquests in Sicily and Spain. There are two concepts used in the term alchemy, namely a mystical and a physical. The mystical (philosophical) considers the transmutation through a Divine mixture of the base metal of the soul into a perfection. Reisman[87] states, "that alchemy entertained such a thought is strongly supported by the fact that Western alchemists made unanimous appeal to Hermes Trismegistus as the greatest authority on the art of alchemy and his alleged writings are undoubtedly of a mystical character." Of further interest is that physical alchemy, though it concerned itself with chemical processes, was not able to divorce itself entirely of mystical elements as is indicated by the alchemical language in which metals are called *noble* and *base*, *perfect* and *imperfect*.

Hermes Trismegistus* is believed to be the mythical founder of alchemy. It is questionable as to whether such an historical personage ever lived, but his name became ultimately the most influential in the entire history of the occult science. "Stories of his literary and scientific powers are almost infinitely various but the theory which finally came to prevail was that which made him a contemporary of Moses in ancient Egypt. Whether he was human or divine remained in some uncertainty. No Egyptian work ascribed to him exists, but Greek treatises un-

* Hermes Trismegistus (Lat. "the thrice greatest Hermes), an honorific designation of the Egyptian Hermes; i.e., Toth (q.v.), the god of wisdom.[88]

der the name of Hermes Trismegistus actually began to be produced about 100 A.D. . . . It is a singular fact that alchemical literature passing under this name is extremely rare in Greek, but in Arabic times something happened to the reputation of Hermes Trismegistus. He emerged into the European Renaissance as the supreme patron of alchemy, which came to be specifically the 'Hermetic Art.' During this period a new method was developed for closing the mouth of a flask in which an alchemical substance or mixture was to be treated with sustained heat.[83] This was quite an innovation since in the old way the opening was closed with some kind of sticky clay called "lute." Now, if the neck of the flask was heated to the point of viscosity and twisted, an air-tight closure would take place. This received the high-sounding name of *"Seal of Hermes"* and such a vessel was spoken of as "hermetically sealed," an expression still in common usage today.

As civilization progressed and religious disciples developed, the attainment of immortality became the great religious concern of millions. Thus, the search for "an elixir of life" was one of the objectives of early alchemy. It became but a short step from mysticism to magic and alchemy.

A study of alchemy in ancient China reveals significant and interesting data about early alchemy. The Chinese believed in certain mythical beings called *h'sien,* closely resembling the Arabic *djinn* (a word perhaps even derived from hsien), who could move unharmed through fire or water, pass instantly through walls or doors to any distant place, or assume invisibility. Such stories were used by the alchemists to set forth the marvelous effects of their medicine. Although the Confucian religion frowned on such beliefs, the Taoists cultivated them and incorporated into their philosophy means of developing alchemical medicines as a supposedly scientific means of attaining immortality.

Another notion which alchemy used but did not invent is that of the *Tao* or Way. This is probably the most influential single idea in Chinese thought. "The Taoist religion" among whose devotees alchemy developed, derived its name from this word. Philosophically, the *Tao* is the great organized structure or guiding principle of the universe. Morally, it is the proper course and conduct of life. In religion, the goal of immortality is often spoken of as the attaining of the *Tao*. It is a multiform word or idea, quite impossible to hold down to a single definition. The alchemists in their writings use it in many of its different senses, and occasionally seem even to mean by it the proper way of process for making their medicine."[83]

"Gold is non-corruptible in its nature and is therefore the most valuable of things. The men of the Art, feeding on it, attain longevity." Thus wrote Wei Po-Yang about 142 A.D., and it obviously holds the key to the whole development of Chinese alchemy, if not even of alchemy in general. Actually, it presents an idea, highly logical, and utterly false, that had been circulating for three to four generations and was destined to reach to the far parts of the world and hold its place in the field of science, pseudo or quasi, for at least a millennium and a half longer.

The value and integrity of gold was probably realized at a very early time in the history of mankind. At first, it was probably cherished because it did not tarnish or rust and did not melt away when melted in the fire. Thus Wei Po-Yang states: "When gold is placed in a hot fire, it is not deprived of the brilliancy of its color. Since the days of the unfolding of the universe (creation), the sun and moon have not diminished in brightness nor has gold lost its weight."

But how could gold be used as a medicament? Wei Po-Yang knew of it, in the form of dust or powder and its therapeutics which he vividly described: The *chin-sha* (gold dust), having entered the five internal organs, spreads foggily like wind-driven rain. Vaporizing and permeating, it reaches the four limbs. Thereupon the complexion becomes rejuvenated, hoary hair regains its blackness, and new teeth grow where fallen ones used to be. If an old man, he will once more become a youth; if an old woman, she will regain her maid-hood. Such transformations make one immune from worldly miseries, and one who is transformed is called by the name of *chen-jen* (true man).*

---

* For further study of Chinese alchemy the reader is referred to Wilson's *Biographies of Early Chinese Alchemists* and *Later Developments of Chinese Alchemy* and *Relation of Chinese Alchemy to That of Other Countries.*[82–85]

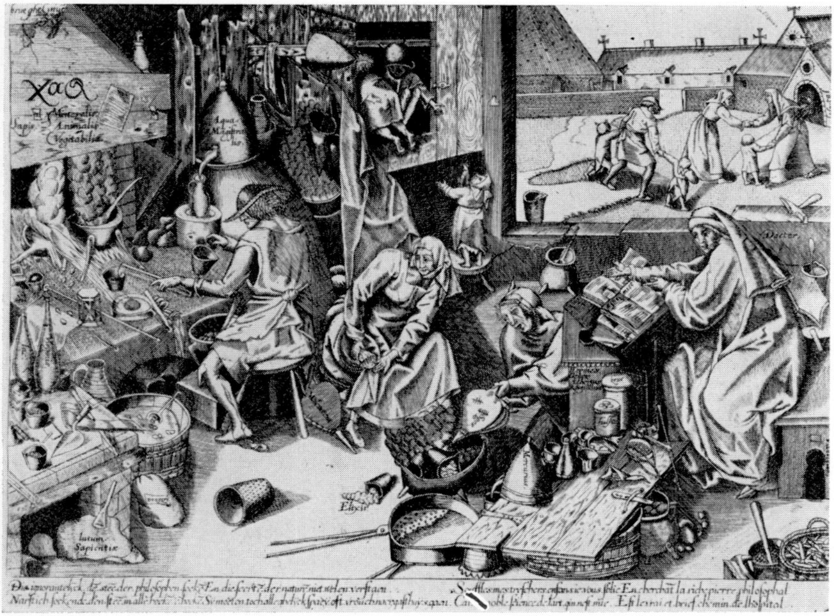

FIGURE 18. Drawing entitled "The Alchemist" by Peter Bruegel the Elder. Original drawing in pen and brown ink is located in the Kupferstichkabinett in Berlin and is dated 1558. This is a print supplied by the Medical Historical Library of the Yale University School of Medicine. The Alchemist, a shaggy and disreputable figure, is shown at his workbench heating a crucible in his search for the philosopher's stone ("Lapis"), an ill-defined object which would catalyze the transmutation of the base metals into gold. The alchemists believed that an initial supply of gold was necessary in gold-making, or multiplying, since bodies could multiply only in their own species. Thus, the Alchemist is shown dropping his last coin into the crucible; meanwhile his wife fruitlessly shakes her empty purse, and his children, one of whom wears an inverted pot on his head, scramble and search in the empty larder.

The multilingual inscriptions below the print allude to the fact that hunting for the philosopher's stone "is the true and short road to the Hospital." In the background, in an example of graphic time travel, the Alchemist, wife and children are shown being received in the poorhouse ("Hospital"). (Reference: Townsend, Gary L.: The Alchemist. *Journal of the History of Medicine,* 21:408-411, 1966.)

Smith,[73] without doubt, one of the greatest of the twentieth century physiologists, gives great credit to alchemists and writes: "It was in alchemy that the uses of urine first began to acquire a truly scientific cast. Earlier alchemical interests had centered on the salts of ammonis: ammonium chloride and ammonium sulfate, collectively called 'volatile salts' to distinguish them from involatile salts such as sodium chloride. Pliny in his *Natural History* refers to *Hammoniacussal,* but how the Romans prepared al ammoniac is unknown, though the name is said to have been derived from the fact that this salt was first made in the vicinity of the Egyptian temple of Jupiter Ammon. Later, alchemists prepared volatile salt for medicinal use by the dry distillation of fermented urine, and this salt was used in many alchemical operations."

Smith[73] also writes of the extraordinary and exciting substrate for alchemy, the element phosphorus. This word in Latin meaning *the morning star* and in Greek *a bringer of light,* was early applied to any substance that glowed in the dark, and it was only after the seventeenth century . . . that it was restricted to the element *phosphorus mirabilisor igneus,* a waxy crystalline solid with a disagreeable odor which possessed the remarkable property of burning, when exposed to air, with a bright flame and great heat. For this reason, it had to be prepared in the absence of air and stored under water.

Pure phosphorus was first isolated by the alchemist Brandt of Hamburg in 1669. He started with microcosmic salt (ammonium sodium hydrogen orthophosphate), so-named by the alchemists because it was obtained from decomposing urine of man. Though abundant in the earth and in all animals and plants, phosphorus is never found free in nature and Brandt was able to sell the secret of its preparation to a man named Krafft, who in 1677 exhibited some elementary phosphorus in England where it attracted the attention of English Chemists. Kunckel, in 1678, and Boyle, in 1680, worked out Brandt's secret of evaporating urine and dry-distilling the residue, collecting the distillate under water. The method was passed on from Boyle to a Mr. Hawkwitz, a druggist of London. Mr. Hawkwitz for more than twenty years prepared phosphorus from urine and sold it to all the natural philosophers of Europe for a fancy price. Urine remained the sole source of this exciting element until 1775 when Scheele developed a method preparing it from bones.

The early years of the eighteenth century saw the advent of the scientific epoch in the examination of urine. Chemistry now was emerging as a quantitative science. Alchemy* had been a mixture of empiric observations combined with astrology, mysticism, and religious philosophy. It had continuously operated behind a cloak of secrecy and expressed itself in esoteric symbolism.† The trend was now to disregard the stars, and for all chemists to work more or less openly only confining themselves to the composition and transmutation of what appeared to be the fundamental substances of nature. Urine was the main source of studying the composition and transmutation of the substance of living matter.

Until nearly the end of the seventeenth century, the diagnosis of disease was accomplished by visual examination of the urine (uroscopy). Van Helmont‡ was the first to inaugurate the quantitative study of urine. He devised a method of examining the urine by weight. He accurately determined the specific gravity of urine by weighing it in a glass vessel with a narrow

---

* In the latter periods of the Middle Ages, and in the seventeenth and eighteenth centuries, many of those that called themselves alchemists were charlatans and swindlers who often deceived both prince and pauper with their hocus pocus.

† Dante in his *Divina Commedia* condemns the false alchemists to Hell (Vaccaro, *Medical Life* (Feb.) 1932, quoted by Reisman, p. 118, foot-note:

> *So shalt thou see I am Capocchio's ghost*
> *Who forged transmuted metals by the power of Alchemy;*
> *And if I ken thee right,*
> *Thou needs must well remember how I aped*
> *Creative nature by my subtile art.*

‡ Jan Baptist Van Helmont (1577-1644) was a wealthy physician who lived near Brussels. He spent most of his life in retirement, carrying out chemical experiments. He considered himself a *philosophus per ignem,* a philosopher by fire, which approximately signifies a professional chemist. Although many of his theories were erroneous, he contributed much to the advancement of chemistry.

Van Helmont rejected strongly the Aristotle theory of the four elements. He felt that neither fire nor earth was a fundamental constituent of substances. Air was an element that could not be changed into any other form, and where it did exert any influence, as in the helping of burning of a fire, it did so only be a mechanical action. This left water as the basis of all chemical substances, and much of Van Helmont's experimental work was devoted to proving the importance of water in nature. This probably accounts for his great interest in urine.

neck and known to hold a certain weight of rainwater; he thus noted the dilute nature of the fluid excreted after the ingestion of water and the concentrated nature of that excreted after no ingestion of water as well as in fever. This was one of the first most forceful measures for eliminating the random examination of the urine as formerly practiced by uroscopists.[77, 87]

In 1674, Thomas Willis rediscovered the sweet taste of urine in diabetes mellitus, but the cause of the sweetness was not determined until one hundred years later, when (1778) Cruickshank, Dr. Johnson's personal physician, showed that this sugar was not milk sugar. All are agreed that because of Willis' observation there eventually followed the distinction between diabetes insipidus and glycosuria.*

The scientific epoch of urine analysis was further enhanced when Lorenzo Bellinni† (1643-1704) discovered that the change in color, taste and odor of urine were due to variations in the relative proportions of water and solids present. Although Bellinni's experiments were primitive when compared to later technique, he describes in his work, *De Urinis,* the evaporation of urine in an earthenware pot, with no cover, placed on an ordinary fire. He noted that the more the solution (urine) darkened in color, it lost its transparency, and by continual evaporation it passed through various degrees of tint from red to brown to almost black. By taking the weight after each of these changes of color, he tried to determine the quantity of water evaporated. He recorded that if an equivalent volume was added to the residue, its color, character, and properties would be restored. He believed that urine was composed of

---

* Doctors of India were careful observers of nature. They were famliar with the sweet taste of urine in diabetes mellitus long before it was suspected and known in Europe. It has been suggested that this discovery may have been made by the observation that ants sought out and enjoyed the urine of diabetics.

† In 1662, Bellinni (Lorenzo) wrote a classical description of the gross anatomy of the kidney. *Exercitatio anatomica de Structura et usu renum.* He is credited with first describing the renal excretory ducts (Bellinni's ducts) and also formulated a physical theory of the secretion of the urine. In 1683, he published, *de urinis et pulsibis, de missione sanguinis, de febribus, de morbis capitis, et pectoris,* in which he stressed the value of the urine as an aid to diagnosis and insisted on its chemical analysis in pathological conditions.

water, salt, and tasteless earth or tartar, and the consistent taste and color depended on the quantity of water which held these constituents in solution.

Bellinni's pioneer efforts were followed by those of Boerhaave* (1668-1738) the famous Dutch physician, who made further advances in the chemistry of the urine. In his first thesis, *De utilitate isprecendorum in algris excrementorium ut Signorum* mention is made that any substance found in the urine previously existed in the blood, therefore an examination of the urine should reveal an increase or decrease of a certain substance in the blood. He also studied the density of urine by adding the mercury hydrometer† to the physician's armamentarium.

The medical student of the twentieth century thinks little of the historical background of albuminuria and accepts with little awe the simple test for the detection of this substance. Yet, early in the history of the chemistry of urine, it was a rare test. Hippocrates noted in patients with kidney disease the presence of cloudiness which in all probability was due to albumin. In 1582, Willichins[89] noted a cloud in urine after it was heated. In 1670, Thomas Willis noted that in some disorders, the urine became cloudy when heated. Dekkers,† professor of medicine for thirty years at the University of Leyden is

---

* Boerhaave had a great reputation as a clinician and his writings had tremendous influence. Haller, Cullen, Pringle, Van Sivieten, and deHaen were among his pupils. His greatest contribution was his *Elementa chemiae,* published in 2 vols. at Leiden in 1732.

† The principle of the floating hydrometer was known to Archimedes, and early in the fifth century Synesius, Bishop of Cyrene, wrote to Hypatia, the famous mathematician and philosopher of Alexandria, asking her to have made for him an instrument which, from his description, was clearly intended for measuring the density of liquids (urines, oils). There is no evidence in Synesius's letter, however, that he intended to use it for urine. (Letter of Synesium of Cyrene, p. 99.) This reference was originally given to Homer Smith, by Dr. James P. Simonds of *Chicago.*

† Frederik Dekkers was born in 1648, in Holland. He stulied at Leyden under Sylvins. He graduated in 1668, and in 1673 he published his well known *Exercitationes practicae circa methodum* (practical exercises in methods of treatment), and in 1694, became Professor of Medicine at Leyden. Dekkers died in 1720.

Major described Dekkers' *Exercitationes* as a "curious work in which the chapters are arranged, not according to disease, but according to the remedies employed." (Reference: Major, Ralph H.: *Classic Descriptions of Disease.* Thomas, Springfield, p. 527, 1945.)

given credit for first detecting albumin in the urine. In his textbook, *Exercitationes practica circa medendi methodum* printed in Leyden in 1694,[90] he discusses the changes in the urine of emaciated individuals and consumptives. He did not link the albuminuria with dropsy and specifically regarded it as an occurrence in wasting diseases.*

Further advances were made by William Cruikshank† in 1798, when on experimenting with urine from a diabetic patient he made several pioneer observations. He noted the action of nitrous acid and other reagents on the urine of healthy individuals and observed that ammonia and fixed alkalies produced a cloudiness. This he believed was due to phosphate of lime, and that lime water produced a still more copious precipitate. From nitrous acid, he noted no precipitate occurred in the urine of a healthy person, but that in the urine of a dropsical patient, it produced coagulation or cloudiness, and he thereby discovered the first chemical test for albumin. Cruikshank made many experiments but the real value of his experiments is that they drew the attention of the medical profession to the importance and value of the chemical examination of urine as an aid to diagnosis.

In 1801, Jarrold described a method of testing for albumin. He placed an ounce of the patient's urine in a glass vessel to which he added a few drops of solution of acetate of lead to precipitate phosphoric and juriatic acids. Twelve years later, Weels used the nitrous acid test for albumin and Blackall in his writing *On Dropsies* in 1813, noted the effect of heat on urine with reference to albumin. "Writers have spoken of the colour of the secretion, its quantity and sediment, and it is a circumstance hardly credible that amidst so much minute labour bestowed on these topics the effect produced upon it by

---

* Domenicus Cotunnius (sometimes called Cotungno, 1736-1822) is sometimes credited with being the first to demonstrate albumin in the urine by boiling it. Unfortunately, he did not publish his findings until seventy years after Dekker.

† In 1779, he privately printed, *Experiments on the insensible perspiration of the human body* in which he demonstrated that carbon dioxide is given off by the skin. With Hunter and Hewson, Cruikshank contributed to the basis of modern knowledge concerning the lymphatics.

the application of heat have been so greatly overlooked. . . . Every practitioner may shortly convince himself beyond the possibility of doubt that in a considerable number of dropsical cases the urine evaporates like diluted serum of blood."

In 1827, Richard Bright definitely established the relationship of albumin in kidney disease.[91] As a matter of fact, the recognition of nephritis as a disease entity was a very late event in the history of medicine. The ancients, according to treatises from Hippocrates, had limited knowledge of kidney disease, confined essentially to injuries and suppuration of the kidneys, and stone formation. Alexander of Tralles, Aetius and Paul of Aegina mentioned inflammation of the kidney, calculous and colic though they had no clear ideas about nephritis. Aetius and Avicenna noticed that dropsy develops in the course of induration of the kidneys as leading to a decrease in the urine passed and a dropsical habit of the body. Although both Blackall and Wells observed in several autopsies definite morbid changes in the kidneys, and Braude at the same date and later Scudamore had demonstrated that albuminous urine contained very little urea, it remained for Richard Bright* to establish the relationship between dropsy and lesions of the kidney.

In 1852, J. Florian Heller presented the nitric acid test for albumin, still known as the Heller test. In 1874, G. Esbach announced Esbach's reagent for the quantitative determination of albumin in the urine.

An epoch-making step as far as urine analysis is concerned occurred in 1820 when Prout, who, by his numerous experiments, placed the chemical examination of urine on a more scientific level, and demonstrated its great value as an aid in diagnosis. He was the first to use litmus paper in testing urine. He confirmed Cruikshank's former observation that the sugar found in diabetic urine was not the same as common sugar, but

---

* Garrison and Morton (p. 200) write: Although the name of Bright is perpetuated by his classical description of chronic non-suppurative nephritis, he made many other valuable contributions to medical knowledge. . . . He differentiated renal from cardiac dropsy and was first to correlate this and the previously observed albuminuria with the nephritic changes observed at autopsy.

more nearly approached that which is found in grapes. For detecting bile, he used a piece of white linen which he dipped in the urine, and on the addition of a few drops of muriatic acid, if bile was present, it turned green in color. Prout also investigated the deposits found in urine, made an analysis of them and arranged them according to the colors. His investigations were of great originality and ingenuity and he attracted much attention to the possibilities of chemical analysis. This stimulated many investigators in Great Britain and on the Continent to indulge in further investigation and experimentation.

One of the earliest textbooks devoted to scientific urine analysis was that written by Rees in 1836, on the analysis of the blood and urine in health and disease. In this extraordinary book, Rees recorded the constituents of the urine as determined from his own researches, together with analysis of urinary deposits, as well as recommending several tests for such examination. Prout's nitric acid test for albumin and excessive urea was advised. He also recommended a solution of caustic ammonia to precipitate earthy phosphates.

Osborne, in his work on the *Nature and Treatment of Dropsical Diseases,* in 1837, describes his method of testing the urine for albumin by heat. He recommended heating the urine in a spoon over the flame of a candle, when a white coagulate will be formed in these parts of the fluid next to the metal, long before the heat was advanced to boiling point.

Markwick, in 1847, wrote a guide to the examination of the urine, which was practically the first handbook of chemical analysis of the urine. He calls attention to the use of blue and red litmus paper, and stresses the importance of taking the specific gravity of urine. It was Markwick who estimated albumin by boiling a given quantity and weighing the residue. To detect bile he added hydrochloric acid and sugar by the yeast test for the copper test of Trommer.

Of interest is the history and antiquity of the copper test which some have traced to the Egyptian priest-physician era who originated the formula of the famous compound known as Unguentum Aegyptiacum. This preparation was used as an application to wounds, abrasions, ulcers and tumors and was prepared by boiling together a mixture of verdigris, honey and vinegar. During the preparation by boiling, the color of the mass changes, due to the chemical reaction between the copper acetate and the glucose. The medication was prepared in this manner for centuries and was included in the *Pharmacopeia Universalis* up to 1833. No explanation of the change in color was made until Baume, the celebrated chemist of the eighteenth century, attributed it to *phlogiston* of the acetic acid which united with the *verdigris* to form metallic copper. Lavoiser subsequently contradicted this theory and demonstrated it to be erroneous.

In 1815, Vogel read a paper in Paris before the French Academy of Science* on research devoted to the decomposition of salts and metallic oxides by sugar. In his work, he demonstrated that the reddish or brown-colored precipitate produced in the reaction was not metallic copper bicuprous oxide, or as it was then known, copper protoxide: He contended that the color depended upon the length of time the mixture was heated, and that the precipitate was only to be obtained from cane, starch, and grape sugar, sugar of milk, manna and honey.

It was not until 1841 that Trommer, under the influence of Mitscherlich, established the fact that this sugar could be recovered with an alkaline solution of copper. Trommer clearly showed that by making the copper salt solution alkaline, it became a valuable reagent in distinguishing between the various sugars and sugar-giving substances. Then followed in rather rapid succession the introduction of various tests for the detection of sugar in urine. Mention should be made of the Polarization apparatus of Mitscherlich in 1847, Barriswill's suggested improvement of Trommer's method in 1844, the liquor potassium test of Moore and Heller in 1844.

Fehling, whose name has been synonymous with the detection of sugar in the urine, did not publish his first paper on the matter until 1848. His technique consisted essentially of

---

* The French Academie des Sciences was organized in 1666, one year after the Royal Society was founded in London, and a similar society in Rome. These Societies met and criticized all important scientific contributions.

working out with greater care the details of Trommer's methods. Actually, the Fehling test is a refinement of the Trommer test for glycosuria.

In 1854, a further step was made toward the quantitative analysis of urine by Davy, who published a method of estimating the quantity of urea in a given solution. Davy's method of estimating urea depended upon the decomposition that occurred from the combinations of hypochlorides of soda, potash, or lime with urea, the urea giving off its nitrogen, which was collected, measured and estimated.

In 1861, Lionel Beale published his well-known work on the urine, which contained over sixty analyses of the urine in disease. He strongly advised and stressed the importance of microscopic examination of the urine. His investigations placed the analysis of urine on a truly scientific basis for the first time.

In 1884, Sir William Johnson re-introduced the picric acid test in urine analysis. This test had first been introduced in 1865 by Braun, but had fallen into disuse until 1884, when Johnson realized its value.

The ancient Eygptian, Mesopotamian and Greek writers mentioned hematuria, and it is obvious that its presence aroused the attention of physicians even in the days of antiquity. This curiosity continued for many millennium, but the first chemical demonstration, however, did not appear until 1853, when Teichmann described the Hernin test. This test was later modified by Symous. Teichmann's test continued to meet with objection and in 1858 was largely replaced by the more desirable test of Heller.

The history of chemistry with particular reference to urinalysis now shows a further advancement, namely the significance of quantitative as well as qualitative analysis of urine. Berzeluis is credited with the first quantitative urine analysis in which he gives quantitative values of: (1) water, (2) urea, (3) uric acid, (4) ammonium lactate, (5) mucus, (6) sodium chloride, (7) potassium sulphate, (8) sodium sulphate, (9) biphosphate of ammonium, (10) hydrochlorate, (11) ca and mg phosphate, and (12) silicon.

Esbach, in 1874, presented his technique for the quantitative determination of albumin. In 1884, Johann Kjeldahl estimated the nitrogen content of the urine and this was followed in 1892 by Hopkin's quantitative analysis of uric acid in the urine. The oxalic acid content of the urine was perfected by Salkowski in 1899 and further advances in quantitative analysis of the urine progressed with the introduction of microchemical and calorimetric methods.

With the almost complete establishment of scientific chemical urine analysis during the nineteenth century, the chemist and clinician now turned to the study of blood. Such an attitude was logical since even in the aphorisms of Hippocrates, it was suspected that certain elements of the humoral system were removed via the kidney and urine.

As knowledge of chemical facts increased, it followed that knowledge of the urine and blood, particularly in the presence of disease, increased. With crude apparatus, the study of chemistry, particularly of organic compounds was a slow and tedious one. Berzelius carried out organic analysis with great care, but it required eighteen months for him to perform twenty-one analyses of seven organic acids. According to Leiscester, credit for perfecting organic analysis and making it a routine procedure belongs to Justus Liebig. "By 1831, he had described the method which remained standard until it was modified by the introduction of microanalysis in the twentieth century. With the development by Dumas of his method for nitrogen analysis in organic compounds in 1833, organic chemistry possessed the basic analytical techniques upon which the greatest advances in this science were made."

The advancement in the field of blood analysis lagged behind the rapid strides made in urine analysis. New methods employing microchemical and calorimetric measures hastened the universal adoption of urinalysis as well as accelerated the basic foundation for the chemical analysis of blood. Thus, with these methods available, Folin, Benedict, Marshall and Van Slyke inaugurated methods which required small amounts of blood (formerly 100-200 cc [modern laboratory needs no more than

10 cc of blood]) and such tests are indispensable to the modern urologist who no longer speculates as to the disease as did his predecessor, the uroscopist.

Mention should be made of the discovery of Rountree and Geraghty of the excretory test using phenosulphathalein. This was followed by the use of other chemical dyes introduced into the circulation as indigo carmine, methylene blue and other similar chemicals. With the introduction of opaque chemicals (Swick) urography became established. Further advances in chemistry fostered urology as an important surgical specialty, ultimately making it one of the most exact sciences in medicine.

Chapter X

Galaxy of the Ancients Leonardo da Vinci (1452-1519)

LEONARDO DA VINCI has been described as the most versatile man who ever lived. He was a painter, sculptor, architect, musician, writer, philosopher, mathematician, scientist, inventor, chemist, metallurgist, biologist, botanist, and a civil, military, mechanical, and hydraulic engineer. Why then classify him in a galaxy of ancients contributing to urology?*

He is included because of his insatiable curiosity, particularly with regard to human anatomy. He contributed much to a better understanding and appreciation of anatomical dissections. Although Leonardo was not a physician, his knowledge of medicine was great. This he learned just as he acquired knowledge of other scientific problems of which he had no basic training.

Elmer Belt[92] in writing about *Leonardo the Florentine,* clearly demonstrates that the period in which Leonardo lived was an era of great mental excitement and stimulation. "The years of his life were marked by an age of spreading scholarship and developing intellectuals, the like of which has seldom been seen. Touching his life were Andrea del Verrocchio, Lorenzo il Magnifico, Machiavelli, Michelangelo, Botticelli, Marsilio Ficino, Cesare Borgia, Lodovico il Moro, Bramante, Titian, Raphael,

---

* In our "Galaxy of Ancients," I have chosen those who have contributed not only to basic science, but also to original and specific advances in urology. These men impressed and puzzled by the formation of urine, investigated its mysteries, first by uroscopy then by anatomical dissection, followed by physiological investigation and finally by clinico-pathological correlation.

Durer, Francis I of France, Guilio de Medici, Pope Julius II and Pope Leo X. Contemporaries, too, were Christopher Columbus, Savonarola, Copernicus, and Benvenuto Cellini."[65]

Of even greater significance, as emphasized by Belt, are two vital factors occurring during Leonardo's formative years which stimulated a wide rebirth of learning—a Renaissance. One year after Leonardo's birth, Constantinople, the largest and most influential European city of the Middle Ages, fell to the Turks. With this conquest, many of its Christian scholars moved into Italy, carrying with them, a great wealth of artistic and literary treasures. New centers of learning now arose, and Florence, Leonardo's city, benefited greatly by this move. Indeed, with the closing of the trade routes through Constantinople to the East, Florence became a great and prosperous trade center.[93]

The second vital factor was the great contribution of Johannes Gutenberg, who in 1446, made it possible to produce books more quickly, more efficiently and more accurately than thousands of scribes. By 1500, as a result of Gutenberg's invention, 17 European cities were engaged in printing tomes, and more than 40,000 different works in editions, totalling 10,000,000 copies appeared.

"The advent of printing," writes Belt, "as a means of communicating ideas, the perfection of the convention of perspective in illustration, and scholarly study of the great accomplishments of earlier civilizations all converged to focus in the Italian cities as Leonardo attained maturity. The brilliant light that they brought to man's intellectual life in Italy burned most brightly in Leonardo's own environment at Florence. Leonardo's special ability to absorb new ideas, his great talent in self-expression both in words and in the graphic arts, and his awareness that of all the impressions experienced by man, it is his own personal experience that counts most soon made Leonardo master of his environment."

Sixteen years after Leonardo's death Giovio[93] describes Leonardo as follows: His mind was of a delightfully brilliant and generous cast, his face outstandingly pleasing; since he was such a marvelous inventor and judge of all sorts of amusements and distinguished pastimes, especially of pageants, as well as an ex-

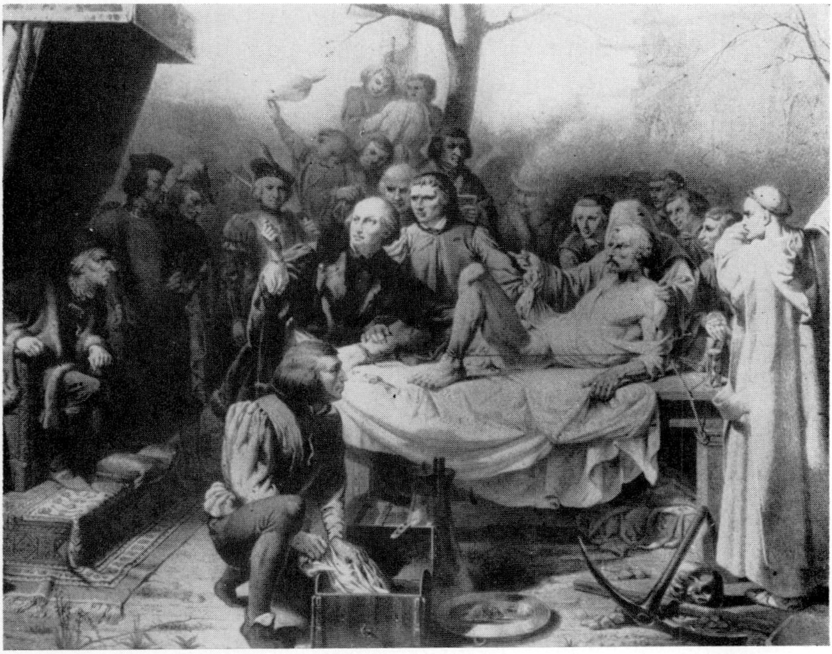

FIGURE 19. Premiere Operation de la Pierre Fait en Presence du Roi Louis XI par Germain Colot au Cimetiére St. Séverine, Janiver 1474. (Photograph courtesy Myer M. Melicow, M.D., College of Physicians and Surgeons, Columbia University Presbyterian Medical Center.)

pert singer who accompanied himself on the lyre, he was a favorite of the Princesses of his time.

In his lecture *Leonardo, The Anatomist,* Belt[94] states: "In Leonardo's drawings of the human body, man lives, functions, changes. Leonardo, the artist, renders these human figures in their most subtile spiritual expression. He succeeds, too, in showing the human form in quick motion, in violent motion, and in dramatic emotion. All depends upon the correct depiction of the human frame. The use of the limbs and their working are to him a mechanical performance worthy of deep study. Leonardo's insatiable desire to know and his penetrating intelligence converted Leonardo the Artist into a Scientist now travelling along unexplored roads."

Leonardo da Vinci was fascinated by riddles and problems.

Thus his notebooks contain scores of unsolved puzzles. Even in his paintings, the figures strangely smile, pointing towards mysteries that were beyond the reach of man's imagination. His own mind had no boundaries and he delved in art, engineering, anatomy, botany, geology and mathematics. His range of imagination is amply demonstrated by his interest in aeronautics, for in 1492 he compiled his note book: *Codice Sul Volo Degli Uccelli*,[95] a scientific study of the mechanics of flight, begun with Leonardo's investigation of birds, undertaken during his attempts to build a flying machine. The original manuscript of this work is now in Rome.

Garrison[96] describes Leonardo as "the greatest artist and scientist of the Italian Renaissance, the founder of iconographic and physiologic anatomy." At his death, Leonardo left over 750 sketches of all the principal organs of the body, drawings which were not reproduced for many, many years.*

The early sixteenth century was unusual by the actual practice of dissection by artists such as Michelangelo and Leonardo to help improve their skill at painting. Singularly, the fabulous drawings of Leonardo, centuries ahead of their time in accuracy of anatomical knowledge, as well as artistic beauty, remained unknown and were not published until the late nineteenth century. In contrast to this, only one generation later, with the further development of the printing press, it became possible for Vesalius' great work on anatomy to be immediately published and hailed as the first real "text" on anatomy in so-called modern times.[98]

The scientific study of the human body by Leonardo was typical of this man's determination to discover the most secret mechanisms of man and this determination plus the audacity of his inquiries made him one of the most important precursors of modern anatomy. Leonardo, himself dissected over thirty bodies, and it was he who inaugurated the technique of making cross sections of the organs of the body. He also introduced the technique of injecting vessels and internal organs to facilitate anatomical study. The great shame is that the world was deprived of this knowledge for so many years.[99]

---

* O'Malley and Saunders have reproduced by photography 215 of Leonardo's most exciting anatomical plates with an excellent introduction and translation.[97]

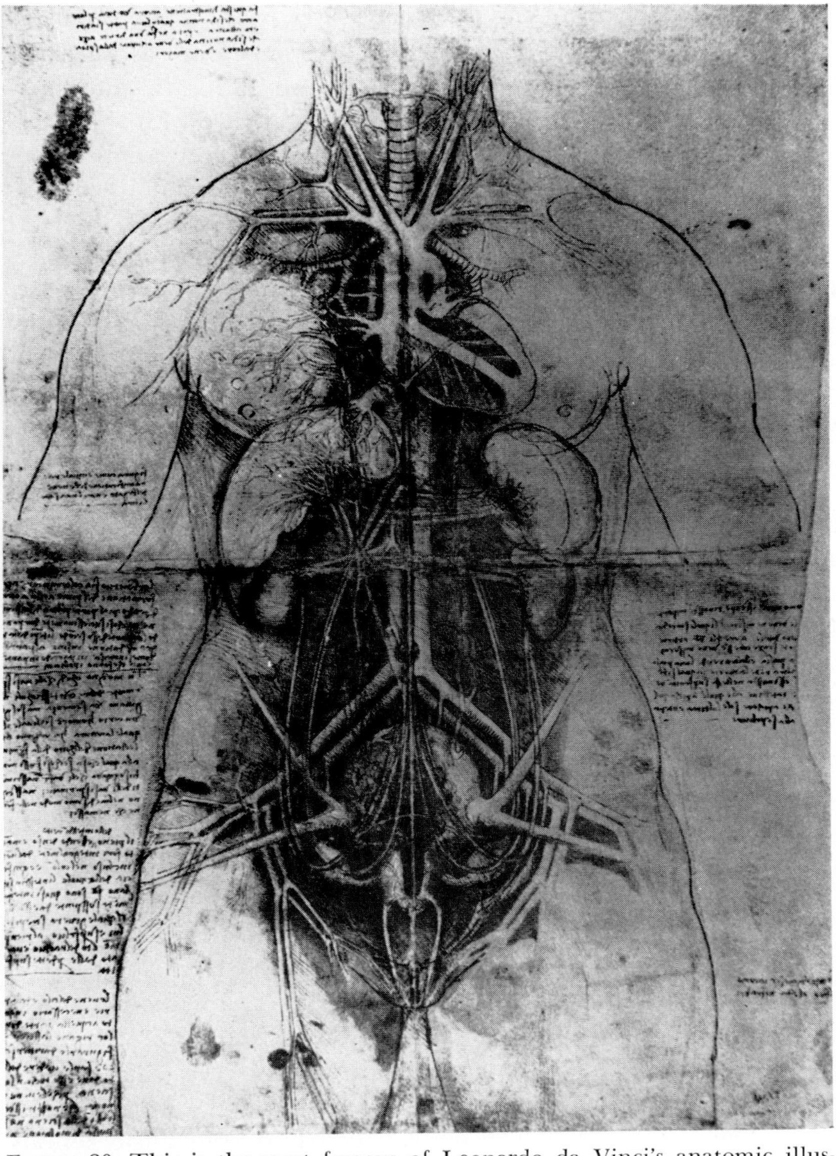

FIGURE 20. This is the most famous of Leonardo da Vinci's anatomic illustrations. Elmer Belt well describes this situs drawing as representing "a mixture of traditional notions and accurate observations. The heart is the two chambered heart of the ancients with a thick ventricle and, as in the ox, moderator bands in both ventricles. . . . Yet, even with its many throwbacks to Galenic authority, Leonardo's demonstration represents an astonishing advance when compared with illustrations current in his day, such as are shown in Magnus Hundt's contemporary book, printed in 1501."

Leonardo da Vinci approached anatomy not only as an artist interested in the human form, but because of his infinite curiosity concerning natural phenomena. Because of his inherent remarkable ability and power of observation, he went below the surface of the body in an attempt to understand the mechanisms and functions of the human body. Fortunately, his unusual perceptive talent was matched by his talent to illustrate. It is possible that this is why he was fond of saying that, "whoever does not draw does not observe." Thus, he saw, described and depicted what earlier anatomists may have noticed casually, but never recorded. Because of his probing mind, he was even able to describe a structure which he never saw, but whose existence he guessed correctly, namely the capillaries.

"The purpose of Leonardo's drawings was to reveal structure and sometimes function through visual demonstrations of the actually dissected material. He said that he combined in each single drawing the experience gained from a number of dissections. He found ingenious ways of demonstration never used before to show simultaneously in one drawing not only what he had experienced in various dissections but also the various layers of the dissected specimen which could not be shown in a straight surface view. He thus maintained the characteristics of a study from nature. He seldom used diagrams but an instance of such use is the drawing of a frog's spinal cord. In another diagram he shows the rotation of the radius in the forearm by the biceps and pronator teres muscles. He drew the entire body in anterior, lateral, and posterior projections as if he were walking around the dissection."[99]

"In Leonardo's bones," continues Belt, "a lifelike portrayal is given to all of his pictures through the presentation of proper carrying and supporting angles which are correctly shown, thus creating realism even in his skeletal drawings. Leonardo illustrated every bone in the body. He demonstrated the actions of the bones as levers when acted upon by muscles. He illustrated for the first time the proper double curvature of the spine, the true tilt of the pelvis, and the proper number of vertebrae, accurately portraying each, especially those of the cervical spine and sacrum."

"He described the teeth, presenting their proper number, strangely a matter of dispute, for as Vesalius a generation later said: 'Anyone can count his own teeth'. . . . As visual aids Leonardo used rope strands to indicate the direction, origin, and attachment of muscles. He realized that in the body, muscle groups are balanced, an anterior group against a posterior group, and he ingeniously used cord and wire in diagrams to represent muscle groups as a means of clarifying their action. This is the first use of this method of illustration in the history of anatomy."[99]

Leonardo's drawings are described as seeming transparencies. He was so gifted that he portrayed several layers of organic structure as if transparent with an overall outline of the parts removed in dissection. Such a system ingeniously anticipated modern principles of didactic demonstration. At a time when x-rays were not known and not even thought of, Leonardo's power of imagination seems miraculous. In the famous drawing of the leg, he indicates (or identifies) for the first time in the history of anatomy the correct position of the femur. "Add to this discovery," writes Belt, "the quality of the drawing as such, a masterpiece of clearness and beauty of line, of distinctness, elegance, and dignity of form, and you have the artistic and scientific phenomenon: Leonardo at his best."

Leonardo was the first to demonstrate the shape and size of a body cavity by injection of a solidifying medium. He utilized an old method familiar to all workers in bronze—"the lost-wax process." In this manner he outlined the ventricles of the brain by pouring hot melted wax into them through a hollow straw, while the ventricular fluid was allowed to escape from a lower opening. He also filled the aortic valve with wax and showed that after systolic closure hardly a drop of blood could return to the ventricle through the valve during diastole.

Keele[100] writes: "Leonardo da Vinci has been described as the man who awoke too early in the darkness, while all the others were asleep. His gigantic efforts in the realm of what we now call science tragically failed to disturb his fellows from their slumbers. Only by his painting did he arouse them to their senses." Thus, his fame today is mainly as the painter of *Mona*

Lisa and *The Last Supper* and more recently, the *Gineora dei Benci.*

In 1505, Leonardo da Vinci described coronary occlusion and its effect in causing death. While Leonardo was talking to an elderly man in the ward of a hospital, the patient died quietly. Leonardo lost no time in opening the body in his search for "the cause of a death so sweet." In his search, he found an occluded artery in the wall of the heart and thus for the first time this pathological entity was described.

Leonardo was the first to call the heart a four-chambered muscular organ. The two-chambered heart was an Aristotelian concept passed on by Avicenna and Mundinus. He was the first to observe persistent foramen ovale, and one of the first to describe in detail, and illustrate the structure and function of the heart valves, which he studied by means of clever glass models. He timed the heart beat, synchronizing systole with the throb of the pulse and with the thump of the heart against the chest wall. This thump had been previously thought to be diastolic and due to an explosion of gases in the heart.

In 1837, Thomas Wilkinson King, of Guy's Hospital in London, drew attention to what he called the moderator band of distention of the right ventricle. This muscle band extending from the interventricular septum to the base of the right anterior papillary muscle and containing the right atrio-ventricular bundle of His, is often referred to as the moderator band of King. Yet, 300 years before King, Leonardo had already seen and drawn the moderator band and singularly had correctly guessed its function.

Leonardo's one weakness, and that which influenced his erroneous concept of the movement of the blood, was undoubtedly due to his knowledge of Galen's *De usu partium.* This, unfortunately, led him to believe that the interventricular septum was perforate and that these perforations would permit the blood to flow through the septum from the right side of the heart to the left.* He describes these channels as "invisible

* Belt, in a personal communication, questions this statement and points out that Leonardo does not demonstrate such pores and in "his picture of the cup septum he shows no single line going thru the septum."[101]

pores." In 1638, William Harvey demonstrated that the blood moves in a circle, but he too had to assume the presence of tiny peripheral channels linking arteries and veins throughout the body. The actual existence of *capillaries* had to await Malpighi's great contribution after the perfection of the microscope (1660) by Anton von Leeuwenhoek. Leonardo also coined the word capillary to describe those hairlike structures, too fine to be seen.

Many of Leonardo's drawings contain inaccuracies, which most da Vinci authorities believe is not because of his lack of observation or anatomical technique but because of the influence of the teachings of Galen and Avicenna. Some of these inaccuracies may be attributed to mere bridging a gap in his dissections. Regardless, the number is not overwhelming, but is of keen historical interest. For example, in an early diagram the urethra is shown as a double channel, the lower one to carry urine and sperm, while the upper conveyed animal spirit to the embryo—the teaching of Avicenna.

Other drawings on the same page, show in the male, the mythical path from the spinal cord to the urethra for animal spirit, and in the female, the imaginary path by which retained menses were thought to pass to the breast during pregnancy to produce lactation. The former is well described by Belt:[102] "As students of the urinary tract, we are drawn to these figures of the brain and spinal cord by two fanciful structures which Leonardo demonstrates as passing parallel to the spinal cord, one on each side, seemingly arising from the substance of the brain. These were probably vertebral arteries, but in Leonardo's coition figure we see them again, this time taking off from the lower end of the spinal canal. They were thought to carry spiritual power to the superior of the two channels through the penis to contribute the more gummy portion of the ejaculate. Leonardo[102] states: 'With great diligence you should make the demonstration of the two vessels which are the depository of the human semen in the penis. Determine which structures are those which constrict these vessels and throw forth the semen. Give the measure and the site of those (structures) in the penis.' "

The notion that the most active and thickest part of the semen comes from the spinal cord and passes by means of vessels from the lumbar region to the testis, dates back to the days of Hippocrates. Actually, Leonardo accepts the Galenical theory that sperm are made from blood within the structure of the testis.

The urologist is further entranced by Leonardo da Vinci's explorations and illustrations of the genito-urinary system. Of interest is Leonardo's depiction of the kidneys. Leonardo's drawings of the kidney are correct with properly placed blood vessels. The vessel seen going upwards from the renal vein is undoubtedly the supra renal vein. The relationship of the renal artery, vein and ureter, and the demonstration of the left spermatic vein into the left renal vein and of the right spermatic vein into the vena cava cannot be disputed. This observation was also recorded by Galen. The drawing of the kidney dates from about 1505, and it is difficult to understand why Leonardo did not transect the kidney and make such a sketch in subsequent years. This is especially puzzling since he notes on this page "cut it through the middle and depict how the passages for the urine are closed and how they distill it." It is possible that such drawings may have been made and were lost. The known anatomic drawings of Leonardo are probably only one-third of the total of his anatomy.[102]

Of special interest to the urologist is Leonardo's struggle similar to Galen's struggle (see p. 64) to understand the passage of urine from the kidney into the bladder via the ureter, and he could only evaluate the ureter as a simple tube with the water flowing through it, influenced only by gravity and by those laws which influence the flow of liquids. Thus he writes: "The urine, having left the kidneys, enters the ureters and from there passes into the bladder near the middle of its height. It enters the bladder through minute perforations made transversely between tunic and tunic. This oblique perforation was not made because Nature doubted that the urine could return to the kidneys, for that is impossible from the 4th (book) on conduits where it is stated: water which descends from above through a narrow vessel and enters under the bottom of a pool, cannot be opposed by reflux movement if the magnitude of the water in the pool is not as great as the magnitude of the vessel which descends, or the height of the water greater than the depth of the pool. If you were to say that the more the bladder is filled the more it closes, to this I would reply that these perforations being confused by the urine which closes the wall, would prevent the entrance of other urine which descends. This cannot be according to the 4th (book) mentioned above which states that the narrow and elevated (stream of) urine is more powerful than the low and wide which lies in the bladder."

The study of the flow of urine through the ureters is continued further by Leonardo. He visualizes the effect of position upon urine drainage from kidney to bladder in a series of diagramatic sketches which shows the patient: (1) erect, (2) upside down, and (3) lying on his side. The dissertation states:

> "The authorities say that the ureter is carrying urine to the bladder do not enter it directly but enter between layer and layer in such a way that they are not opposed, and that the more the bladder is filled, the more they are closed. They say that Nature has done this solely because when the bladder is full, it would return the urine back whence it came. Hence on finding its way between membrane and membrane to enter the interior (of the bladder) through a narrow passage not corresponding to (the point of entry in) the first membrane, the more the bladder is filled, the more it forces one membrane against the other, and thus has no cause to reverse and turn back. This proof is not true for the reason that if the urine in the bladder were to rise higher than its entrance, which is near the middle of its height, it would follow that this entrance would be closed immediately, and it would be impossible for urine to enter the bladder, and it would never exceed half the capacity of the bladder. Therefore, the rest of the bladder would be superfluous, and Nature makes nothing superfluous. Consequently, we shall state, according to the 5th (section) of the 6th (book) 'On water,' how the urine enters a long and tortuous passage into the bladder, and then when the bladder is full, the ureters remain full of urine. The urine of the bladder cannot rise higher than their surfaces (of the intramural portion of the ureters) when man is standing

> erect. But if he remains lying down, it can return back through the ureters and even more so, if he places himself upside down which occurs infrequently, although, recumbency is common. Whereas if a man lies on his side, one of the ureters remains above, the other below, and the entrance of that above opens and discharges the urine into the bladder. The other duct below closes because of the weight of the urine. Hence a single duct gives its urine to the bladder, and it is sufficient that one of the emulgent (renal) veins purifies the blood of the urinary chyle mixed with it, since the emulgent veins are one another and do not proceed entirely from the vena chilis *(vena cava)*. And if a man lies with his back to the sky, the 2 ureters pour urine into the bladder. They enter through the upper part of the bladder (when prone), since the ducts are attached to the posterior part of the bladder, the part which when the body is lying downwards, remains above. Thus the urinary entrances can remain open and contribute to the bladder as much urine as required to fill it."

When one accepts Leonardo's brilliant interpretation of the heart chambers and the action of the heart muscle, it is difficult to understand his basic error concerning bladder mechanism. His theory, that once the fluid level of the bladder reaches the level of the ureteric orifices, no further urine can enter the bladder, was postulated approximately nine years earlier than his studies of the heart. This may be of some significance.

The sketch of the male genitalia reveals the testis with the spermatic vessels coiling on its upper pole. Here the epididymus is not well defined and the vas passes to one end of the vesicle, from the other end of which emerges the ejaculatory duct. The ureter is shown in a much more normal position relative to the bladder neck than in the earlier diagram, but is incorrectly placed in relation to the vesicle.

On the same sketch page, and on the right is a sketch showing two ejaculatory ducts opening into the urethra. "See which is the first in the urinary canal, either the mouths of the spermatic vessels (ejaculatory ducts) or the mouth of the urinary vessel. But I believe that that of the urine is first so that it can then clear and wash out the sperm which makes the urinary anal sticky."

Belt, who in addition to being one of the world's authorities on Vinciana, is an outstanding urologist, and has therefore carefully studied Leonardo's contribution to urology. Thus, in evaluating Leonardo's attempt at functional approaches to anatomic problems, he (Belt) quotes Leonardo's remarks on the penis. "The origin of the penis is situated upon the pubic bones so that it can resist its active force on coition. If this bone did not exist, the penis, in meeting resistance, would turn backward and would often enter more into the body of the operator than into that of the operated."

For many years, the erectile power of the penis had been contributed by the ancients to be the result of a pneuma or vital spirit. This theorem became corrupted in the Middle Ages by the belief that air under pressure produced the hardness of the penis. Leonardo objected to this theory by stating: "Of the virile member when it is hard, it is thick and long, dense and heavy, and when it is limp, it is thin, short and soft, that is limp and weak. This should not be adjudged due to the addition of flesh or wind but to arterial blood. I have seen this in the dead who have this member rigid. For many die thus, especially those hanged of whom I have seen an anatomy, having great density and hardness, and these are full of a large quantity of blood which had made the flesh very red within, and with others, without as well as within. And again, one observes that the rigid penis has a red gland (testa) which is a sign of an abundance of blood and when it is not rigid, it has a whitish appearance."

Modern geneticists would be impressed by Leonardo's early belief in genes. Although he did not use this term, he did not believe that the female merely incubated the germ cell of the male, but believed that the genetic responsibility was equally divided between the male and female. Thus he wrote, "the black races in Ethiopia are not the product of the sun; for if black get black with child in Scythia, the offspring is black but if a black gets a white woman with child its offspring is grey. And this shows that the seed of the mother has power in the embryo equally with that of the father, whether in Scythia or Rome."

It is strange but the prostate gland is not definitely shown in any of Leonardo's drawings. This could be due to the fact that most of his anatomic studies were made on the bodies of oxen. These animals are castrates and hence have small atrophic prostates. Human bodies for dissection were hard to obtain and like Galen, Leonardo frequently transposed knowledge gained from his animal dissections directly into his sketches which aimed to present the anatomy of man.

In Leonardo's drawing the "Great Situs" figure, Leonardo begins his intended series of graphic presentations. It presents a blend of medieval concepts and of original, accurate observations. It represents a striking advance over the crude and highly schematic drawings by Leonardo's contemporary, Magnus Hundt, of Leipsig, current and typical of the time (1500).

Belt[102] stresses the keenness of thought, philosophy and speculation of Leonardo with regard to conception, the human embryo and its habitat, the uterus—"Observe in the uterus where its spermatic vessels originate. The child generated by the fastidious lust of the woman and not of the will of the husband will be of small, vile and crude spirit. . . . The man who uses coitus with contention and with depreciation makes irritable and untrustworthy children and when the coitus is made with great love and great desire of the partners then the child will be of great intellect, spirited and lively and lovable. . . . Different foods produce different blood and different blood makes different kind of sperm and different sperm have different influences on children."

One of the most famous of Leonardo's sketches is his masterly presentation of the pregnant uterus. Murphy[103] points out that when this and other drawings were seen by William Hunter, about the time he was to publish his *Atlas of the Gravid Uterus* in 1774, he stated that Leonardo was 300 years ahead of his time. Thus, Leonardo's ideas of the placenta as the source of fetal nourishment, of the circulation and of the method of separation of the placenta were indeed the product of an extreme scientific, investigative extraordinary mind.

O'Malley and Saunders[97] who have so brilliantly helped to bring Leonardo da Vinci into proper historical perspective state:

"It is essential that his biological contributions be viewed as a whole. It is not enough to examine his illustrations alone, but if we are able to understand this extraordinary figure as a unified personality and historical phenomenon, it is necessary to study the many notes and observations which accompany the drawings. We may excuse the incompleteness and disorganization of his writings on the grounds of their haphazard informality, and we can make allowances for the uncertainty which surrounds their chronological sequence but we cannot ignore them and the imperfections which they reveal without gravely distorting the true historical picture. Without the notes (which accompanies the sketches), it would be impossible to perceive beneath the genius of his art the groping of his mind as it sought emancipation from a debased medieval Aristotlianism, through a corrupted Galenism to the achievement of a position of relative scientific independence."

"We would fail to see him" continues O'Malley and Saunders,[97] "as part of the contemporary growth, and we would lack an appreciation of the difficulties which he had to surmount. It has been this failure to consider the notes and illustrations as one which have been responsible for the many specious and unjustifiable claims that have been made on his behalf such as the all too frequent assertion that Leonardo had knowledge of the circulation of the blood."

With regard to Leonardo's section on the genito-urinary system, O'Malley and Saunders[97] confirm Belt's speculation that almost all Leonardo's studies on the kidneys were carried out on animals. This is further evidenced by his primitive views regarding the physiology of the kidneys. As stated above, this is especially vivid in his description of the passage of the urine from the kidneys to the bladder via the ureter.

The traditional theories of the male and female reproductive organs are treated with a curious blend of fact and fancy. But the significant thing is that in earlier sketches, this brilliant man reflects primitive "medieval theories of generation" whereas in later sketches and notes he reveals predominantly Galenical theories and philosophy. Thus, in his early studies, he puts down as pictures what he read in the older texts. He frees himself from these errors as he proceeds with actual dissections. As he keeps on dissecting and drawing, his drawings and his expressed ideas grow more and more correct.

It is unfortunate that Leonardo's influence on the course of anatomy was spread only by his personal contacts. How great it might have been if his researches and drawings had been published during his lifetime or soon after his death, instead of being scattered and practically lost for more than two hundred years, is a fascinating speculation.*

No more fitting tribute can be written of Leonardo da Vinci than that of Sir William Osler:[104] "Insatiate in experiment, intellectually as greedy as Aristotle, painter, poet, sculptor, engineer, architect, mathematician, chemist, botanist, aeronaut, musician and withal a dreamer and a mystic, full accomplishment in any of one department was not for him! A passionate desire for a mastery of nature's secrets made him a fierce thing replete with too much rage. But, for us, a record remains—Leonardo was the first of the modern anatomists and, fifty years later, into the breech he made, Vesalius entered."

---

* Leonardo bequethed his notebooks to his disciple and friend Francisco Melzi, after whose death, in 1570, some manuscripts were given away or sold, and others stolen. Some were bought by Charles I of England, who kept them in a large strong box. In 1690, they were shown by Queen Mary II to Christian Huygens and from all sources were not seen again until about 1760. In that year Robert Dalton, librarian at Kensington Palace, found them in a locked chest whose key had been lost. Dalton showed the drawings to William Hunter who was amazed at their accuracy. It is only within the past fifty years or so that Leonardo's writings and sketches have become available so that his work could be evaluated and enjoyed by many.

Chapter XI

Galaxy of the Ancients, Continued
Paracelsus (1493-1541)

PARACELSUS is one of the most unusual medical figures of antiquity. He was the first of the ancients to lecture in the vernacular instead of in Latin. Paracelsus disagreed with Galen and Avicenna. Osler speaking of Paracelsus said he was "the Luther of Medicine, for when authority was paramount he stood out for independent study."

His two great contributions were *Paramirum,* a treatise dealing with the causes and nature of disease; and *Paragranum,* considered by Karl Sudhoff (the greatest of all medical historians) to be of great importance since it expounded the general principles of medicine.

What Paracelsus meant by the word *Paramirum* or for that matter *Paragranum* has puzzled many scholars. It is obvious he was fond of utilizing the prefix Para—as for example in his even more popular chosen name—Paracelsus. His true name was Philippus Theophrastus Aureolus Bombastus von Hohenheim, and after completing his studies in Italy, he followed the humanist fashion and adopted the Latin name Paracelsus but what it actually means we do not know.

Paracelsus worked on the *Volumen Paramirum* for many years and completed it around 1530. It was not published until 1562. "It is the ripest fruit of Paracelesian thought, a philosophy of medicine as challenging today as it was then. It is not easy to read," writes Sigerist.[106] "It is written in the terminology of the day, but if we take the trouble to interpret it, the book impresses us as very modern."

In still other writings, Paracelsus elaborated more specifically on the material process of health and disease. Thus, he repeatedly emphasized that the human body does not consist only of four elementary humours; blood, phlegm, black and yellow bile, which everyone accepted. Paracelsus insisted that they do not play the significant role attributed to them by Galen and his followers.

Paracelsus was the first to write on minors' diseases, to establish the relationship between cretinism and endemic goitre, and to note the geographic differences in disease. He has been called by some "the pioneer of modern chemists" and by others "uncouth, boorish, vain, ignorant, and pretentious." In his treatise, *De Gradibus,* can be found many innovations in chemical therapeutics. Paracelsus suggested the hereditary transmissions of syphilis and advocated mercury internally, as an antisyphilitic. He called the disease "French gonorrhea" and thus started the confusion which lasted until the nineteenth century.

Paracelsus was doctor, chemist, lecturer and reformer. His novel doctrines gained him many followers. His *Chinegia Magna* went through many editions and translations—like Paré he did not believe in the use of boiling oil for the purification of gunshot wounds.

Charles Singer[105] describes Paracelsus as, "a person of violent, dramatic, and repellent temper, a born rebel whose iconoclasm doubtless did something to deter men from the worship of the old idols. His symbolic act of burning the works of both the Greek Galen and the Arab Avicenna, as an introduction to his lecture course at Basel, typified the position of the independent investigators of the generation that immediately followed him."

Sigerist[107] states that in the Renaissance, Paracelsus never tired of postulating the necessity of studying disease conditions in foreign countries. "He lived what he preached, travelled all over Europe and the near East, and when accused of being a man without a residence, he answered in the fourth of his famous *Defensiones,* pointing out that 'diseases wander hither and thither throughout the breadth of the world, and stay not in place. If a man wish to recognize many diseases, let him travel: if he travel far, his experience will be of great and he will learn to recognize many things.' "

Perhaps the true nature of Paracelsus can best be evaluated when it is realized he was born in a most interesting time, a most propitious time when Europe awoke from her slumber in the darkness of almost one thousand years. He was born into the world (1493) after Columbus had discovered America and during his lifetime Luther was to cleave Catholicism in two and Copernicus was to recast and reorganize astronomy.

Thus, he emerged in an era of revolution and progress, and he matured despite his outlandish and almost unbearable deeds, he became more and more deeply concerned with the stagnation that characterized medical thought and education. He was a knight of the Renaissance and he launched himself into a war against sterile dogma and opposition to progress. This was his creed all through his life.

Two years after Paracelsus died, Vesalius published the *Fabrica,* a revolutionary anatomical atlas, which minimized Galen's former authoritative position in anatomy. This war against Galen actually was started by Paracelsus when on St. John's Day, June 24, 1527, Paracelsus accompanied by students at *Basel* carried the heavy, venerated *Canon* of Avicenna, and hurled same into the fire, which prompted Paracelsus to write: "Thus the realm of medicine has been purged." (See Chapter IV—Avicenna and Islamic Science.) In addition, he made no friends nor allies with the powerful acadamecians, who abhorred his lecturing in German instead of conventional Latin, and considered him crude, bombastic, and unreliable. Unfortunately, the Council as well as the student body did not approve of his methods of teaching, his mannerisms and boastful claims and he was forced to leave a position which he had long sought for comfort, security, and opportunity to write and publish.

How did "bombastic" Paracelsus obtain this desirable position in the first place? About 1526, Paracelsus was practicing in the city of Strasburg, not far from Basel and the famous University of Basel. Although none of Paracelsus' books had been published, his reputation for successful treatments of surgical diseases and gout had reached Basel. Singularly, Frobenius, the great printer, had successfully been treated by Paracelsus for gangrene in his right foot thus avoiding an amputation recommended by the attending surgeons. Similarly, Erasmus of Rotterdam who was living in Frobenius' house was also successfully treated by Paracelsus. Thus, with the recommendation of these two powerful men, the Town Council offered Paracelsus the position of municipal physician. Paracelsus eagerly grasped the opportunity of putting an end to his ceaseless wanderings and also the possibility, if through the gratitude of Frobenius, of publishing his theories and opinions. Unfortunately, at the time of his expulsion from Basel, Frobenius had died, and Paracelsus had few friends. In view of a pending court suit from a canon of the cathedral, who accused Paracelsus of charging an excessive fee (this being customary at the time), he left the city in February, 1528.

Paracelsus violently opposed the Galenic-Arabic concepts and the philosophy upon which they were based. Instead, he offered as a substitute a system deeply rooted in chemistry with an abundant mixture of cosmology and astrology. No one can deny his great interest and contributions of chemistry and particularly in its association with pharmacology and medicine. It was Paracelsus who introduced tin as an anthelmintic; introduced antimony as a preparation; and utilized zinc and zinc salts to medicine. As mentioned above, he recommended mercury compounds instead of metallic mercury for syphilis and made every effort to establish definite doses and course of therapy. He was familiar with the pharmacologic actions of lead, arsenic, copper and iron compounds. Despite the opposition of his contemporaries to his then called revolutionary suggestions, he continued with his work so that succeeding generations of medical men became cognizant of such chemicals with ultimate utilization of them.

Of interest is that a generation before Paré (see Chapter XIII) Paracelsus condemned the practice of cauterization of wounds. His sympathetic attitude towards mentally disturbed patients clearly reveals an unusual insight into psychiatry and psychomatics. Thus he wrote: "Nobody can be cured by faith, unless the disease was imaginary in the first place," and "the curing power of medicine consists not so much in the spirit that is hidden in them but in the spirit in which they are taken."

For many academicians, it was basic to separate medicine from surgery. This Paracelsus bitterly opposed and did all he could to weld the two disciplines together. He personally practiced in medicine and surgery and signed himself *"beyder Artzney Doctoru"* (Doctor of Both Medicines). He did not recommend elective operative surgery and in wound management, followed Hippocrates theory, that "healing was solely the property of nature, and that the doctor could only assist the natural forces, primarily by supplying nutrition and in preventing complications. The integument was likened to the shell of the egg, the bark of the tree, or the skin of the apple, when breached, it permitted the noxious contact of the internal tissues with the outside air, whence arise all complications. The early closure of the wound with bland and nutritive substances was thus clearly indicated. The use of sutures for this purpose was deplored."

The medical student of today would undoubtedly be amazed were he to have one of his professors lecture to him in the following bombastic manner, as did Paracelsus when he addressed the students at the University of Basel.[108]

> "Students, I greet you. Medicine alone, of all the intellectual disciplines is a necessity and since few doctors today practice it with success and to the advantage of their patients, it seems necessary to reinstate it in its original exalted position. It is my desire to rid medicine of its most glaring errors and to teach, not according to the rules of the ancients, but on these principles which derive from the nature of things and which I have reached through my own reflections and have formed valuable in long use and experience. I am permitted by the generous honor of the council of Basel to teach according to my own methods and to lecture daily on practical and theoretical medicine, both internal medicine as well as surgery. I shall read with diligence from text books of which I am the author, those things of greatest value to you. You may judge me only after you have heard me.

"I should like to lecture to you on surgery, but first, you must understand certain things concerning medicine as a whole and the practice of surgery in particular. I have repeatedly attempted by constant observation and diligent work to determine the basis of medicine. Many things have compelled me to this. Firstly, the uncertainty of the practice, because so little honor and praise is attached to it, so many sick are made worse, killed, maimed, and entirely forsaken, not just in one disease but in almost all diseases. So uncertain is treatment that even in my times scarcely a physician must be a doctor of both medicines. Secondly, you should know what medicine is not based on science alone, but in science and experience, and experience is what has been proved right and true.

"Thirdly, medicine is changing and growing daily and the physician must know not just one disease or know how to care for one wound, but he must know all diseases and how to cleanse and treat all wounds. You must use your eyes and observe, look about, travel and ask questions. Do not be ashamed to ask questions even if you are a doctor.

"You will not find everything written in the books of Galen and Avicenna, all of surgery has not been written, for new times bring new diseases and new books will outmode the old. . . . You should know the make-up of man, where the bones and other structures lie and their relation to each other. If you do not know these things how can you diagnose injuries or know how to put them right? It is not enough that you know the externals, you must know the internals better than the externals; you must know all the veins and arteries, nerves and bones, their length, number, form, location in every limb; also, where the emunctoria are and how they are to be turned aside and what lies in each and where the intestines lie—the surgeon should know all this just as the carpenter knows the construction of a house. The surgeon must know anatomy and not be like the barber or bather who knows no more than the butcher who cuts, trims, and separates his meat.

". . . Learning and experience are the basis of surgical knowledge, so do not try to fly until you have learned how. Haughtiness, arrogance and feigned knowledge are of no avail;

> only real knowledge and skill. A serious fault with learning today is that it is not followed to completion but that each student wishes to become a master before the pupil has grown up.
>
> "Medicine has become a field for the dishonest to plow, the nobleman and the merchant have much money, therefore they are cultivated. Not just the apostates, but other light-fingered folk have taken to medicine, the hangmen, poachers and others without honor. But just as there are true physicians and false ones, and the false patients seek the fake physicians and the true ones the true physicians."

There is no question that Paracelsus was a prolific writer but unfortunately he was unable to persuade anybody to publish his writings. Much of his work did not appear until some years after his death. This, unfortunately, raises the issue what actually was his, and what was revisions and interpolations of over-zealous disciples, or even antagonists, who took this means of discrediting him.

Nevertheless, we know that Paracelsus believed that medicine rested on four pillars. First, astronomy in which man was the microcosm and the universe was the macrocosm. To fully understand man, it was essential to understand the workings of the cosmos. The second pillar was natural science which included geography. This was probably the result of his extensive travels which convinced Paracelsus of the importance of regional variations in disease. The third pillar was chemistry, in which there is recourse to the refinement and application of natural substances for purposes of treatment. The fourth pillar, according to Paracelsus, was love and he strongly believed that only a virtuous, unselfish man, could hope to be a good physician.

Paracelsus could well have established himself as did Galen, but unfortunately he failed to be impressed by his contributions to the *materia medica*. Instead, he continued experimenting without rhyme or reason. He rejected the use of polypharmacy, only using drugs in emergencies and in their simplest forms: "apothecaries are my enemies because I will not empty their boxes. My recipes are simple and do not call for forty or fifty ingredients. I seek not to enrich the apothecaries, but to cure the sick." Being a strong follower of Hippocrates, he believed that in nature's battle against disease the physician is only the helper, who furnishes nature with weapons and that nature actually is the physician.

"Unlike Hippocrates, he was not content simply to seek for ways to enable the life force to operate more freely. There must, he felt, be some way to stimulate it; and the best way, he came to the conclusion was through love. He was himself a truculent, cross-grained man without, so far as can be judged, much charity in his character; but he realized objectively that here was a potent therapeutic force, operating through faith, and 'capable of making for itself every herb an invisible nettle, an invisible celandine, an invisible triold, everything that grows is terrestrial nature, the power of belief can likewise bring'—with its counterpart: 'the power of belief can likewise create every sickness.' "[108]

In 1538, three years before his death, Paracelsus settled down for a few years in the Austrian province of Carinthia. It was here, at the age of forty-five, Paracelsus wrote a defense against the attacks that had been made upon him. The following is the Seventh Defense, as translated by Tempkin:

The Seventh Defense

How I Too Know Not All, Cannot And Am Not Able To Do What Each One Needs, Or Might Need

"This I must confess, and I am not able to grant and fulfill everyone's desire; as they certainly and undoubtedly would have it from me: this I cannot do, nor is it in my power. For God did not create medicine thus according to their will, that it might act immediately according to the will of all comers. If then God will not grant nor give such people anything, how can I help it? For I cannot master nor overpower God, but He me and all others. Thus are all answered alike: if they were agreeable to God or pleasing to him for healing, He would not have withdrawn nature from them. It is the same thing as one who thinks himself a fine, handsome fellow and wants to stand out before all others and wants all women and maidens to favour him. But he was born crooked, has a hump on his back like a lute and in other respects too he has no comeliness of body. How can women favour one whose own nature does not favour him, but spoiled him in his mother's womb and made nothing good of him? In order, however, that I may intsruct you the better, know ye that if God bestow no good on a man, how then should nature bestow good on him? Where both favours are absent, of what good is the physician? And who can blame him? Now they say when I come to a patient, I know not immediately what ails him, but I need time to find it out. It is true. That they judge immediately is the fault of their foolishness; for in the end the first judgment is false and from day to day they know the longer, the less, what it is, and make liars of themselves. Whereas I desire to approach from day to day, the longer, the closer to the truth. For with hidden diseases it is not as with the recognizing of colours: in colours one sees well what is black, green, blue, etc. But if there were a curtain before it, thus also would not know. To see through a curtain requires effort where there has been none before. What the eyes see can well be judged hurriedly, but what is hidden from the eyes it is in vain to conceive as though it were visible. . . .

"Why do you throw it in my face if I cannot cure impossible things when you cannot cure the possible? But rather you ruin it, so that I must build it up again. How can I cure a cut-off heart, put a cut-off hand back on? Who has ever been able by the light of nature to join death and life and unite them, so that death should receive life? Indeed, it is not natural but divine. How should I do such things, when you cannot heal wounds in which there is no death, except what you invite? You are longsighted, you see into the distance, but not yourselves nearby. I will prove it with your conscience, that it teaches and instructs you, that you do an act against it, and would glorify yourselves with that which brings you to shame. For you have medicine from God, with which to drive out all things possible; you could do it, and are incapable. Why then do you accuse me of doing nothing for impossible diseases and that for them no medicine is given me, nor created? . . .

"With this I desire to have defended and protected myself for the last time until further provocation, which, if God will, will also be returned blow for blow.

"And herewith too I desire only to beg that the pious and

just of true conscience should not bother themselves with my writings. For necessity required that I answer. For Christ too replied and was not silent. For everyone should know that answering is just and fitting, in order that those do not stagnate completely nor blind themselves with idle talk, who live on and enjoy idle talk. If they were not answered, they would win the argument and would consider themselves right, and there would afterwards be even more error, rubbish, disaster and corruption. Wherefore is answering equivalent to anticipation of present and future corruption and revelation of what the ranters are. For such reasons as these then I have been pleased to answer and to protect myself from all those whose hearts are full of ill will, that both sides may stand revealed. For it is necessary that vices come; but woe unto him through whom they come! That is to say, that liars speak contrary to the truth; but woe unto them, for truth reveals the lies. If they were silent concerning their vices, truth too would be silent. But since it is necessary, lies and vice cannot, and may not, be silent: it must be uttered, but woe unto them. Thou, reader, however, shouldst consider and measure all things most justly, that the reading may bear the fruit, profit and good."

Paracelsus founded no specific school. Nevertheless, he reexamined and re-evaluated the basic problems of the healing art. He clearly and forcefully made a distinction between physicians who cured through medicine and those who cured through miracles. He replaced the ancient shotgun preparations with simple essences and tinctures. Above all, he helped raise the ethical standards of the medical profession with his famous dictum: "The most precious thing we physicians possess is our art, and next comes love for our patients, hope being the keystone of both." He thus deserves a place in our "Galaxy of Ancients."

Chapter XII

Galaxy of the Ancients Continued
Andreas Vesalius (1514-1564)

ONE could not possibly write a galaxy of ancients and omit the name of Andreas Vesalius. He was a paradoxical man brought up in a paradoxical time. It is now over four hundred years since the death of this great physician (October, 1564), yet there are few great names in the history of medicine better known. He came on the scene when the credulity of tradition, ecclesiastical or scientific, was being questioned. His contribution was the astonishing enlistment of graphic art in the service of biological structure in general and particularly of anatomy.

It was a period of time difficult to describe. Despite some advances it was a revival of, with unquestioning obedience to, past systems. The aphorisms of Hippocrates, the voluminous dogmatisms of Galen and the Canon of Avicenna formed the basis of medical instruction. Fetish-worship of ancient authority was paramount. If Avicenna said that a disease was cold and moist, and that such a remedy must be used because it was hot and dry, so it was believed. If Galen had announced that such and such a disease was incurable, no further effort at treatment was made. This attitude extended even into the seventeenth century.* It is easy to assign the principal reason for this servility to the ancients. When, through the activity of the

* In spite of the advances in anatomy since the twelfth century, especially since the sixteenth century, physicians continued to accept some aspects of the Galenical tradition of medical treatment with great persistence. Thus, even to the end of the eighteenth century, followers of Galen wrote books, monographs and dissertations devoting much space to philosophic Galenic principles of Medicine.

Medici and the capture of Constantinople, Greek literature was given to Europe, the quickened minds of the time could not fail to notice the vast superiority of the classical writings in form and substance over the uncouth and thought-restricted productions of many manuscripts. The medieval writings were not the work of monks. They acknowledged this with enthusiasm and so everything Greek or moulded upon Greek models was eagerly received and obediently adopted.

The foundation of early sixteenth century medicine was basically Galenic or Hippocratic, for medicine in Renaissance Europe was slow and far behind the awakening of thought in the arts and letters. Actually, there were only three men who challenged the status of medicine. Paracelsus was the first who challenged the authoritative medical view by burning Galenic texts in 1527; the second was Andreas Vesalius who published his authentic findings in human dissection; and thirdly Ambroise Paré, who challenged therapy and classical surgical procedures, by publishing his observations on the treatment of gunshot wounds in 1545.

Vesalius' great contribution was his break with tradition as to the study of anatomy, and the need of human dissections. His text was ultimately accepted (although not immediately) and served as a stimulus for further observation and study by others in the following centuries. Singer[105] describes Vesalius' *De humani corporis fabrica* as epoch making and a milestone in the history of thought, since it was the first great work of science in the modern manner. It is the accepted foundation of the modern disciplines of human and comparative anatomy and physiology. It introduced a sound and positive basis into medical education. Because of the skill of the woodcutters craft, it established exact graphic treatment as an essential adjunct of biological research.

"Much visual energy has been expended on study of the illustrations of the Fabrica and considerably less on its text," writes O'Malley.[110] "Some have disputed learnedly over the question of which portraits of Vesalius are genuine, even though all have the shakiest of provenances or are obvious copies of the woodcut portrait in the Fabrica. Some have contrived to make Vesalius a man of explosive temper, which in

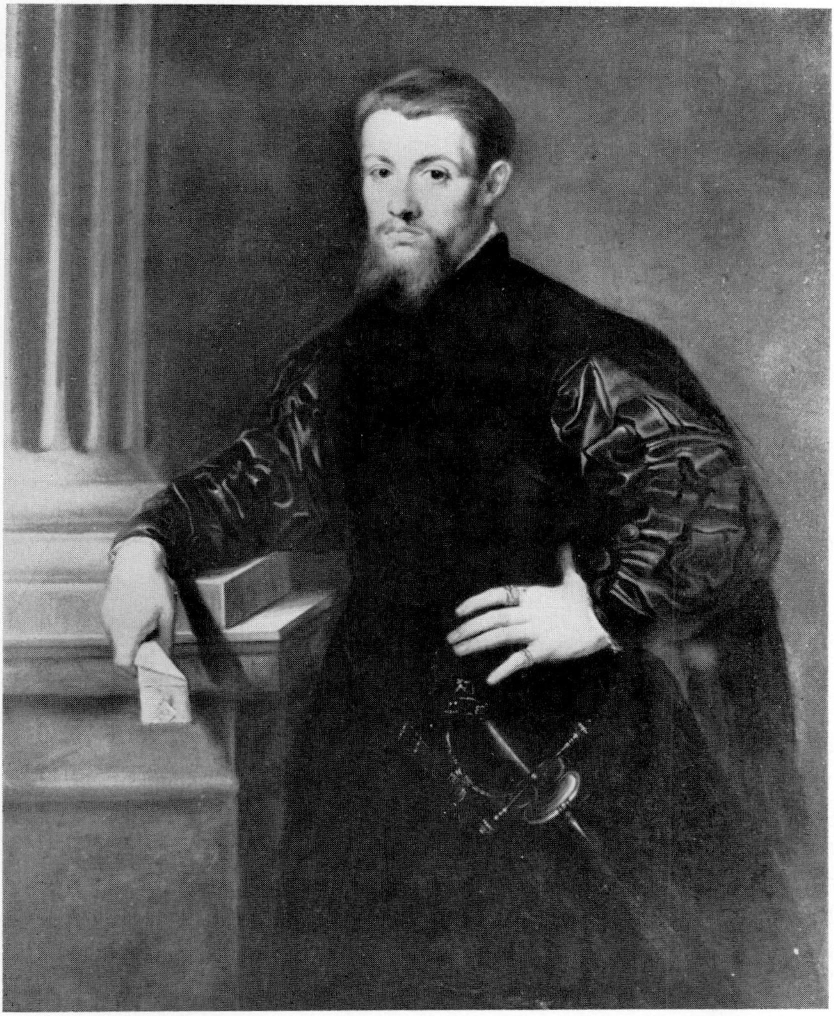

FIGURE 21. A portrait in oil attributed to Jan Stephen Van Calcar (1499-1546?) purchased at Oxford in 1918 by Harvey Cushing and bequeathed by him to the Yale Medical Library in 1939. In his Iconography of Andreas Vesalius (1925), M. H. Spielman calls it a "repetition of the portrait in the Louvre" and says: "It is well indeed, that a reputable version of this celebrated and much-discussed work should find a home in America, where it may be seen by students and scholars." Discussion has centered chiefly on the identity of the sitter. The exemplar in the Louvre is now listed as "Portrait of a Young Man." (Photograph courtesy of Yale Medical Historical Library.)

turn led to the decision that he must have had red hair. One writer, by accepting the legend that Vesalius the anatomist as a child dissected small animals, discovered indications of sadism, and by mistranslating the word "lend" as "borrow" in a German text, this same person also contrived in a somewhat tortuous fashion to make poor Vesalius a manic-depressive. All these things have their amusing side, but are also to be regretted since once such distortions have reached print, it is always very difficult, if not impossible, to expunge them completely."

According to Singer,[111] even until a few years ago, "Vesalius was a mysterious figure around which had gathered certain legendary tales, some of which only robust faith could accept. Despite his exceptional learning and accuracy, the great biographer of Vesalius, Roth, wished the reader to believe in a being of almost limitless intelligence and virtue." Fortunately, researchers of modern scholars particularly O'Malley and Saunders give us a more accurate and more human picture of this outstanding ancient.

The following facts, though historical in nature, are universally accepted as authentic. Vesalius was born on December 31, 1514. His father, also named Andreas, was the illegitimate son of Everard van Wesele, a member of a family already distinguished in medical circles for several generations. The father was an apothecary of Emperor Charles V.

Young Vesalius received his preliminary education in Brussels. In February, 1530, at the age of sixteen, he matriculated at the University of Louvain, in the arts course, a prerequisite for admission to any professional school. In 1531, the Emperor legitimized the father's birth, and some believed that this may have encouraged young Vesalius to consider medicine and to carry on the tradition of the family.

Since the University of Louvain was not an outstanding school of medicine, Vesalius journeyed to Paris, where in September, 1533, he entered the more illustrious medical school, at the University of Paris. There, Vesalius studied with Jean Fernal, Guinter of Andernach, Jean Tagault, and possibly, although there is no definite proof of this, for only a brief time, with Jacobus Sylvius.

Like other young students of the times, Vesalius accepted

Galenic anatomy. But, he continued to dissect whenever possible and in this manner acquired considerable knowledge of anatomy. He surreptitiously visited old Parisian cemeteries and the gallows and thereby gathered an abundance of material.* Vesalius remained in Paris studying for the degree of Bachelor of Medicine until 1536, when because of the outbreak of war between France and the Empire, he became an enemy alien and returned to Brussels without his degree.

He enrolled in the Medical School of the University of Louvain, where as a result of his studies in Paris he obtained the degree of Bachelor of Medicine, late in 1537. By this time, he knew he had to do something to correct anatomical theories, based entirely upon Galenic structure and thought. In all fairness to Galen, it should be pointed out that because of the then prevalent law Galen could not dissect human bodies. His opinions were therefore formulated from available dissection material of monkeys and of pigs. Unfortunately, Galen believed anatomic structures of animals to be identical with man.

Dissatisfied with methods of obtaining material for dissection and study, Vesalius decided to go to Padua for the Degree of Doctor of Medicine. In December, 1537, he successfully passed his examination and received the degree of Doctor of Medicine with "highest honors." On the following day, he was appointed to the then relatively unimportant chair of surgery, but which carried with it the duty of lecturing on anatomy.

Padua, as the center of the scientific Renaissance, was then at the peak of its glory. While religious wars raged over Europe, sparing no country, hundreds of foreign students were grouped

---

* A word about Anatomy at Paris. The early history of anatomy at the University of Paris (Faculty of Medicine) is meagre and incomplete. The building which housed the medical school in the Rue de la Bucherie was completed in 1477. It had no anatomical dissecting room. When such dissections were performed, and rarely so, they were usually held in a cellar of some available building, not in the Hotel-Dieu. Although as early as 1483 a formal anatomical knowledge was demanded of the candidates for the baccalaureate, no dissection was held until 1493. In 1526, the medical faculty made an appeal to the Parliament for more dissections, which remained comparatively rare until 1536, after the departure of Vesalius. The advent of the renaissance element came to Paris later than to Padua, and Paris had little contact with the great Italian Universities. Above all, there was no authoritative Parisian anatomical text and this undoubtedly was a perplexing problem to Vesalius.

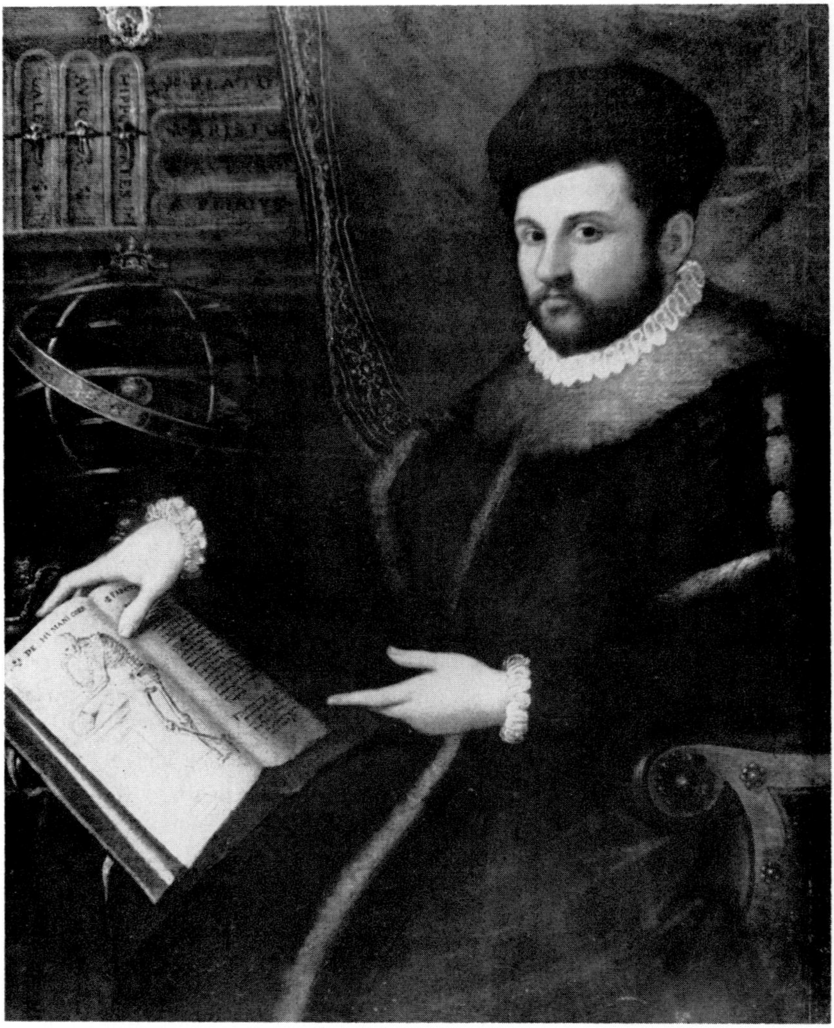

FIGURE 22. Italian, late 16th Century, North Italian School. Portrait of a physician, for many years believed to be portrait of Andreas Vesalius, now identified as one of Juan de Valverde de Amusco, an anatomist contemporaneous with Vesalius. (Reference: Guerra, Francisco—Juan de Valverde de Amusco—Evidence for the identification of his portrait—claimed to be that of Vesalius—with a reappraisal of his work. *Clio Medica,* 2:339-362, 1967. Pergamon Press Ltd. Photograph courtesy of the Walters Art Gallery, Baltimore, Md.)

in the *nationes,* which offered hospitality to the newcomers and were organized with perfect discipline, as centers of friendship and of learning. In this respect, Castiglioni[112] writes: "in the second half of the sixteenth century, the German *Natio,* which comprised the Flemish students, had an enrollment of 977 members, attending the medical school. In occasional fierce competitions with other universities, of which we possess records, the Venetian Senate tried to engage the most famous teachers for the school, and according to the new trend of medical doctrines, anatomy was evidently intended to have an important part in the medical course."

The course in anatomy at Padua was no different than that which Vesalius had experienced in Paris, and no different from the mode of teaching anatomy elsewhere. The professor of anatomy would sit apart from the cadaver, reading from the anatomical text of Mundinus* in Latin, and the dissector who rarely understood Latin, would do the dissection.

---

* Mondino de Luzzi, better known as Mundinus (1275-1326) is credited as the first to break away from the avoidance of dissection of the human body, which had been shunned for so many years. Mundinus was the first to reintroduce systematic human dissection, since the time of the great Alexandrians, Erasistratus and Herophilus, 1500 years earlier. Mundinus is supposed to have been born in Bologna in the latter part of the thirteenth century and to have received his medical degree from the University of Bologna in 1290. Up to the time of his death in 1326, he was professor at the university and practiced in his native city. Of interest is that he held two chairs at the University of Bologna; one in anatomy and one in surgery, an arrangement which persisted for 250 years, until separate chairs were established at the end of the sixteenth century. This holding of conjoint chairs of anatomy and surgery existed in other Italian schools. Indeed, Vesalius held a similar dual chair at Padua two hundred years after Mundinus. Unlike Vesalius, Mundinus tried to prove the veracity of Galen and other traditional anatomical authors. Thus, his description of the liver is a true Galenic description yet he begs the issue when he says, "the intrinsic and integral parts are five lobes. Yet in man these lobes are not always distinct." The medieval description of the liver always presented it as a five-lobed organ, based on Galen's dissection of animals.

Mundinus' *Anatomia* was used as a compendium of anatomy for the student and also as a dissection manual. The book was first printed in 1478 and had many subsequent editions, serving as the standard textbook of anatomy for more than two hundred years, and then replaced by Vesalius' *Fabrica.* "The volume is one of the classics of medicine, even though its contents contain no strikingly new material; its author ranks among those who fundamentally influenced the growth of the medical sciences. He is one of a large group of men, surgeons by training and vocation, who made important contributions to the basic sciences as part of their specific professional interests, experiences, and capabilities."

Garrison and Morton, describe *Anatomia,* as the first book devoted solely to anatomy; "it was written for his students in 1316. The medieval anatomical vocabulary, well set forth by Mundinus, was derived mainly from Arabic." The reader should not overlook the fact that even though the *Anatomia* is based on human dissection, in actuality Mundinus relied largely upon such of Galen's and Avicenna's writings that he was familiar with or as O'Malley so well puts it, "He dissected merely to experience for himself what they had written and cretainly with no thought of putting his authorities to the test."

In 1521, Berengario Da Carpi (Giacomo) an eminent anatomist corrected Mundinus in "*Commentaria cum amplissimus additionibus super anatomia Mundini una cum textu ejusdem in pristinum et verum nitorem red acto.* This volume is the first to mention the vermiform appendix, the larger pelvis of the female, and the first good description of the thymus. In the *Isagogae,* an epitome of the *Commentaria* (1522), he includes a description of the valves of the heart.

Although Andreas Vesalius is now recognized as the founder of modern anatomy, a few others rather often overlooked deserve some mention of this honor. As mentioned above, the dissection of the human body, which is the only means of an accurate understanding of human anatomy became possible when it was no longer believed that such a procedure would provoke the wrath of the dead upon the investigator. Thus, from the fourth century B.C. onward, a new attitude developed toward human dissection. Herophilus of Chalcedon, born in the last third of the fourth century B.C. is considered "father and founder of modern anatomy." His writings as well as those of Erasistratus have been lost, but fortunately what we know of them is gleaned from later writers, particularly Galen.

Herophilus was a very successful teacher. He was the author of a work, *On Anatomy,* a special treatise *of the eyes,* and a popular handbook for midwives. According to Singer, he definitely recognized the brain as the central organ of the central nervous system, and contrary to the views of Aristotle's belief on the primacy of the heart.

He distinguished between motor and sensory nerves, described the cerebrum and cerebellum (torcular Herophili). Herophilus noted the fourth ventricle and the calamus scriptori, which he named. The term *rete mirabile* is a Latin translation of the name which he gave to that structure at the base of the brain, which does not exist in humans but only found in animals. The terms *prostate* and *duodenum* were coined by Herophilus.

Erasistratus of Chios (290 B.C.) was the younger contemporary of Herophilus. He differed from Herophilus in that he could be called a physiologist rather than an anatomist. Indeed, he has often been referred to as the "Father of Physiology." The physiology of Erasistratus was based on the belief that every organ is equipped with three-fold system of tubes, vein, artery and nerve. He believed that these divided beyond vision, and continued on and on. The minute division of these vessels, plaited together then made up the tissues.

Erasistratus believed that blood and two kinds of pneuma were the essential sources of nourishment and movement. The blood is carried by veins and the air is taken in by the lungs and passes to the heart, where it becomes changed into a peculiar pneuma, which he called the vital spirit, which is then sent to the different parts of the body by the arteries.

Vesalius quickly changed the technique of anatomical dissections and instead of remaining seated in a lofty chair while assistants demonstrated and barbers cut, he descended into the operating theatre to dissect and to demonstrate personally as he lectured. This was contrary to custom. To many, it appeared faulty for a physician to actually touch a cadaver. Vesalius soon introduced other changes in the curriculum which ultimately made his course a major attraction for university students as well as townsmen who came in swarms to the anatomical amphitheatre.

In the development of medical teaching throughout the centuries, the history of the anatomical theatre has a particular importance. It is closely connected not only with the history of medicine and of teaching, but also with the history of art. The purpose of the theatre was to offer a performance because an anatomical dissection at that time was really more of a theatrical performance than a lesson. To the dissection were invited all the outstanding personalities and the authorities of the town. Later, the theatre became the center of anatomical teaching; it was the first laboratory, the first place where objective scientific research was carried on. At first, anatomical instruction was given in the homes of the teachers; then rare dissections were done in cellars, sometimes in a cemetery or in other hidden places. Only later did it become evident that in order to make it possible for a large audience to attend the dissection, it was necessary to have a place where many people could be present at the same time and still be able to follow the demonstration of the dissector. Still later, about the latter part of the sixteenth century, this early anatomical theatre which at first had been built very plainly of wood, was now transferred to the universities, where appropriate buildings and sometimes quite splendid ones were erected as anatomical theatres.[113]

Of great historical value is the excellent preservation of a student's notebook of dissection carried on from December 6th to December 24th. In these notes, Vesalius (like Mundinus) was still fitting the animal anatomy of Galen to the human cadaver. Nevertheless, the time was approaching when he would be unable to reconcile what he observed in the human body with

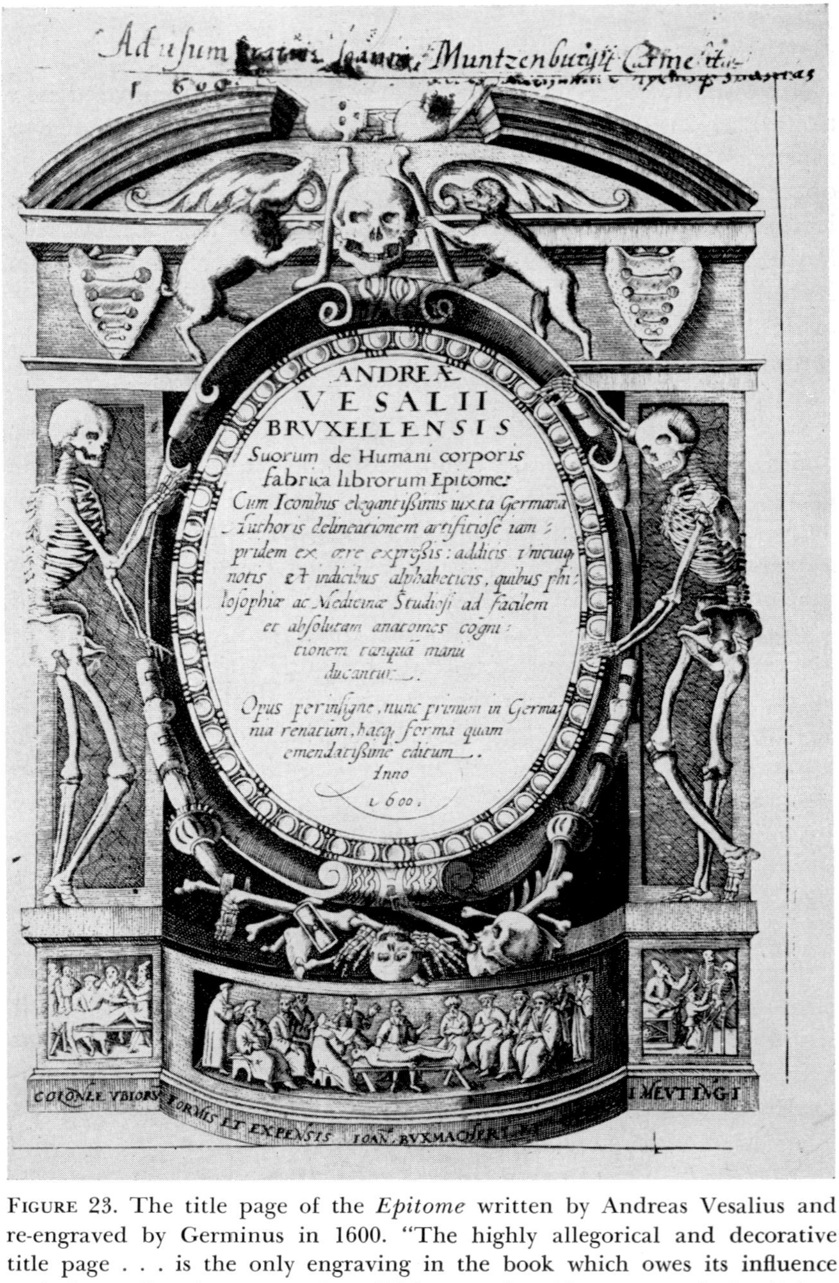

FIGURE 23. The title page of the *Epitome* written by Andreas Vesalius and re-engraved by Germinus in 1600. "The highly allegorical and decorative title page . . . is the only engraving in the book which owes its influence entirely to Germinus. . . . In addition to the title page and the 'Adam and Eve' figures, Germinus included in his engravings all the large illustrations from the *Fabrica* and the majority of the important smaller ones usually in almost the same size as Vesalian figures." (C. D. O'Malley. Photograph courtesy Rare Book Room, Library, New York Medical College.)

what he read in Galen's text. Galen's hold on anatomic knowledge was so strong that when Vesalius demonstrated that Galen's description of the hip bone was wrong; he apologized for deviating from the master's teaching by stating that since Galen's time, man had changed his shape by wearing tight trousers.[114]

At the age of twenty-four, Vesalius introduced another didactic novelty. He had very large charts made on which he depicted in minute detail the anatomy and physiology of the body, so detailed that one could easily observe his errors. A study of the charts, which were roughly copied in the above-mentioned student's notebook, reveals a predominance of Galenic or animal anatomy. But they also demonstrated independent observation and hence accurate portrayal of human anatomy. Students were enthusiastic about these charts, and to prevent use and distribution of inferior copies, Vesalius was forced to publish his drawings. To his own sketches of the vascular system were added plates of his skeleton, drawn from three standard aspects by Johannes Stephanus from Calcar in the Netherlands, and at that time a student in Titian's studio in Venice.

Singer and Rabin,[49] in discussing certain anatomical elements in the Tabulae (PLVII), elaborate on Vesalius' consistency in representing the right kidney as higher than the left, as it is in most animals but not in man. In this interpretation, Vesalius follows Galen's *De anatomicis administrationibus* and Aristotle's *De partibus animalium.* "In man," write Singer and Rabin, "the right kidney is lower than the left. This is said to be related to the great size of the right side of the human liver. The renal vessels in man are correspondingly connected with the aorta and the vena cava respectively at a somewhat lower level on the right side than on the left. In the domestic animals —cat, dog, sheep, ox, as well as in the ape and rodents (though not in the pig)—this relation is reversed. In all these creatures, the level of the left kidney and its vessels is considerably lower than the right . . . the lower level of the right kidney and its vessels is evident at any autopsy of a human body. To make the right higher as he always does, Vesalius must have had his anatomical picture fixed from the bodies of animals before he attacked the anatomy of man. Estienne makes the same error.

He and Vesalius have accepted the statement of Galen that "in all animals the right kidney is at a higher level than the left," which is itself a repetition of Aristotle." O'Malley[116] points out that in the *Fabrica* Vesalius wrote that he had also found the reverse.

Of equal interest to the urologist is the earliest representation of the prostate gland. This appears in Tabula I of Vesalius' *Tabula Anatomicae Sex*. This structure was first described in 1536 by Niccolo Massa but without sketches. Since Massa's book was printed at Venice, it is more than likely that Vesalius was familiar with it. In *Tabula I,* the prostate is represented as having two lobes in front. Vesalius does not give this gland a name in the *Tabulae,* but in the *Fabrica* he alternates by calling it *corpus glandulosum* and *assistens glandulosus.* The gland was first called "prostate" by Casper Bartholin in 1611. It seems that Vesalius must have seen the prostate in the human body, for his figure could not have been obtained from the ox, sheep or carnivor, for these animals have a small circular prostate. Neither could it have been drawn from the ape, which has a well-developed gland, but does not extend in front of the urethra. It more likely was the prostate of a dog.

Again, in *Tabula I* (organs of generation, above of the man, below of the woman), the student of urology will note that the third figure (male) shows the implantation of the *vasa* carrying down the semen *(deferentia).* The term *vasa deferentia* is a modern one, and is believed to have been introduced by Jacopo Berengario da Carpi in his *commentaria . . . super anatomia mundini,* Bologna, 1521, and therefore during the time of Vesalius who used the term in both editions of the *Fabrica.* Strangely, Vesalius does not credit Jacopo as its author. In a somewhat similar neglect, Vesalius does not mention Niccolo Massa of Venice, who in 1536, wrote an excellent account of the generative organs, and quite thoroughly described the prostate.

In *Tabulae I* of Vesalius' *Tabulae Anatomicae Sex,* there is a reproduction of the generative organs. In this figure, the inferior vena cava is seen greatly expanded and obscuring most of the aorta. This is similarly shown throughout the *Fabrica* and the *Epitome*. Of interest is the course of the veins from the gonads, correctly shown for both sexes, that of the right entering the trunk of the vena cava and that of the left the renal vein. Gunther gives credit for this anatomical lesson to Vesalius, whereas actually this anatomical relationship was a medieval commonplace. "In 1536," write Singer and Rabin, "the very year of publication of Guenther's *Institutiones,* Massa (c. 1480-1569) issued his *Anatomicae liber introductorius*. It devotes four and a half pages to a correct account of the distribution of the seminal vessels. These had already been well described by Berengario in 1522 and by Mundinus in 1316. Mundinus refers Guenther's very point to Avicenna. Doubtless Avicenna himself derived it from a passage in Galen's *De vent. art. diss.,* which Guenther missed. . . . But apart from all this, an interesting connection here arises. Avicenna's knowledge of the asymmetry of the renal veins can be traced to Book XIII of Galen's *De Anatomicis Administrationibus*. Now this thirteenth book was unknown to Guenther though he had printed a Latin translation of the first nine at Paris in 1531. The last seven books were early lost from the Greek text. They survived only in an Arabic translation and were recovered in the twentieth century. Thus, "on this particular point," emphasize Singer and Rabin,[49] "the sources of Mundinus and the medieval Arabists were actually better than those of the renaissance scholars for they went back through Avicenna to elements in Galen that were otherwise inaccessible."

The six plates were issued in 1538 *(Tabulae Anatomicae Sex)*. They were instantly popular and immediately plagiarized in many countries. In addition to the unusual accuracy and clarity, the woodcuts set a new standard in the printing art, and have been called an excellent pioneer example of typography and format. "It may be difficult today to understand the novelty of this venture. Few anatomical works up to this time had been illustrated, and of those that were, the illustrations were little more than symbols or decorations. Indeed, many of the leading physicians of the day were actively opposed to the illustration of the printed word on the grounds that this had not been done in classical times and would degrade scholarship." Up to this time, Vesalius was a follower of Galen, but from now on there occurred a definite change, for he now became increasingly perplexed by the discrepancies between Galen's descriptions and what he found by human dissections. Sigerist believes that when Vesalius realized that what Galen was describing was not human anatomy at all, but the anatomy of lower animals, brought to Vesalius a sense of liberation—the fetters of tradition had been broken.[107]

Singer and Rabin[49] stress the character and purpose of the *Tabulae* and verify that in the original form of this work of Vesalius, there was no title. In 1538, it became known as the *Tabulae Anatomicae Sex*. These researchers believe "the *Tabulae* is confessedly no more than a preliminary effort. Vesalius had a larger enterprise in mind even when its sheets were passing through the press. He ends his dedication with the words: 'Should I find it acceptable to the learned, I hope to add something more considerable thereto.' " "But the same preface," write Singer and Rabin,[49] "introduces an element of the Vesalian problem."

> "Not long since," he writes, "when appointed at Padua for the course of the Surgical part of medicine, in discussing the treatment of inflammation, I had . . . made a drawing of the veins . . . this . . . so pleased the professors and students of medicine that they pressed me for a similar delineation of the arteries and nerves. Since the conduct of dissections was part of my duty, and knowing this kind of drawing to be very useful to those attending the demonstration, I had to accede to this request. Nevertheless, I am convinced that it is very hard—may be futile and impossible—to obtain real anatomical . . . knowledge from mere figures . . . though no one will deny them to be capital aids to memory."

The defense of the use of drawings as a means of teaching requires some explanation. It follows that by the sixteenth century there had come in scientific disciplines, great respect for the written word. In the middle of this century (1530-40-1550), there waged a ridiculous war against the use of illustrations. Thus, the great contemporaries of Vesalius, namely Sylvius

(1478-1555), Fernel (1485-1557), Guenther (1487-1574), Massa (c. 1500-69), Colombo (1516-59), Falloppio* (1523-62) avoided the graphic method of teaching anatomy.[117] These men opposed such a method for it would be a break with classical tradition, at a time when everything dealing with antiquity was authentic. Sketches were believed to be symbolic of charlatanry, quackery and vulgarism. Some of the predecessors of Vesalius, such as Berengario da Carpi, Charles Estienne and Eustachio were brave enough to utilize graphic anatomical methods in their works. Most of the Eustachio drawings were not published until long after his death (1574).

In 1538, Vesalius published the *Venesection* Letter. It should be recalled that from remote antiquity venesection had been established as a standard therapeutic measure, emphatically recommended by Hippocrates and subsequently by Galen. In medieval times, and particularly under the influence of Arabic Medicine, these practices had become corrupted in their use and particularly in their indications. With the recovery of classical learning at the beginning of the sixteenth century, a new approach to venesection took place. Pierre Brissot, a Paris physician became a strong advocate of the procedure and condemned the Arabic procedure of bleeding a patient from a point on the body as far away from the region of the ailment as possible and removing no more than a mere token of a few drops of blood. He recommended the removal of a sensible quantity of blood, particularly in the treatment of pleursy, and that it did not matter whether the blood was from the right or left side.

A dispute of almost international magnitude now arose and the issue of the *Venesection* Letter placed Vesalius with the champions of the purified classics and adherents of the Hippocratic-Brissot School. This Vesalian contribution was significant since contrary to previous theories, he (Vesalius) introduced an entirely new thought, namely the findings of direct observation. Indeed, it went further in that he emphasized the

---

* O'Malley[117] informs me that Falloppio mentions his preparation of a fully illustrated anatomical text. Falloppio is best remembered for his account of the tubes named after him.

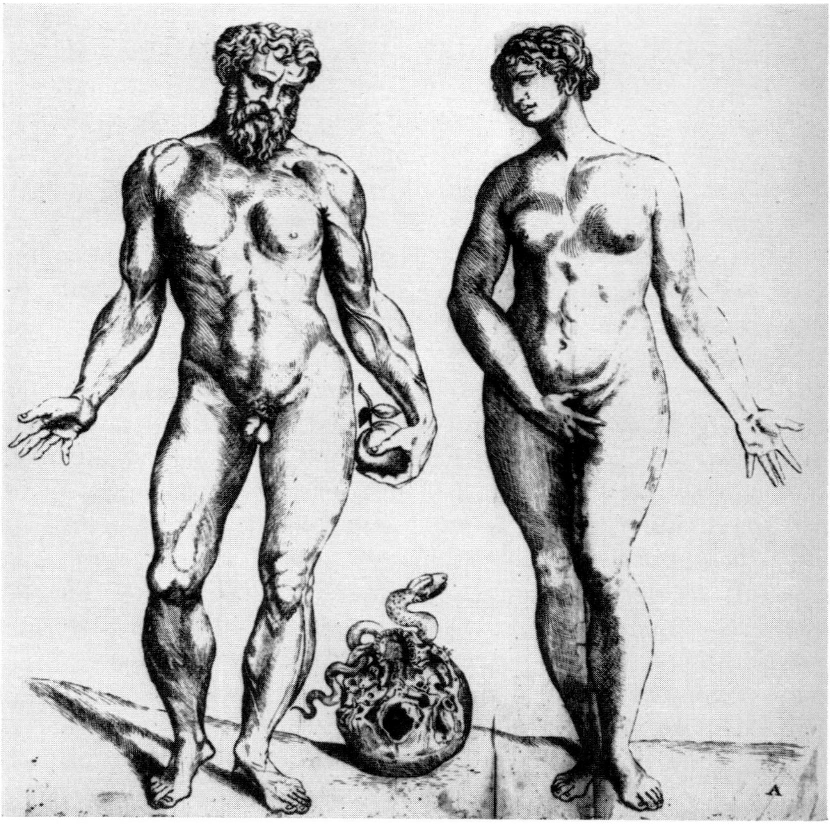

FIGURE 24. In the *Epitome,* this composition of the naked man has the symbols of Adam and Eve, i.e., an apple, serpent and skull. In the *Fabrica,* the male does not have an apple in his left hand, but instead holds a skull. The female figure is the same in all editions. (Photograph courtesy Rare Book Room, Library, New York Medical College.)

importance of the venous system and subsequent discovery of the venous valves which ultimately provided William Harvey with the key to unlock the mystery of the circulation.

As more bodies became available to Vesalius for careful dissection and study, it became more and more difficult for Vesalius to present Galenic theories to his students. Indeed, as more opportunity for extensive dissections became available, he (Vesalius) could no longer attribute his findings as anomalies from the writings of Galen. His first declaration was accepted as heresy but the students cheered him. News reached the students at the University of Bologna, where he was promptly invited to give a series of lectures. This he did in January, 1540, when he proved his theories dramatically by articulating side by side the skeletons of a man and of an ape, clearly showing that Galen's osteology agreed with the simian skeleton but not the human.

And now commenced the writing of his masterpiece, *De Humani Corporis Fabrica,* which has survived to this day, in its accuracy and superb presentation. Vesalius must have realized that his vast anatomical treatise would have epochal significance for he denied it no amount of energy, attention and material resources. For example, the illustrations came from Titian's studio, the finest Venetian block cutters were utilized and, above all, the best printer, Johannes Oporinus* of Basel.

Despite the long trek to Switzerland, Vesalius chose Oporinus and supervised the proofreading and other changes needed. He had the plates transported on mule-back on a long and hazardous journey through the Alpine passes to Basel and to Oporinus. But why, this long trek, when the great Italian printing center was in Venice?

Vesalius had developed a good relationship with Oporinus, and knew that the Swiss printer would spare no sacrifice in order to produce the book in the highest standards of book production. Indeed, most authorities agree that the second edition of the work in 1555 was an even greater example of the sixteenth century typographers art than the first one, and it has

---

* Johannes Oporinus (1507-1568) the Latinized form of Herbst, was the son of an unsuccessful artist. He was born in Basel where he received his elementary education under his father's guidance since the family could not afford to send him to school. He subsequently went to a private school at Strasburg, where he spent four years in the study of the classical languages. He was exposed to printing while copying manuscripts and as a corrector for the great printer Johann Froben. He then spent a hectic life in the household of a bombastic Theophrastus von Hohenheim, better known as Paracelsus. He gave up the thought of medicine and entered a more serene academic life, first as Professor of Latin and later of Greek in the University. He subsequently entered the printing business, first with a partner and later by himself, and remained in this business until 1566 when he retired. On July 6, 1568, he died and was buried in the Cathedral of Basel.

been difficult to understand how Oporinus could have expected any returns from the venture.

Although the text of the *Fabrica* should be of primary interest, all who write of this great contribution concern themselves mostly with the illustrations. This may be explained on the basis that the text has not always been available to all but rather confined to a few. In addition, many scholars found the text to be written from a philosophic rather than a specific point of view. Regardless of all criticisms, the *Fabrica* is, without question, one of the great accomplishments of the human spirit.

Vesalius in his *Fabrica* gives a correct description of the structure and physiology of the kidneys. This did not soften the anger aroused by Galenic followers. Actually, this is the first accurate anatomical description of the kidneys ever recorded and although there are some minor inaccurate descriptions, it is indeed indicative of the tremendous strides made in renal anatomy and physiology as compared to Galen's renal anatomy. With regard to the kidneys he wrote:

> "I have tried to find an explanation of the urinary secretion according to the descriptions of the ancients. The Galenists have tried to study the function of the kidney mistakenly and with negligence, without observing the course of the vessels and affirming that they had seen I don't know what kind of filtering membrane. Some others like Prometheus, very satisfied with themselves disdained to dissect the kidneys and, aloft on their chairs, believed to have accomplished their duty attributing to man the structure according to their own imagination. And therefore, the most important doctors of our times have taught and written that we may imagine three ways through which blood may be separated from urine in the kidneys. They don't give any descriptions of what is to be found in the kidneys, but speak according to their ideas of sinuses and channels, and so everybody believes and accepts that there are two sinuses, the one above and the other below placed the long way in the organ and separated by a transverse membrane. Into the upper sinus the renal vein and artery open, which carry the serous blood which passes very slowly through little and very narrow holes of the membrane

of the sinus. The blood cannot pass, being too damp, but only the serum. These passionate architects of human nature in order to construct a work more elegant than nature itself did, teach that the urinary duct starts from the inferior sinus and receives the filtered urine."*

With the publication of *De Humani Corporis Fabrica,* a storm of anger and abuse was hurled at Vesalius, by his contemporaries.† Sylvius, his former teacher, turned against his brilliant pupil, calling him a madman.‡ Vesalius, only in his twenty-ninth year, and perhaps still with youthful impetuousness, decided to end his days as an anatomist. Since his family had a long tradition of imperial service, he applied to the Emperor and received the post of physician to the imperial household. This was unfortunate, for anatomical advancement would no longer have his untiring support. Some idea of the zeal with which Vesalius had previously devoted to his anatomical studies, as well as his bitterness, is well recorded in the following statement quoted by O'Malley:

"No longer shall I willingly spend hours in the cemetery of the Innocents in Paris turning over bones, nor go to Mont-

---

* "The *Fabrica,*" writes Corner, "was published at the climacteric period of the Renaissance, only twenty-five years after Luther nailed his thesis to Wittenberg Cathedral door and in the same year in which Copernicus revolutionized astronomy with the book *De revolutionibus orbium coelestum.*"

† Bartolemeo Eustachio (1520-74), a great anatomist, had published some extraordinary plates (not published during his life time) among which were those of the kidney. These are accepted by anatomists as being superior to those of Vesalius. Indeed, Eustachio severely criticized Vesalius for having represented the kidney of a dog in place of that of a man. The fine plates by Eustachio remained unprinted and forgotten in the Vatical Library, until discovered in the early 18th century, and were then presented by Pope Clement XI, to his physician, the famous Lancisi. Lancisi and others are of the opinion that if these plates had appeared in 1552, Eustachio would have ranked with Vesalius as one of the founders of modern anatomy.

‡ Jacque DuBois Sylvius (1478-1555) asked Vesalius to renounce his heretical utterances and to confess his mistakes and his sin in departing from the footsteps of Galen. When Vesalius refused, Sylvius called him a madman and a two-legged ass, and went so far as to ask Charles V, at whose court Vesalius was appointed physician, that "Vesalius be punished and in every way restrained lest, by his pestilent breath, he poison all of Europe."

faucon to look at bones—where once with a companion I was gravely imperiled by many savage dogs. Nor should I care to be locked out of Louvain so that, alone in the middle of the night, I might take way bones from the gibbett to prepare a skeleton. I shall no longer bother to petition the judges to delay an execution to a time suitable for dissection, nor shall I advise the students to observe where someone has been buried or urge them to make note of the disease of their teacher's patients so that they might later secure the bodies. I shall not keep in my bedroom for several weeks bodies taken from graves or given me after public execution."

War broke out in 1544, and as a military surgeon Vesalius was able to apply his great anatomical knowledge to surgery. He became well versed in gunshot wounds, and abhorred the practice of using boiling oil. In 1562, his main contribution to surgery, was the success of surgically induced drainage of empyema, which he reported and recommended to other surgeons, only after many trials and errors personally supervised by Vesalius. Thus, his reputation as a surgeon became so well established that when in 1559 Henry II of France was injured in a tournament, Vesalius was called to Paris, and placed in charge, in the presence of Ambroise Paré, who had great esteem for Vesalius. Ambroise Paré made up the anatomical section of his great text of surgery by borrowing freely from the *Fabrica* condensing it and putting it into French and thus making Vesalian anatomy available to the barber-surgeons.

As time went along, and Vesalius' experience became greater, he realized that there were many errors in the first edition of *De Humani Corporis Fabrica.** It is probable that the revised text was written by Vesalius during a long stay with the Emperor in Augsburg from August, 1550 to October 1551.

---

* Along with *De Humani Corporis Fabrica,* Vesalius had published a smaller companion volume, called the *Epitome.* This was written in simple style and as an introduction to the more formal and advanced *Fabrica.* It in no way enhanced Vesalius' reputation but was extensively used, in fact read more than *De Humani Corporis Fabrica.* The illustrations appearing in this chapter are direct photographs of a copy of the *Epitome,* now in the Rare Book Room in the library of the New York Medical College, Flower and Fifty Avenue Hospitals.

Complete publication of the full seven books, after some delay, occurred in August, 1555. The second folio edition of *De Humani Corporis Fabrica* was more elegant than the first edition. The paper was heavier and the type larger. A new title page appeared as well as many improvements in the text. Of singular interest, the original woodcuts from which these editions were printed, remained and were utilized for over 400 years in Europe, and finally destroyed by the bombing of Munich during World War II.*

With the abdication of Charles V in 1556, Vesalius, for reasons unknown, took service with Charles V's son, Phillip II, King of Spain. In 1559, he was transferred to Spain with his wife and daughter. In Madrid, he built up a large practice among the foreign embassies. From this point on, little verification of Vesalius' career is available other than to point out that it was neither significant or happy. In 1564, he went on a pilgrimage to the Holy Land and stopped off at Venice where he learned his friend Falloppi† had died. This left the chair of anatomy at Padua vacant, and many think Vesalius would have cherished this appointment again.

---

* In 1934, under the editorship of Doctors Weigand Lambert and Archibold Malloch, a magnificent edition, struck from the original wood blocks, the *Iconea Anatomicae of Andreas Vesalius,* was published jointly by the New York Academy of Medicine and the Library of the University of Munich. These illustrations were reproduced by Drs. Saunders and O'Malley in their *Illustrations From the Works of Andreas Vesalius of Brussels* in 1950.

† Gabriel Falloppi's (c. 1523-1562) early education was first directed towards the classics, later in an ecclesiastical direction and finally toward medicine, studying under Nicolo Machella in Modena, toward the end of 1551, he was appointed to the famous chair at Padua, as a successor to Realdo Colombo, who had succeeded to Vesalius' anatomic chair. Falloppi's name is universally associated with his description of the uterine fallopian tubes. He is of singular interest to the urologist because of his accurate account of the kidney. In addition, he is credited with perhaps the first record of a case of bilateral duplication of the ureter and renal vessels. He also was among the first to observe the straight tubules now named Bellini, who gave a more minute description of them in 1662. He also noted multiple calyces of the kidney as well as renal corpuscles, now usually associated with the name of malpighi. Fallopi criticized Vesalius for his description and illustration in the *Fabrica* of the unipapillary kidney of the dog instead of that of a man. Falloppi was also the first to describe the three layers of the bladder: "it possesses three tunics, as do the stomach and intestines."

The ship on which Vesalius was returning ran into a severe storm and was wrecked. Vesalius managed to get to the shores of the island of Zante, where he shortly died, the cause of death unknown.

It was a miserable ending for a man of international distinction. Almost every ambassador thought the news of Vesalius' death to be of sufficient importance for dispatch to his court. International recognition of Vesalius' contributions to anatomy and medical science, became more significant and more evident with the passing of century after century.

Chapter XIII

Galaxy of the Ancients Continued Ambroise Paré (1510-1590)

AMBROISE PARÉ is the most celebrated surgeon of the Renaissance. He is included in our "galaxy of ancients" because, like Vesalius, he contributed to the advancement of medicine, particularly the practice of surgery.* He was a great admirer and follower of Vesalius, and in the preface of his *Anatomie Universelle* acknowledges his great debt to Vesalius, his teacher. Indeed, Paré did much to popularize the *Fabrica* and teachings of Vesalius by writing an epitome of them in the vernacular of Parisian French.

The history of surgery during the sixteenth century is dominated by the outstanding figure of one man, Ambroise Paré.

---

* Sigerist writes, "In Italy during the thirteenth century, there had been a great development of surgery, which had spread thence to the adjoining land of France. Surgery must always keep in close touch with life, and can never be so theoretical as internal medicine. Only by practice does a man learn how to operate. A suture holds the edges of a wound together, or it fails to do so. One thing or the other; there can be no dispute about the matter, that was why, even during the heyday of scholasticism, there had been noted practitioners of surgery . . . to the surgeons of these days, when most wounds were made with cold steel, 'healing by first intention,' that is to say a primary, non-suppurative growing together of the edges of a wound, seemed the most desirable. A change came, however during the fourteenth and fifteenth centuries, when the increasing use of firearms imposed new tasks upon army surgeons. Even small arms were then of large calibre, their bullets ranging up to nearly an inch in diameter. These projectiles must have inflicted horrible wounds, most of which, doubtless, were infected from the onset. We can hardly be surprised, therefore, that by degrees the idea gained ground that suppuration was a normal stage in the healing of wounds, and that gunshot wounds were poisoned by the gunpowder. As for suppuration, you may still hear the expression 'laudable pus.' "

He alone among the surgeons of Europe possessed those qualities which ensured preeminence. Indeed, his survival as a Huguenot in Paris during the turbulent years of his maturity revealed qualities which fitted him to be surgeon to four kings of France and sometimes their counsellor as well. It enabled him at the same time to make important contributions to the advancement of his profession.[118]

To fully appreciate and evaluate Ambroise Paré, as a great scholar and surgeon, it is well to first understand the environment in which he lived and the status of the medical profession during Paré's career. Hamby[119] in writing of Ambroise Paré, calls him the "Surgeon of the Renaissance," but emphasizes that although the Renaissance bloomed in France in the sixteenth century, it arrived almost a century later than in Italy, from which it came. Actually, the influence of the Renaissance did not reach its peak in France, until the nineteenth century."

Paris of 1530, the time when Paré lived in this ancient city, had a population of about 150,000 people. "Historians estimate that six or seven thousand of them were paupers. The bubonic plague was raging, as it did periodically within the close confines of all the old walled cities; the mortality was high. Under the stimulus of the young king, Francois I, the face of the city was changing. The Louvre was being converted from a medieval fortress, into a Renaissance palace. The Hotel-de-ville and St. Eustace's great church were under construction. Notre-Dame the Sainte-Chapelle, the Hotel-Dieu and the Grand Chatelet, the grim fortress-prison on the north bank of the Seine, were the major landmarks of the city. . . . The streets of old Paris were narrow, only six to twenty feet in width. They were usually unpaved, although some of the major ones were cobble-stoned. Sewage disposal was elementary. Wastes usually were thrown from windows into shallow ditches along the curbs. In wet weather, the streets were filthy quagmires, and in hot weather the city literally stank. Paving was being extended as rapidly as possible, but the Parliament had many demands on its funds, and taxation was exorbitant. The nobility lived largely out of town; in inclement weather, they deserted the city completely.

. . . Travel was usually on foot or on horseback. No carriages were allowed in Paris until its streets had been gradually widened. . . . Chairs supported on poles toted by porters carried the frail, the infirm and those adverse to horseback."[119]

Now what about the status of Parisian medicine during the life of Ambroise Paré? The reader will recall that prior to the tenth century medical knowledge was meagre and based mainly on folklore. In the eleventh century, beginning with the School of Salerno in Italy, schools arose under church protection, support and control. By the thirteenth century, Italy was the land of several universities, but in the next century, lost the support of the church, because the Popes had moved to Avignon, France. This created a rapid surge in the development of French universities, particularly Montpellier and the university at Paris. Because of the closer proximity to the Holy See, French school became more affluent and could afford more manuscripts which stimulated progress in medicine and surgery. Thus, Guy de Chauliac became a leader in surgery, stimulated mainly by the "new" ideas now made available by translations of the ancient Greeks, Hippocrates and Galen.

Of further importance is that by the fifteenth century, rag paper making and printing from movable type was invented in the West. This eliminated the possession of important manuscripts to only those wealthy universities who could buy these tomes. Printed copies of these important manuscripts were made in French and Latin translations and widely distributed throughout western Europe.[120]

Hamby[119] believes that the discovery of America by Columbus had an indirect impact upon medicine in the fifteenth century. Prior to this epoch making discovery, all recourse had been to authority, and it followed that the oldest authority was considered necessarily the best. When Christopher Columbus defied the oldest authority and established a new one, others began to question previously established authoritative beliefs. This attitude influenced experience and rationality to challenge precedent and authority.

Despite this sign of rebellion, those in authority still defended their positions and this is best exemplified by the status of medicine in France, in the early sixteenth century when Paré was born. Thus, the medical profession in Paris at this time was under the nominal control of both the Crown and the Parliament, and was divided into three classes. The medical schools were controlled by the physicians who guarded the rights and privileges of the *Faculté de Medicine.* Medical candidates desirous of studying medicine came from the universities and consisted in the main of churchmen who had learned the classics, Latin, Greek, mathematics and church matters. It followed that their medical instruction was in reading the classical writing of Hippocrates, Galen, Avicenna and others. Such students had no contact with patients but had all the questions and answers (when possible) in their Latin texts. Anatomy and surgery were entirely theoretical and direct from the text and many students graduated without ever witnessing a dissection. Of singular interest is that these French students did not study in French, for a real basic French had not as yet been established. Indeed, it was frowned upon to speak in the vernacular for this would avail information to the uneducated. The educated person would not care to write in the vulgar tongue, which had its own dialect in different districts. In addition, the *Faculté* had the legal authority to prevent the publication of medical writings not in Latin, as will be seen by Paré's first significant publication.[118]

The physician who answered university requirements and graduated had a high position in society. He wore the "Long Robe" and conducted himself in an exalted manner. He kept his distance from the patient and often would not even see the patient but would make a diagnosis from an observation of a sample urine (uroscopy) and from reported symptoms, which he would compare with the writings of the ancients. At times, he might even resort to astrology. He never touched the patient and never handled an instrument. If surgery was indicated he called in a barber-surgeon who operated under his supervision. Surgery was despised and avoided and it can readily be understood why this attitude was assumed, in a time when asepsis and anaesthesia had not been developed.

The so-called barber-surgeon, frequently wandered from

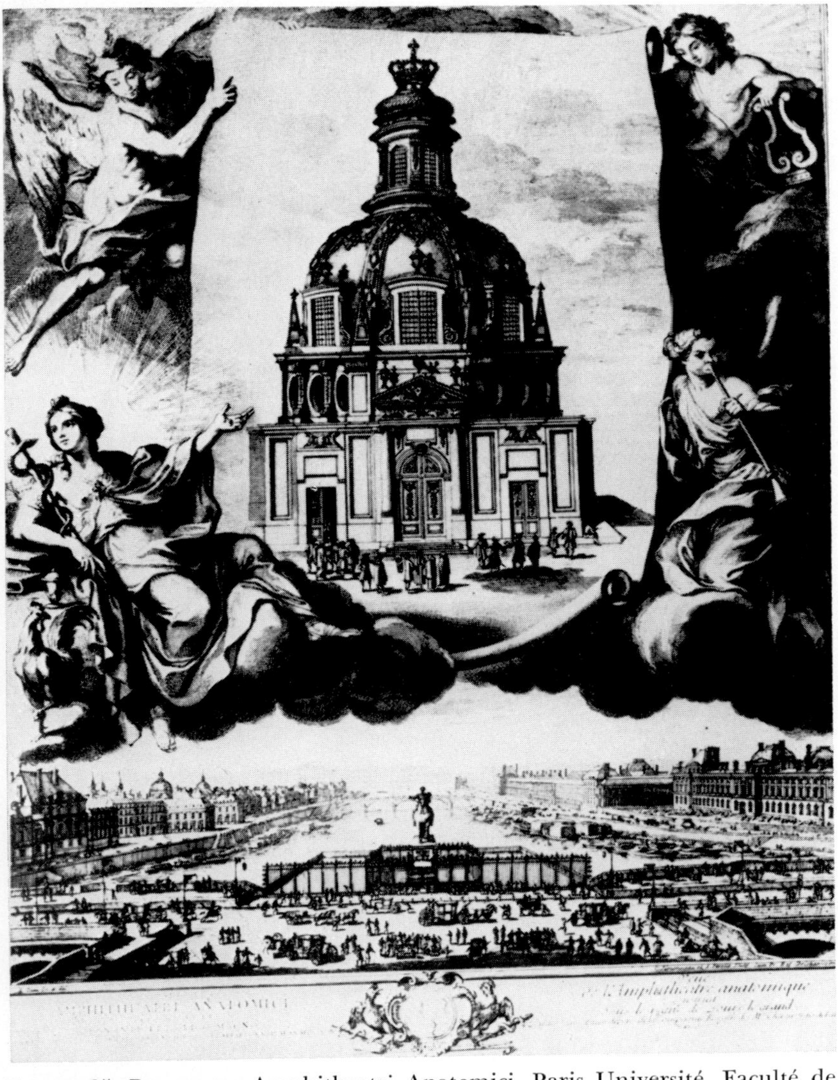

FIGURE 25. Prospectus Amphitheatri Anatomici. Paris Université, Faculté de Médicine, College des Maistres Chirurgiens Jurez de Paris. Etching and engraving—exterior view and vignette of Paris below—1694. Engraved by A. Perelli after C. Simongreau. (Courtesy National Library of Medicine, Bethesda, Maryland.)

town to town, selling his wares, for there were not sufficient people in one community to require such services. They most often frequented fairs where people in greater numbers congregated periodically. Thus, there developed outside the universities a group of primitive surgeons with whom the educated physician, steeped in the writings of Hippocrates, Galen and other ancients, would have no dealings. In time, these barber-surgeons banded together to form guilds to protect their interests. Thus, by 1301, the Corporation of Barber-Surgeons of Paris had become established. When Paré arrived upon the scene, it was a strong organization. Its members were licensed to practice only after serving an apprenticeship and passing two examinations. The guild was led by the King's Premier Barber-Surgeon and they made their vows and annual respects in the church of St. Sepulchre in rue St. Dennis; their patron saints were Sts. Cosmas and Damian (see Fig. 17), martyred medieval surgeons, who were shared with the true surgeons as well. Finally, to earn the title of Master Barber-Surgeon, a candidate had to pass examinations and pay a fee to the *Faculté de Medicine,* do the dissections for the physicians, and renew their vows annually on St. Luke's Day.

Hamby[119] writes, "those who aspired to be licensed as barber-surgeons were not educated people. They served apprenticeships under barber-surgeons, and their lives were hard ones. They slaved in the barber shops, shaving patrons, trimming beards, clipping hair, dressing wigs and assisting their masters in their crude surgery. Their masters were not eager to have these potential competitors learn much or progress rapidly; they were kept at their menial tasks as rigorously as possible. Apprentices with ambition, intelligence and energy to learn and to progress in surgery had few literary resources. Unable to read Latin, they had to depend upon word-of-mouth instruction and whatever French translations of earlier authors were available to them. It is unlikely that many apprentices were able to afford them. . . . In 1491, the surgeons complained to the *Faculté* that some of the instructors were teaching barbers apprentices in French. Three years later the *Faculté* got around to replying; on 11 January 1494 they declared that the instructors henceforth would be ordered to read Guy de Chauliac* and other authors in Latin; would 'give certain explanations in the familiar French tongue as they judged proper' and also would teach the apprentices anatomy . . . to avoid taking apprentices away from their master's shops during business hours which ran from dawn into the night, the professors 'out of the goodness of their hearts' gave the lectures to these tired lads at four o'clock in the morning." Ambroise Paré served most of his apprenticeship in the provinces.

In addition to the university doctor and the barber-surgeons, there existed a third class of surgeons who undoubtedly in many instances originally were university-educated men. Many were simply more ambitious barber-surgeons who took advantage of the courses offered at the university. These men were known as *Chirurgiens-juré,* sworn-surgeons, and were given the title of Master surgeon. From this group emerged the confraternity of Saint-Côme, who subsequently set up their own school of surgery, which they called the College of Surgery of St. Côme, in connection with the church of St. Côme. This college was never admitted to the University rank with the *Faculté de Médicine* and ultimately never accomplished its objectives.

Ambroise Paré came of lowly origin, and, by standards of his day, was not well educated. Yet, his name was the first great name of European eminence in French medicine. He acquired skill and knowledge through the great school of experience.

---

* According to Castiglioni (p. 345 *A Hist. of Med.*), Guy de Chauliac (c. 1300-67) was the most famous surgeon of the Middle Ages; his authority remained for about 200 years. He studied at Montpellier, then at Bologna, where he heard the anatomical lectures of Bertuccio, whose teachings from the cadaver he has described. At the time of the great plague, he was physician to Pope Clement VI and later to his successor at Avignon, where he came in frequent conflict with Petrarch. His best known book was his *Chirugia,* a scholastic work of great importance, which held the same classic position for surgery until the time of Paré that Mondino's treatise held for the field of anatomy. There have been many editions of this work, the first of which was published in French in Paris in 1478 with the title, *Le Pratique en Chirurgie du Maitre quidan de Chauliac.* He distinguished the various kinds of hernia from variocoele, hydrocoele and sarcocoele. He described in detail an operation for the radical cure of hernia. In his book, originally written about 1363, Guy de Chauliac, presents his views on fractures and writes an excellent section of dentistry of that period.

Despite his background, he came to know intimately the great men of his century. This was made possible by his reputation for honesty and sagacity which unfailingly encouraged those who came in contact with him, regardless of whether king, prince, courtier or the common soldier. Thus, during the bloodiest massacre of Huguenot's Paris' history, Paré was sheltered by the King in his private chamber.

In 1536, at Turin, Paré saw an old sergeant cut the throats of three helpless wounded men, "gently and without malice" to put them out of their misery. There is no doubt that witnessing this incident had a great influence on Paré, and from then on history recorded, for the first time, an army surgeon went out of his way to help a wounded soldier. This he did effectively at Perpignan (1543), at Boulogne (1545) and on the march through Germany (1552).

Paré loved his fellow men and enjoyed their company. He was gentle, humble, and always willing to comfort his patients even though he realized the prognosis was poor. As befitting a man with limited cultural background, his writings, all in French, were in simple language, but significant because of portrayal of exact observation and accurate recording.

Ambroise Paré was born at Bourg Hersent, a little village near Laval in the year 1510. This made him a contemporary of Bernard Palissy, the potter; of the theologians Luther, Erasmus, Calvin, and Knox; of the artists Raphael and Titian, and of the medical reformers, Paracelsus and Vesalius.

He worked as an apprentice to a barber-surgeon in the provinces before coming to Paris in 1532 or 1533. This was brief and in Paris he became *compagnon* chirurgien at the Hotel-Dieu, a position comparable to that of today's "house surgeon." The Hotel-Dieu was an ancient monastic foundation which was the only public hospital in Paris at the time.* Here he re-

---

* The Hotel-Dieu was first found by St. Landry, the 28th Bishop of Paris around 660. Around 1227, St. Louis (Louis IX) enlarged its area, and although always receiving Royal support, was constantly overcrowded. Actually, the Hotel-Dieu was a collection of several old buildings on the south side of the island, adjacent to Place Notre-Dame. Indeed, some old engravings show that the Hotel-Dieu actually overlapped the corner of the western facade of the cathedral (Hamby). The building was completely destroyed by fire in the 19th century. Since the site was in-

mained until about 1536, when he commenced his career as a military surgeon.

In the sixteenth century, no provision was made for military doctors. Instead, a medical practitioner was attached to the person of a general or noble leader. Paré, in his first campaign, was surgeon to Mareschal de Montejan, colonel-general of the French infantry. This gave Paré a tremendous opportunity for medical practice and he immediately applied himself to the treatment of gunshot wounds and the performance of dreaded amputations. In the 1536 campaign, he made his first great surgical contribution, namely, that the application of boiling oil not only was of no value, but actually was harmful in the treatment of gunshot wounds. Until then, all authorities on gunshot wounds taught, that in order to counteract the poison, the wound should be treated with boiling oil applied locally.† In the *Apology and Treatise*, in *The First Discourse Wherein Wounds Made by Gunshot Are Freed From Being Burnt or Cauterized According to Vigo's Methods,* Paré describes his observations as follows:

> "Now all the soldiers at the Chateau, seeing our men coming with a great fury, did all they could do to defend themselves, and killed and wounded a great number of our soldiers with pikes, arquesbuses and stones, where the surgeons had much work cut out for them. Now I was at that time a fresh-water soldier, I had not yet seen wounds made by gunshot at the

---

adequate and any new construction would interfere with the view of the cathedral, it was rebuilt on the mainland in its present location. Originally, it was managed by a group of Catholic lay-brothers and sisters. In 1535, a new Parliament order changed the supervision assigning two physicians to make daily visits to the sick and also assigned a number of medical students as assistants. It is quite reasonable to assume that most of these students were young barber-surgeons apprentices. Since Paré had completed his apprenticeship in the provenance, it is not clearly known just how he obtained this appointment.

† Garrison and Morton include in their medical bibliography Paré's treatise on gunshot wounds and state it to be one of Paré's most important works. They describe him as one of the greatest of army surgeons before Larrey, and to be particularly remembered for his abandonment of boiling oil and the cautery, for his revival of podalic version, his re-introduction of the ligature and his invention of many new surgical instruments. He was the first to suggest that syphilis is a cause of aneurysm. He popularized the truss, introduced artificial limbs and reimplantation of teeth.

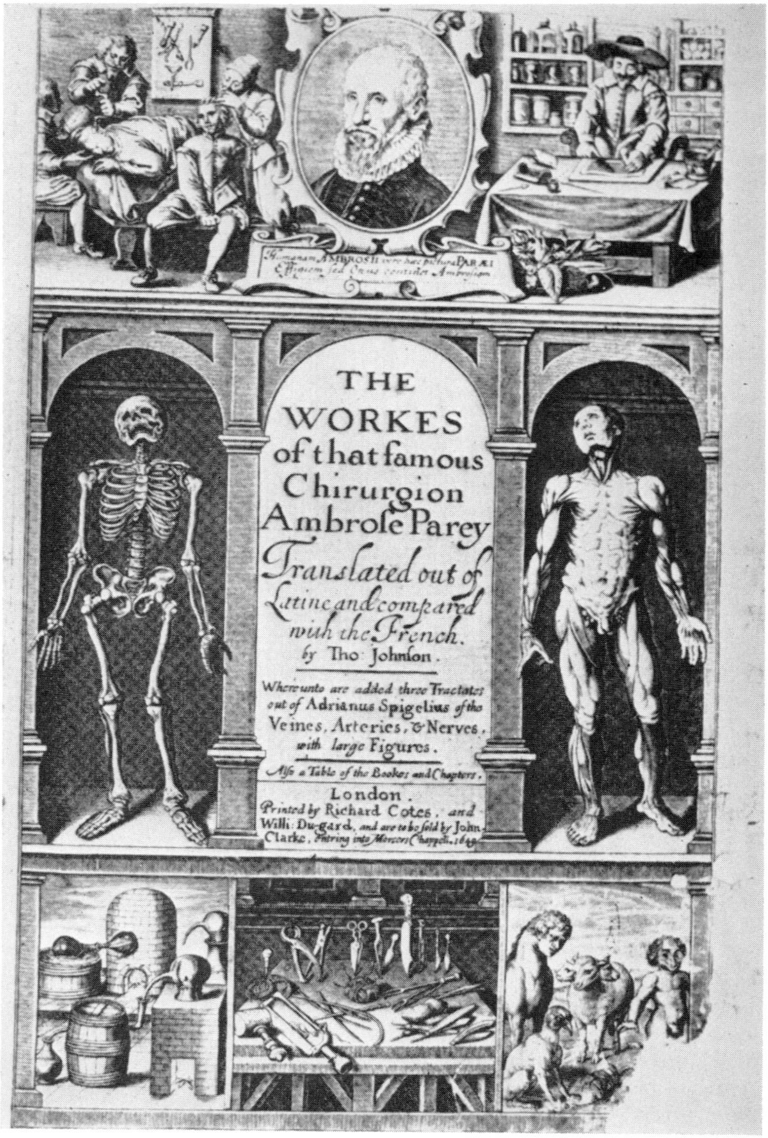

FIGURE 26. Ambroise Paré: (1510-90) The works. . . . Translated by Thomas Johnson. London, 1649. (From the copy in the Wellcome Historical Medical Museum and Library. By courtesy of "The Wellcome Trustees.")

first dressing. It is true that I had read in Jean de Vigo, first book, 'Of wounds in general,' chapter eight, that wounds made by firearms participate of venemosity, because of the powder, and for their cure he commands to cauterize them with oil of elder, scalding hot, in which should be mixed a little theriac; and in order not to err before using the said oil, knowing that such a thing would bring great pain to the patient, I wished to know first, how the other surgeons did for the first dressing, which was to apply the said oil as hot as possible, into the wound with tents and setons, of whom I took courage to do as they did. At last my oil lacked and I was constrained to apply in its place a disgestive made of the yolk of eggs, oil of roses and turpentine. That night I could not sleep at my ease, fearing my lack of cauterization that I should find the wounded on whom I had failed to put the said oil dead or empoisoned, which made me rise very early to visit them, where beyond my hope, I found those upon whom I had put the digestive medicament feeling little pain, and their wounds without inflammation or swelling, having rested fairly throughout the night; the others to whom I had applied the said boiling oil, I found I resolved with myself never more to burn thus cruelly poor men wounded with gunshot."

When de Montejan died, Paré refused to continue in the Army and returned to Paris. Many believed that the young surgeon had now accumulated sufficient money to permit him to study anatomy and take his examinations. In 1541, he passed his examinations for admission to the Community of Barber-Surgeons.

The recognition of Paré's work and skill could not be ignored. Thus that august and pretentious surgical guild, the College de St. Côme, conferred fellowship on him in 1554, regardless of his lack of formal education. Because of his intimacy with high ranking army officers, and his subsequent appointment as surgeon and counselor of successive kings, he was placed in a position so that he could challenge the authority of the Faculty of Medicine, who had unfortunately suppressed surgery for many years.

As would be expected, when Paré's collected works were published in 1575, the Faculty of Medicine attacked Paré because of his use of French instead of Latin. They uncovered an old statute that no medical works could be published without the approval of the Faculty. Thus, to gain for them (Faculty of Medicine) wide acceptance among the learned circles of medicine and surgery, *Paré's Opera* was eventually (1582) translated from French into Latin.

Encouraged by the anatomist, Sylvius* (also the teacher of Vesalius), Paré wrote a classic volume on the treatment of men with wounds made by arquebuses (gunshot wounds). Paré also described his method of locating balls that inflicted the wounds. Thus, when confronted with a difficult case, he would have the victim reassume the position in which he was at the time he received the wound, then with careful search in the direction of entry the ball might be located.

The Apologie and Treatise, Containing the Voyages Made into Divers Places, was Paré's reply to the criticisms of the Faculty of Medicine. It was written when he was 75 years of age and is considered a classic. Paré's courage, ingenuity, intelligence and humanity grows with the record of his adventures and achievements.

Geoffrey Keynes,[118] in his edited issue of Paré's *Apologie and Treatise Containing the Voyages Made into Divers Places* states:

> "The reprinting of this treatise in English is the main object of the present volume, since it contains what amounts to an autobiography covering fifty years of Paré's life from the age of twenty-six to seventy-five. The *Apology and Treatise* was first published in the fourth editions of Paré's collected works. It was written not long before this in answer to an attack by a physician, Etienne Gourmelen, in his book, *Chirurgical artis, ex Hippocrates and Aliorum Veterum Medi-*

---

* Jacques du Bois Sylvius (1478-1555) born at Louvilly, near Ammiens, studied anatomy under Tagault and graduated in medicine at Montpellier. In Paris, he was appointed Professor of the Faculté and became famous as an anatomist. Vesalius studied under him when at Paris, but the two men quarreled violently (see p. 189) since Sylvius was a traditional Galenist and could not accept Vesalius' anatomy. Nevertheless, when Paré visited him and told him about his experience with wounds, Sylvius encouraged him to write even if in the vernacular.

> *corun* Decretis, Libris III, Paris, 1850, in which he tried to prove that Paré's method of treating wounds and his use of ligature to control hemorrhage in amputations were bad practice."
>
> "Even today," continues Keynes, "it is often believed and stated that Paré invented the ligature of large arteries, though he himself made no claim to this. His only claim, as he makes clear in the *Apology,* was that he first applied, in performing amputations, a technique used by many of the ancients in other operations. . . . His main object was to crush his opponent with the weight of his knowledge gained by direct observation and experience, and to point the contrast with Gourmelen's dependence on knowledge derived from books. Paré addresses Gourmelen scornfully throughout as *mon petit maitre,* and has no difficulty in disposing of his arguments, but, although in his seventh decade, Paré is still so full of zest and aggressiveness that he lets his pen run on long after his enemy's defences have been demolished. The result is one of the most entertaining surgical treatises ever written."

Significantly, though Paré did not practice lithotomy himself, he describes the technique. Of further interest are the unusual illustrations accompanying the section "Of Cutting for the Stone" in which he portrays the position of the patient to be cut for stone; probes with slits in their ends; Guiders of two sorts; the effigies of an instrument called a Ducks-bill; the figure of a Dilater shut and opened; crooked Forcipes like a Ducks-bill; winged instruments to hold the stone with the Ducks-beak, "a cleanser or scoop whereby you may search whether there be any more stones behind, as also cleanse or purge the bladder from gravell, clots of blood, and other such bodies, as use to remain behind after the drawing forth of the stone; effigies of a tooth Crowes-bill made neatly to break greater stones, with a screw to force it to-gether."

Paré alternated between military service, in one war after another, with brief periods of private practice in Paris. In 1552, he entered the service of King Henry II as surgeon-in-ordinary, and then served Kings Francois II, Charles IX, and Henry III. Under Charles IX, Paré was promoted to the office of first surgeon to the King, January 1, 1562, and held a similar responsible position while in the service of Henry III.

In 1552, he made his most important contribution to surgery. It was also the most controversial. At the siege of Danvilliers, Paré amputated the leg of an officer but did not apply the traditional hot cautery irons to staunch the bleeding. Instead, he used ligatures to tie off the large blood vessels. This technique had been used by the ancients but had been abandoned and replaced, through Arab influence, by cautery as a means of hemostasis. Actually, the criticism that followed the announcement of this technique provoked Paré to write his *Apology and Treatise* (see above).

Paré died December 20, 1590, at the age of 80 years. During his life time, he had eliminated the fallacious methods of amputations, and treatment of wounds; invented new surgical instruments; trusses for hernia, artificial limbs and artificial eyes. He had published four editions of his collected works, where he inserted his philosophical summary: "I dressed him, and God healed him" *(Je le pensai, Dieu le guarist).*

"Malgaigne,"[122] quoted by Hamby, "said in his Introduction Paré was the first writer of his generation to fertilize the sterile surgical dust of the centuries. After the ancients, only Guy de Cahuliac and Jean de Vigo had preceded him in writing classical surgical treatises. He went far beyond them. When he died, he left animated by his precepts a splendid surgical school faculty including Guillemeau, Portial, Pigray and Severin Pineau; he left the college of St. Côme on a high plane of brilliance and effectiveness. His influence fired the surgeons of Flanders, England and even Germany, where it contended with Paracelsus' doctrines and inspired them to more rapid advancement. Yet, within two generations French surgeons again were under the heavy Hippocratic yoke, and surgery in France was at a low level as it had been when he appeared upon the scene."

Unlike Paracelsus and Vesalius, Paré did not oppose Galen—how could he, a barber-surgeon by training, and with no academic background, attempt to contradict the great master. Nevertheless, a characteristic of Paré, typical of the man's scientific learning, was that when he found disparity between theory and experiment he ignored theory. Paré was an extremely modest and religious man. Like Paracelsus, he believed the foundation of the healing art must be love.

"Je le pensai, Dieu le guarist" is the well known quotation of a brilliant surgeon of long ago but never to be forgotten.

Chapter XIV

Galaxy of the Ancients Continued Giovanni Battista Morgagni (1682-1771)

HISTORY remembers many names and forgets many. Some are remembered because of the lasting contributions they made to medical science. Such a man was Giovanni Battista Morgagni who is frequently referred to as the "Father of Pathologic Anatomy." Most urologists and medical historians are familiar with the name Morgagni. The former know of him because of his many contributions to the anatomy of the genitourinary tract, and the latter know of him because of his significant role in medical history.

It is probable that by now the reader has developed enough interest in Giovanni Battista Morgagni to welcome a brief account of his life and work, and why we include him in our "galaxy of the ancients."

Giainbatista Morgagni (which is the way he usually signed his writings) was born February 25, 1682, in Farli, capital of a small Papal state, southeast of Bologna. From childhood, he showed a natural aptitude for study and at the age of fourteen composed poems and discussed in public ancient philosophical texts. At sixteen, he commenced to study medicine at the university, in the neighboring city of Bologna, but continued at the same time, his work in the field of classic literature. There is no doubt that the humanistic form of his education had a great influence on his clear, concise manner of reasoning, so important in his later medical writings.

For years, he devoted much time in study and writing on archeological subjects. This attracted the attention of Antonio Maria Valsalva, then professor of anatomy at Bologna. It was Valsalva, a fine anatomist who gave to the world the first complete description of the organ of hearing. Valsalva was greatly impressed by the intelligence and enthusiasm of the young medical student, who was nineteen years old when he took his degree. The great Bolognese anatomist deserves much credit for a great deal of his illustrious pupil's fame rests on Valsalva's own accurate notations on morbid anatomy. Indeed, Morgagni himself makes this clear in all his writings, and in his edition of Valsalva's works he indicates the great regard he had for his master. In the *De Sedibus et Causis Morborum per anatomen indagatis libri quinque*—five books concerning the seat and the causes of maladies anatomically studied—Morgagni invariable began with the necropsies of Valsalva, at many of which, as a matter of record, he had himself performed.

The books* printed in Venice, over two hundred years ago (1761) laid the foundations of modern pathology. For the first time, a definite step of progress was made whereby characteristic symptoms and physical signs could now be accurately associated with pathology of individual organs such as the heart, lungs, liver, kidneys, brain and other important structures. Morgagni was then over eighty years of age.

It is revealing to learn some things about this man's mode of life. It was the life a man of science lives, entirely remote from the world of affairs. Sigerist[124] writes: "His hours were filled with conscientious teaching, indefatigable labors in the dissecting room, consultations and an extensive correspondence with his professional colleagues. There did not yet exist an abundance of periodicals eager to publish the most trifling observations, to make the most seemingly inconspicuous ideas widely known. In the eighteenth century, an investigator who believed himself to have discovered something new began its dissemina-

---

* The work was based on 640 post-mortems for Morgagni had diligently searched for the causes of disease. *De Sedibus* went into many editions, was translated into French, German and Italian, while a three-volume English version by Benjamin Alexander was printed in London in 1769.[123]

tion by communicating with his colleagues, subjecting his observations to their criticism. A letter of the kind, swelled to the size of a monograph, was read aloud in a friendly circle, was passed from hand to hand, gave rise to discussion and to control experiments. There was no thought of publication until matters had ripened. The letters exchanged by the scholars of these days are stimulating reading. They give us a lively impression of the workshop of research. People disclose their personality much more freely in letters than in printed publications. If we know the history and geography of learned men of the eighteenth century better than those of their fellows belonging to earlier epochs, this is because of the innumerable letters which have been preserved in MS., and some of them in print.

Prior to the medical Renaissance, the thought that disease processes might originate in localized areas of the body was as yet unknown. As medical men commenced to perform autopsies and began systematic examination of the dead, it soon became apparent that in the beginning disease usually involved one organ or an organ and adjacent tissues, and could remain so for a considerable length of time. Morgagni is the father of this school of thought.

Of course, there were previous contributions to this phase of medicine, in which an effort was made to ascertain the seats and causes of disease. Even Schnenck von Grafenberg's *Observations,* and Bonet's* *Sepulchretum,* had the main purpose of illustrating diseases in terms of anatomic alterations. But, Morgagni's contribution is to be regarded as the culmination of a gradual evolution of pathologic anatomy as well as the beginning of a new concept of pathology as it developed in the nineteenth and twentieth centuries.

---

* Theophile Bonet (1620-1689), a Genovese physician, published in 1697 under the title *Sepulchretum* a comprehensive work comprising all the pathologico-anatomical observations he had been able to gather. Unfortunately, Bonet was not an anatomist, yet he recognized the value of his collection. The sub-title of the book was *Anatome practica* which actually was a compendium of applied anatomy directed towards the practice of medicine. Although he failed in many instances to draw sound conclusions, this was not because he was an ignorant man but because of the available limited knowledge of his day. He differed from Morgagni who had greater skill in knowing what to accept and what to reject from current opinion.

It is quite probable that Galen too, suspected such a modus apparandus when he wrote: "There are very few essential symptoms of disease which do not point to the affected part. Indeed, the alterations of functions indicate only the affected part." In short, it was believed for a long time that anatomic investigations would lead to a better understanding of the causes of disease. As described in our previous sections, such dissections and investigations were hindered by a powerful taboo against contact with the dead body, and only permitted in emergencies when a search was made for a specific cause of death as in plagues with extensive devastation of the population.

In his first book, published in 1706,* one finds an excellent description of the urethral lacunae which today are still named after Morgagni:

> "Several years ago I noticed many peculiar *Foramina,* or small excretory openings, within the upper wall of the male urethra, openings which are distributed in a straight line along the length of the urethra. In most cases they begin to be seen a thumb's breadth from the end of the urinary path and stop seven or eight fingers breadth from it. And as there rarely are more than ten or eleven, so there rarely are found fewer than three or four. . . . Their size is as variable as the distance between them; but most frequently the foremost are also the largest. The largest ones, however, never were so big that I could not cover their orifice with a grain of corn, and seldom have I seen them so small that I could not introduce a bristle. They are of elliptic shape, though sometimes I saw them almost triangular; but their configuration is always extended lengthwise along the urethra. Upon pressure they yield drops of a whitish, thickish, and viscious liquor. . . ."

In his first lecture in Padua, entitled *Nova institutionum medicarum idea,* Morgagni affirmed clearly his program of

---

* Morgagni was promoted to the chair of anatomy in 1715 at Padua, the same chair made famous by Vesalius, Fallopio, Fabricus, Casserius, and Spigelius. He was first called to Padua in 1711, when he taught theoretical medicine. Prior to Morgagni's arrival at Bologna, quiet times had befallen this university city of ancient renown. Foreign students were no longer going south but instead were travelling to Leyden.

teaching, and the methods of study required to train the best students. He requested that the young be instructed first in the principles of mathematics, then in the study of chemistry, botany, and zoology, and finally initiated into the study of anatomy, which is "the indispensable premise for the clinician." . . . "The young man should always propose to himself to reach the highest peaks of science, without resting on the way, and he should strive to surpass his master, even though the greatest, and never believe that the last words in science have been spoken by them or in their books."

Like Vesalius, Morgagni complained often of the scarcity of anatomical material.* In 1719, in a letter to a friend, he tells he was compelled to begin his lectures with great solemnity, but without a cadaver and that sometimes he had to be satisfied with demonstration of the bones of a skeleton. Nevertheless, he would not leave Padua, where he taught for sixty years, never missing a lecture.

Morgagni's great book, on which his fame is essentially founded (on the seats and causes of diseases explored by the anatomist), was published when he was almost eighty years old. Castiglioni describes the book in this manner: "It is the work of a man who in his serene old age collects the sum of his experiences and of his studies, and lays it before a young friend in the form of letters. . . . One must remember the origin of the book in order to explain its form, its style and its success. The author is not a scientist who wanting to sustain his theses or to win a scientific or social position, tries to demonstrate the truth of his discoveries or the importance of his studies, but an expert, an impartial old man, who, having reached the end

---

* There seems to be some difference of opinion in this respect. For example, Sigerist writes, "Morgagni was lucky enough to have extra-ordinarily abundant material at his disposal. Indeed, the supply of bodies from the hospitals were so large that he could not deal with them single-handed. Many of the post-mortems had to be entrusted to his assistants and students, and he had to content himself in such cases with their reports concerning the pathological conditions they found." Sigerist explains this abundant material, that in Italy at that date, there was no prejudice against post-mortem examinations. Persons of all classes, including noblemen of high rank and dignitaries of the Church, were subjected to post-mortem examination by Morgagni. In fact, it is reported that a great many patients gave permission and a wish to have their bodies examined by him after death.

of his active life, desires to confide his intellectual heritage to a young friend, who had asked him insistently and repeatedly to collect and write the prints of his observations and of his experience. . . . In the preface, the author writes that following the advice of his friend, he wanted to correspond with him familiarly, intermixing the different things which they had discussed in their conversations and these remarkable letters followed one another rapidly, addressed, as Morgagni declares, neither to the very erudite nor to the beginners."

All are agreed that Morgagni was the first to lead medicine back to its real source, that is to say to pathology. The followers of the Hippocratic school had superficially touched on this belief but had not gone far enough. Indeed anatomical pathology had not existed as a true science, prior to Morgagni. It now became an exact science with an extraordinary completeness of correlation between clinical detail and post-mortem findings.

To understand the thoroughness of his work, it is well to remember that in his earliest student days, Morgagni made a practice of correlating clinical symptoms with organic change, and this point of view he continued to cultivate all his life. In addition, one must realize that in the days of Morgagni, the standard printed work on the subject was the great *Sepulchretum* written by Theophile Bonet. The more Morgagni read this text and studied it carefully the less pleased he became with it. This undoubtedly was a great influence in his writing of seventy letters, which ultimately spelled out the unintended oblivion for the *Sepulchretum.*

Modern pathology properly begins with Morgagni, but it would be a mistake to consider *The Seats and Causes of Disease* a modern text. It is not a book on pathology in the modern sense at all, but is as such a clinical work, with anatomic explanations of symptoms. The method of organization is the ancient one by parts of the body,* and symptoms referable to

* It is interesting to note, that though Morgagni's essays were published 101 years before discovery of the famous surgical papyrus by Edwin Smith, Morgagni follows the same order as did the ancient document (1550 B.C.) i.e., conditions found in the head were discussed first, then in order, those of the chest, of the abdomen, and of the extremities.

them. Renal symptoms and gastric symptoms in the same patient split a single case report by one hundred pages. A search for tumor pathology leads the inquirer into every section of the book. . . . His inestimable service to the science of pathology was his emphasis on detail and thoroughness. He was never hurried in a description. He introduced nothing new in the way of method and made few out and out discoveries. In no way did he revolutionize pathology as did Bichat and Virchow, but he improved existing knowledge in every field he touched. After Morgagni, pathological anatomy would never again be slipshod or cursory. The new standard was too high.

Castiglioni is kinder toward Morgagni and writes, "it is difficult to realize how many discoveries we owe to Morgagni and for which facts it is necessary to claim priority for him. It is sufficient to point to the pages where he describes the anatomical phenomena which accompany angina pectoris and myocardial degeneration, those brilliant observations on the fibrinous clots which are found in the heart after death and which hitherto had been regarded as pathological conditions. . . . The section of aneurysm* of the aorta remains, as Osler said, one of the best ever written, exhibiting a masterful combination of clinical experience and anatomical observation. . . . The scientists of Europe had such respect for him that he was called, His Anatomic Majesty.† In 1769, the *Natio Germanica* of the artists at the University in which all German students were inscribed, proclaimed him *"Anatomicorum totius Europae princeps,"* the Prince of all European Anatomists.

In his discussion of retention of urine by an enlarged prostate Morgagni writes: ". . . you will observe that they were all from old men: and in like manner, if you examine all my observations

---

* Morgagni's interest in aneurysmal pathology could possibly be because Morgagni's teacher Valsalva, and Valsalva's teacher Malpighi, and Morgagni's friend Ramazzini, all died of stroke.

† To the modern urologist, the name Morgagni is common and of frequent usage. The name is attached to many structures, particularly those encountered in the male genitalia. Thus, the middle lobe of the prostate, especially when enlarged is frequently referred to as Morgagni's caruncle. The urethral fossa navicularis is also known as Morgagni's fossa. Italian anatomists refer to the glands of Littre as Morgagni's glands. The term Morgagni's sinus refers to the prostatic sinus.[125]

in which there was the beginning of a caruncle, you will find that this was found to grow out in the very middle of the internal, and upper circumference of the gland, posteriorly; but whether all these things happened by chance, or otherwise, future observations will show."

Morgagni repeatedly speaks of "Scirrhus" in the prostate, but makes no differentiation between hypertrophy and malignancy. Like any author of the 18th century, he showed great interest in calculi as to various kinds and locations. Equally interesting is his logic about reflux of urine reasoning that with the enlargement of the ureteral orifices, the ureters lost their oblique insertion between the coats of the bladder, so that urine could pass backward when the bladder contracted. In addition, he was familiar with the trabeculated bladder caused by visual neck obstruction, and in one case speaks of resemblance to "the strong bundles of fibres in the heart."

In 1770, when almost ninety years of age, he continued with his course regularly in winter, despite the cold and lack of heating at the University. In 1771, his death was mourned nationally and internationally, and everywhere the greatest honors were paid to his memory. Although he had not created a totally new science, he had definitely emphasized the significant correlation between anatomy, disease and clinical observation.

Chapter XV

Endoscopy and Roentgenology Its Impact on Urology

OUR story would indeed be incomplete without mention of the role of *endoscopy* in the evolution of urology. The word endoscopy comes from the Greek *Evdov* within, plus *Okonelv,* to examine. Literally translated it means an instrument for the examination of the interior of a hollow viscus.

The rise of clinical urology in the modern sense of the term began in the early nineteenth century when Bozzini,[126] in 1806, realized the value of inspecting body cavities with the aid of artificial light. Bozzini soon learned by trial and error, how important it was to have a very bright, steady, non-movable light, which would penetrate easily through the in-and-outgoing conductives.

At first, he used wax candles enclosed in a vase-shaped tube made of tin, covered by cardboard and leather. The round opening through which the light shone was made of brass. Where straight rays could not be used, a mirror was attached to a reflecting conductor. Bozzini used such an appliance in examinations and operations on the uterus and rectum.[127]

In 1860, Voltolini[128] reported his success in applying a new technique in rhinoscopy. He used a mirror attached to an end of a long spatula. Here, the source of light is described as a photogenic lamp in the inside space of which a gasometer discharges oxygen in order to brighten the light as much as possible.

Dosormeaux,[129] to whom has been given the title, "The

Father of Endoscopy" (1867), described an endoscope for the examination of the genito-urinary passage in which he used an indirect method of lighting with a plano-convex lens between the light and the mirror, thus concentrating the rays of the light from the parts of the distal speculum. It was the first apparatus to receive practical recognition and added greatly to the gradual perfection of endoscopy.

Twelve years later, Cruise of Dublin improved the reflecting apparatus, and this kept endoscopy alive. Further studies continued and served as a bridgehead for improvements in endoscopy, far beyond the imagination of early workers in this area.

Until 1867, the source of illumination was wholly without the tube, or speculum. At this time, Julius Bruck,[130] a dentist of Breslau, conceived of the possibility of placing the source of light in the distal end of the instrument. He produced the light by using an exposed electrically heated platinum loop. Strange as it may be, this extraordinary advance did not receive proper recognition for another decade.

In 1862, Haken[131] had devised a glass window at the vesical extremity of a tube allowing visualization of the interior of a water-distended bladder. This principle was adopted in 1874 by Grunfeld, who, by passing a small bougie alongside of the tube, was able to pass it into the ureteral orifice. This is probably the first recorded ureteral catheterization.

Unquestionably, the most outstanding and most vital contribution to urology was made by Max Nitze[132] of Berlin in 1877. Nitze, in cooperation with Beneche, an optician of Vienna, produced what can definitely be called the "first cystoscope" in that it employed the same basic principles of modern cystoscopes, namely: (a) the electric source of illunimation; (b) the placing of the source of light adjacent to the area or field to be examined, and (c) the employment of a lens system.[133]

Max Nitze was born in Berlin, September 18, 1848, and died when he was only 57 years of age, on February 22, 1906. He studied at Heidelberg, Wurzburg, and Leipzig. When Nitze was studying medicine in Heidelberg, Gustav Simon was doing his spectacular kidney operations (see p. 273) and some believe that it may be that Nitze's interest in urology began at that time. Nitze recognized early in his work that the problem of exact diagnosis of bladder and kidney disease before surgery was an urgent one. Nitze's revolutionary idea was to illuminate the bladder from the inside rather than to conduct the needed light from a source outside the bladder. In his own words, he stated "in order to light up a room one must carry a lamp into it."[134]

In 1880, the incandescent lamp of Edison was invented. Mark[135] writes: "While the value of its application to other forms of endoscopy was immediately recognized, it was not until three years later that David Neuman[136] of Glasgow made use of a cystoscope so equipped. Its use was practically limited to the female bladder. The general use of the incandescent lamp in cystoscopy was deferred for four years, i.e., until March, 1887. Working separately, but with the same end in view, Hartwig of Berlin constructed a cystoscope containing such a lamp following the suggestions of Nitze and at the same time a similar instrument was produced by Leiter." Mark[135] emphasizes that this development was characterized by: (1) the discarding of the previous cumbersome cooling device necessary in the exposed platinum loop period; (2) the enlargement of the lens system with a consequent enlargement of the cytoscopic field, and (3) the greater reliability of the illuminating source.

The final decisive step in the development of endoscopy came about by Charles Preston, an electrician of Rochester, New York, who invented the "cold" or low-amperage mignon lamp in 1898. This was first used in the urethroscope presented by Ferdinand Valentine in 1899 and its use in all forms of urologic endoscopic instruments soon followed.

"Urology (American)," states Bandler,[137] "has been most fortunate in having the optical genius of Reinhold Wappler and the mechanical skills of his illustrious son, Fred, at the disposal of all the American urologists, who have given us so many instruments of precision. The scientific knowledge and cooperation of Frederick Wallace has completed an era of invention unexcelled in any other branch of medicine. In fact, the genius displayed by these men in assisting in the manufacture of so many urologic instruments has made possible the application of the principles involved for the production of accurate diagnostic instruments employed in many other special fields of surgery."

But how did this all come about? Reinhold Wappler, a German instrument maker, came to America in 1890 and after working eight years on various types of electrical and optical instruments founded his own firm then known as the Wappler Electric Controller Company. He first produced electro-medical equipment for muscle and tissue stimulation and various types of electrical control equipment. This was first reported in 1898 by Dr. George W. Jacoby.[138]

At this time, American urologists depended entirely on cystoscopes brought over from Germany and Austria. These were extremely delicate instruments and required frequent repairs. Dr. F. C. Valentine, one of the early New York pioneers in urology, was one of the first to seek Mr. Wappler for the repair of his cystoscopic instruments. He was so pleased with the prospect of having available an American source for the repair and maintenance of endoscopic instruments that he soon spread the good news to all his associates. Thus began the establishment of the "American Cystoscope Makers" as a division of Wappler Electric Controller Company.

During the period between 1898 and 1902, a considerable amount of work was done in connection with Dr. William K. Otis[139] in the development of a new optical system. The new system eliminated the difficulties often encountered in the German made instruments due to leakage of water past the right angle prism. In addition, the new optical system contained a hemisphere with a silvered plano side which combined an objective lens and a reflecting prism in one system. This system was patented in 1902 and the cystoscope was described by Dr. Otis in 1905.

During the period 1905-1908, work was undertaken in cooperation with Dr. F. Tilden Brown[140] in the development of a catheterizing and operating cystoscope. Many experimental models were made. The final model was presented by Dr. Brown at the American Association of Genito-Urinary Surgeons, Hot Springs, Virginia, April 2, 1908.

A direct viewing cystoscopic tube without a telescope or optical system was presented by Dr. S. H. Elsner. This system had provision for catheterization. A similar instrument, that is a direct cystoscopic tube without optical system, was described by Dr. Bransford Lewis, in the *Journal of the American Medical Association,* November 8, 1902. Later, Dr. Lewis attempted to apply optical systems to his direct viewing cystoscopic tube.

Of interest is the controversy which developed between F. Tilden Brown and Bradsford Lewis over the priority in the development of the double catheterizing cystoscope. This instant dispute resulted in the publication of several exhibits, papers and circular letters, one of which was entitled, *Some Fact and Fancy in Cystoscopy.*

During the early part of 1908, Dr. Leo Buerger commenced work on the standardization of a double catheterizing cystoscope. One innovation consisted of an optical system which would permit examination of the deep urethra. Some of the features of the Buerger composite instrument were modifications of the original F. Tilden Brown instrument. By mutual agreement, the composite double catheterizing cystoscope became known as the Brown-Buerger Cystoscope. This instrument was thoroughly described in 1909,[141] and the cysto-urethroscope in 1910.[142, 143]

In the latter part of 1909, work was commenced with Dr. Joseph F. McCarthy on the development of an improved composite cystoscope. McCarthy, noting the advantage of the Luys instrument with its extremely small lens system, ultimately after many trials produced his "panendoscope." Subsequently, McCarthy's Resectoscope opened a new era in prostatic surgery and many other instruments for transurethral prostatic resection followed in rapid succession.

During the latter part of 1909, work was undertaken with Dr. Edwin Beer to develop equipment suitable for the removal of neoplasms from the bladder by means of high frequency current through a catheterizing cystoscope. It followed thereafter that many new endoscopic instruments were developed and perfected. Such instruments played an important role in the urologists diagnostic and therapeutic armamentarium, beyond the usage originally planned and certainly far beyond the wildest speculative thoughts of the ancients.

Higgins* writes that "a review of the development of urologic instruments would not be complete without some reference to the origin of the American woven catheters." Few readers will recall that prior to 1930, all woven catheters used in this country were manufactured in Europe, principally in France and Germany. "These were delicate, fragile and easily broken" writes Higgins, "their coating deteriorated rapidly, and they could not be sterilized by autoclaving or boiling: their lumens were small compared to their outside diameter and the drainage properties were frequently inadequate. It was realized that these catheters might not be procurable from Europe in the event of war or other emergency, so a program of research and development was undertaken (by American Cystoscope Makers Inc.) to produce a superior catheter."

This required the manufacture of special machines designed to weave the tubing. An ingenious machine was developed to weave the catheter eyes into the tubular form. Instead of woven silk, nylon was selected because it possesses great tensile strength, and permits the formation of a woven base with a relatively large lumen. To coat the catheter, a synthetic resinous coating was developed which, when applied to the catheter and properly treated, resulted in a catheter which was resistant to aging and could be more easily sterilized. In 1939, just prior to the outbreak of World War II, and after five years of experimental work, the first American catheters were produced. Later, with similar technique, all types of filiforms, bougies, and similar

---

* I cannot leave this historical recording of endoscopy without referring the reader to the brilliant review of Charles C. Higgins, *Urology from 1905 to 1955* and to the prior publication of Hugh H. Young, *Fifty Years of Progress in Urology,* published in 1941. Both articles are exceedingly well documented with an extensive bibliography and well worth reading.

accessories were manufactured in the United States for American use. The importation of such material was never resumed after the war.

* * *

In all of our previous discussions from the very onset of man's interest in urine, it followed that abnormal changes in the appearance of the urine would attract attention. Thus, in 1895, when Conrad Rontgen† discovered the x-ray, another valuable means of diagnosis was brought to the urologist. Prior to this epoch discovery, diagnosis of kidney stone and other abnormalities of the urinary tract depended entirely on the symptoms and examination of the urine. Now fortified with Nitze's cystoscope and Rontgen's ray, rapid strides were to be made in urological procedures and diagnosis.

In 1896, Meadowcroft[147] states that: "A great many experiments have been tried and much thought expended in the direction of obtaining clearly defined radiographs of the heart and other organs, but as these are not sufficiently opaque to the rays, it cannot be said that entire success has yet been achieved in this direction. A cable from abroad announced that a radiograph of the stomach and intestines of a person has been successfully obtained by having the person first drink a quantity of harmless solution of a chemical nature impervious to the x-ray and then making the usual exposure."

A new method of diagnosis was now available. It had to be

---

† William Conrad Rontgen was born March 27, 1845, in Lennep, a small town on the edge of the Ruhr Valley. His early education was irregular and informal but at the age of 23 he received his degree in mechanical engineering from the Polytechnical School in Zurich, and in 1869 obtained a doctorate in philosophy at the University of Zurich. At the age of 43, he was appointed Professor of Physics and Director of the Physical Institute at the University of Wurzburg. In 1895, or at his 50th birthday, Rontgen had become well known and admired by his peers for his accomplishments in research. In describing Rontgen, Brogden writes, "Besides the ray that perpetuates his name, Wilhelm Conrad Rontgen left the scientific world another great legacy; the example of stupendous results obtainable through disciplined, intelligent and observant individual research. An American magazine correspondent reported an interview with Rontgen after his discovery. He asked the great physicist what his thoughts were upon perceiving the first fluorescent glow in the dimly lit laboratory. "I did not think," said Rontgen, "I investigated."[146]

perfected. With increase in the power of the x-ray apparatus and improvement in the construction of the tubes plus increased clinical experience and accumulation of valuable data the "new" diagnostic procedure soon became a valuable part of the urologists armamentarium.

The first recorded attempts to render the urinary tract opaque to the x-ray was made by Tuffier in 1897 in France. He at-

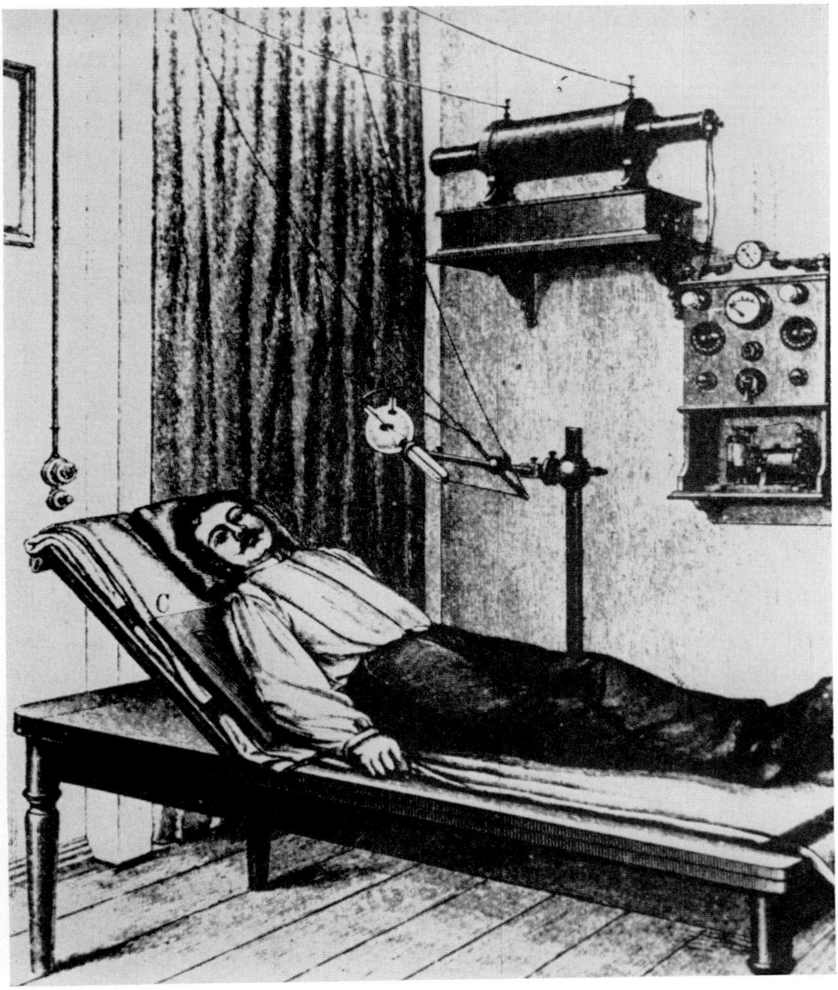

FIGURE 27. Early roentgenography.

tempted to first determine the position of the renal pelvis and to outline the course of the ureter by means of an opaque catheter.

In 1909, Cunningham[148] wrote: "Previous to the employment of the roentgen rays as a means of detecting calculi, the error in diagnosis between stones in the kidney and the ureter was great because of the similarity of the symptoms. The employment of the roentgen ray has been of the greatest value in the diagnosis. This method, however, involves a considerable error, the error being twofold: first, the inability to detect pure uric acid or urate calculi; and the second, the presence of questionable shadows in or near the course of the ureter. These may be due to faulty plate, calcified glands, sclerotic artery, phlebolith, calcified bodies in the muscle fascia, or accentuated calcification in the transverse processes of the vertebrae, pelvic bones, etc."

Actually, the era of pyelography in urology was introduced by Volker and Lichtenberg in 1906.[149] They injected into the renal pelvis 2 per cent solution of collargol, and the solution unexpectedly filled the ureter and renal pelvis. Three years later, Keyes[150] suggested argyrol for this purpose and described definite architectural changes in the calyceal arrangement, significant of disease. In 1910, Braasch[151] described the various alterations in renal pelvis as recorded by pyelography and indicative of hydronephrosis.

Uhle and Pfahler[152] did considerable research looking for a safe, painless and effective contrast media. In 1910, they recommended the use of silver oxide, and later silver iodide as contrast media. The young urologist of today will be interested in the following description of the technique recommended by these researchers: "The injections are given by means of a syringe of 10 cc capacity and injected slowly so as not to cause sudden distention of the kidney pelvis, a condition which will provoke renal colic. To prevent over-distention, or the too rapid distention, we have devised the following technique: The buttocks of the patient are raised and warmed solution allowed to flow by gravity from a graduated burette which is held about two feet above the level of the patient. This method of examination determines the size of the kidney, pelvis, the amount of destruction of the kidney substance, and the position of the kidney in its relationship to other structures. It also determines the position and alterations in the size and shape of the ureter."

Higgins writes, "The development of urologic roentgenology was rapid from 1910 to 1920. In 1913, Braasch described inflammatory changes within the kidney, as shown by pyelography, and from 1910 to 1925, he made 11 reports on the roentgen anatomy, congenital anomalies, and pathology of the urinary tract . . . the decade of 1920 to 1930 saw enormous advances in roentgenologic diagnosis in which the ground work for most of our present practices was laid; the culmination of this period was the advent of intravenous urography. . . . From 1929 onward, this method has occupied an extremely important part in roentgenologic diagnosis of all diseases of the urinary tract. The early investigators of intravenous pyelography recognized its value as a renal function test; they also recognized the limitations of the method in certain pathologic cases, and realized that it could not entirely displace retrograde pyelography and the catheter in the determination of the source of blood and pus, or in the segregation of urine from the two kidneys." With successive years of experimentation, a less toxic contrast media was developed which further enhanced the value of intravenous pyelography more frequently now referred to as excretory pyelography.[153]

A word about the procedure of perirenal insufflation of oxygen in the study of the kidney. This procedure was almost simultaneously but independently introduced by Carelli and Sondella[154] and Rosenstein in 1921.[155] General acceptance of this procedure was delayed mainly because bilateral visualization necessitated separate injections for the two sides, and partly because instances of fatal air emboli were reported. With its value as a means of detecting adrenal tumors clearly demonstrated, an increasing interest in and usage of the procedure occurred. In 1935, Cahill, known for his great interest in pheochromocytoma, made the first report on the use of air insufflation to verify suspected adrenal disease. In 1944, he[156] listed the following contraindications to this procedure: acute infections in the region to be injected, evidence of large renal tumors, with the possibility of marked superficial venous hypertrophy and the possibility of fascual plane malignancies, such as retroperitoneal lymphosarcoma with adhesions and vascularity. To neutralize the fear of air embolism, Cahill volunteered the opinion that if all cases of air embolism be carefully investigated they will show that bleeding was present and that often air was injected in a case in which its use was contraindicated.[157]

Renal arteriography was the next great advance in roentgenologic diagnosis in urology. In 1929, dos Santos Lamas and Caldas[158] first described their technique of injection of the abdominal aorta, to delineate the arterial circulation.

A word about "Fiber Optics" which was not included in Higgins 1955 report since the actual release of this new armamentarium of the urologist did not occur until May, 1960. Fiber Optics has been applied to a revolutionary new system for transmitting images and light around corners or through uneven contours, by utilization of long thin fibers of optical glass. Again, the American Cystoscope Makers, Inc., under the brilliant guidance of Fred Wallace, have added further refinement in diagnostic acumen for the American urologist.

The development and clinical testing of medical diagnostic instruments utilizing fiber optics has been under way for several years. Wallace,[159] in 1963, states: "Fiber Optics is a term applied to a system for transmitting light and images through thin fibers of optical glass by total internal reflection. The development of methods for producing thin, flexible, optical fibers and their application to flexible or rigid optical instruments for image or light transmission represent a major scientific breakthrough in the field of endoscopic instrumentation. . . . The fiber optic sheath consists of 2 metal tubes, with the ends fenestrated and the distal portion formed into a concave or convex beak as required. A layer of optical fibers is placed between the 2 tubes, the distal end formed into a circular rod which exists at a right angle to a connector. Water inlet and outlet and a cone fitting are provided at the proximal end. The cystoscope sheaths have been made in 24, 21, 18, 16, and 12 French sizes. This sheath accepts the standard operating and examining telescopes." Similar techniques have been applied to the urethroscope and resectoscope sheath. The superiority of illumination provided by fiber optics in endoscopic instruments is now generally accepted.

Marshall,[160] in writing on this subject in 1964, states: "Would it not be useful to be able to look down a flexible tube and see clearly out the other end while the tube was being bent in various directions? This ancient dream has become possible during the past 10 years because of the development and great improvement in fiber optic instruments. . . . These fascinating instruments, developed by Mr. Frederick J. Wallace and his associates at American Cystoscope Makers, Inc., represent a major advance in urological and general surgical equipment. The rigid endoscopes and cystoscopes with illumination via fiber optics appear superior to the instruments now in general use."

Radioisotope Renograms and Renal Photoscanning in Urology

The advances made in the roentgenological development of urology have far surpassed the original views of Rontgen and those engaged in x-ray research at the beginning of this century.[161] One of the most recent of such advances is the radioisotope method of determining individual kidney function. This was first developed and almost immediately put into clinical use in 1955 at the University of California Medical Center in Los Angeles.[162]

At first, experiments with Urokon (Urokon-I^{131}) and Diodrast-I^{131} were used. This produced in rabbits and dogs similar characteristic renograms but only Diodrast could be used in human beings. Even Diodrast was not the chemical of choice for it is also excreted in small part by the liver, and because of its rapid passage through renal tissue is not ideal for kidney studies. Since the original experiments, other radioisotopes have been successfully used.

The principle of the radioisotope renogram is radiation projection analysis possible because the material injected is selectively excreted by the kidney, and thus continuous radiodetection over the organ dramatically reveals a characteristic rise and fall of the radioactivity as the material is secreted and excreted by the renal tubules. Both kidneys can be tested individually and simultaneously by using two radiation and recording units. A third unit over the upper chest is used to reveal the blood clearance rate.

Kaufman[161] believes the renogram has great advantage in its ease of performance, lack of hazard, trauma or pain to the patient and the rapidity in which it is performed, plus the immediate availability of results for interpretation. The cost still remains high and is probably the main reason for its lack of universal adoption and present confinement to large medical centers equipped with adequate grants for its further study and evaluation.

Equally of recent vintage, historically speaking, is radioisotope photoscanning of the kidneys with a radioactive tracer. This is a technique for graphically recording a clearly delineated spatial image of the kidneys. According to Pearman,[162] this technique fits into the diagnostic armamentarium of the urologist, for it fills the gap, where other procedures are unable to detect the variant arterial blood supply and other poorly demonstrable kidney disorders. He (Pearman) believes the renal photoscan has proved valuable in localizing renal cysts and tumors, and in delineating horse shoe kidneys, duplex kidneys, polycystic kidneys, ectopic kidneys, and atrophic kidneys. The procedure is also claimed to be of diagnostic value in patients with suspected renovascular hypertension, especially those with segmental ischemic renal lesions. The future role to be played by the urologist trained in the fields of nuclear physics, electronics, and radiopharmacology, is indeed more than speculative in nature.

Great urologic progress has indeed taken place since the days of uroscopy. Many of the advances in urologic diagnosis have been made possible by the radiographic and cystoscopic techniques only recently developed. As a result of these advances, urology has become one of the most accurate of all surgical specialties. No longer are such disorders obscure and dimmed by the mists of antiquity that bewildered our ancestors.

Chapter XVI

Urologic Surgery from Antiquity to the 20th Century

Part I

The External Genitalia

THE surgery of primitive people, though limited in scope, possessed an astonishing degree of technical efficiency. Even today, there are primitive people with amazing knowledge of anatomy and surgical techniques. Thus by analogy, if nothing else, Paleolithic peoples must have been at least as proficient.

The most ancient operation of which we have objective evidence is trephining of the skull. This procedure dates back to the Neolithic period.* Sigerist describes the Neolithic man as a skillful craftsman and one who could readily apply his skill to surgical operations, as evidenced by the findings of skulls with trepanation. Prehistoric trephined skulls have been found in France, in the Western Mediterranean basin, in Spain, Portugal, Algiers, Italy, Great Britain, Switzerland, Germany, Bohemia, Austria, north of France, in Belgium, Denmark, Sweden,

* The transition from the Paleolithic to the Neolithic period, from a food-gathering to a food-producing economy, marks perhaps the greatest step in the history of civilization. It is still controversial whether this development took place slowly and gradually or whether it was initiated or at least accelerated by the invasion of foreign tribes from the East. Suffice it to say that the stone was polished now and tools were articulated, man lived in huts he built, close together forming villages which were frequently protected by a wall. Of surgical interest was the castration of the wild bull into a docile domestic animal (the ox).[106]

and as far as Poland and Russia. Primitive trephining was also practiced in America, particularly in Peru and Mexico. The operation is still used by lay practitioners in the Balkans, among the Cabyls of the Atlas, and a number of primitive tribes of the South Pacific.

It is difficult to believe that such a delicate operation could be performed with crude tools* and with a meagre anatomical and surgical knowledge. Nevertheless experiments performed on cadavers showed that the procedure could be easily performed using only a sharp flint. This was accomplished by either scratching the bone, or by making a circular incision that was gradually deepened, or finally by drilling a series of small holes arranged in a circle and then cutting the bridges between them.

Castiglioni and others believe that trephining among the ancients owes its origin to a demonic or magic concept. Nevertheless, one finds in many ancient manuscripts, particularly that of Constantinus Africanus, great understanding of head and brain injuries. Such manuscripts give the differential diagnosis of injuries of the skull and the indications for trephining. The

---

* The materials most commonly used by the ancients for making surgical instruments were iron, steel, tin, lead, copper and bronze. Gold and silver were used occasionally but it is quite possible that the few gold forceps unearthed may have been boudoir instruments rather than surgical instruments.[163] Many of the instruments (catheters and sounds) found at Pompeii were made of brass. Hippocrates mentions pessaries made of horn and Galen speaks of sounds, dilators and ointment spatula made of wood. The ancients used a crude syringe made of horn. The word "horn" was frequently used as the name for syringe.

During the time of Hippocrates, the smelting of iron and tempering of steel were understood as is shown by the following Hippocratic statement:

> "In like manner iron is derived from stone and earth burnt together. In the first exposure to the fire stones and earth mix together with scoria, but at the second and third burning the scoria separate themselves from the iron, and this phenomena meets the eye, that the iron remains in the fire fallen apart from the scoria, and becomes solid and compact."[164]

Even in remote antiquity, the process of hardening steel was known. For example, approximately five-hundred years before Hippocrates, the Greeks of the Homeric Age must have known something of tempering as is hinted in the Odyssey (the blinding of the one-eyed giant, Polyphemus, by Ulysses:[165]

> "As when the Smith and hatchet or large axe tempering with skill, plunges the hissing blade deep in cold water (whence the strength of steel) so hiss'd his eye around the olive-wood."

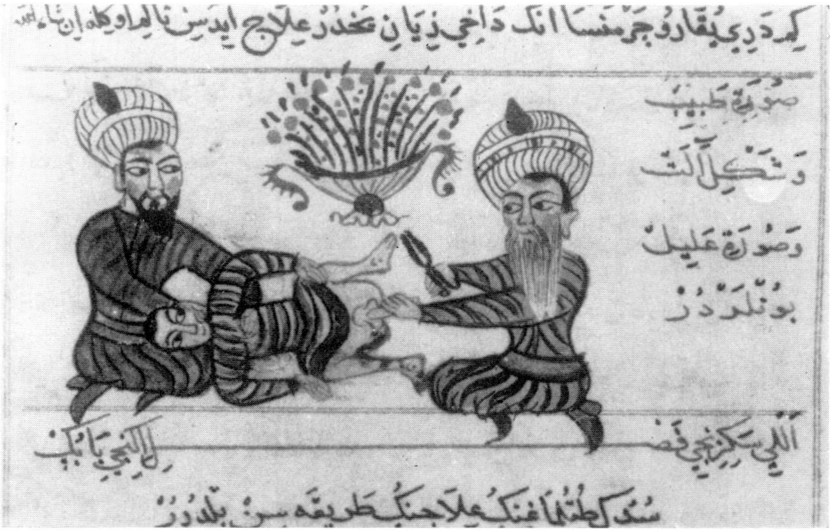

FIGURE 28. Circoncision du garconnet avec des ciseaux. (Photograph courtesy Rare Book Room, New York Academy of Medicine.)

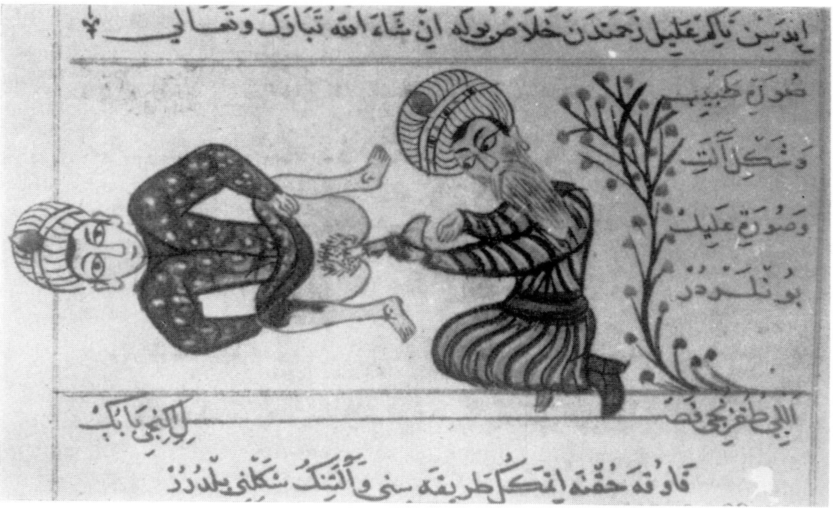

FIGURE 29. Traitment de la retention d'urine. (Photograph courtesy Rare Book Room, New York Academy of Medicine.)

subject of trephining is included in this chapter *not because of any urologic significance, but as an interesting testimony of the awakening of the ancient with regard to surgery and an attempt to protect and restore health.*

According to Brim, the most important operation mentioned in the old testament is that of circumcision. Much has been written upon this subject, yet insufficient information has been derived from its Biblical source which curiously enough, does not describe its modus operandi. The details are supplied by the rabbis of the Talmud . . . "the first divine commandment in the Pentateuch is embodied in the covenant between God and Abraham. 'This is my covenant which you shall keep, between Me and you and your seed after you: Every male child among you shall be circumcised.' "

Circumcision can definitely be traced to antiquity. It was prescribed by the Mosaic religion and was common among all primitive peoples of the orient, Africa and Polynesia. It was originally performed with a sharp stone. Among the Jews, a sharp stone was used even when bronze instruments were available, for the procedure was a sacred one and it was important to preserve the traditional form of the ancient rite.

Circumcision was prevalent in Egypt. Yet, it would appear that only certain males were subjected to this procedure as evidenced by archaeological and literary sources. Many mummies, particularly those of royal blood, have been unearthed without evidence of circumcision. It follows that at no time in Egyptian history was circumcision practiced on all males. During the Roman period, all priests were required to be circumcised. The Romans tried to discourage this practice but failed to suppress it because certain religious acts could only be performed by those who were circumcised. The operation was not performed by physicians but by priests, who avoided the use of a bronze knife and used instead a stone knife. This would seem to indicate that the Egyptians also tried to follow a ritual that undoubtedly was an old one.

* * *

When we come to surgery of the scrotum and its contents, we find little data or source material in ancient medical literature. Rathbun[167] believes that this is due in part to the fact that many of the ancient races, particularly the Egyptians and the Hindus, looked upon the external genitalia as sacred and containing the center of life from which all physical and psychic power emanated. Thus, for generations, it was believed that any mechanical or surgical interference with this part of the human anatomy was both dangerous and sacrilegious. Circumcision as described above was the only exception to this mystical belief.

Complete emasculation was another exception to the avoidance of genital surgery. Thus, among some of the ancients, particularly the Chinese, total emasculation was frequently performed in order to prepare the young male to function as a guard or servant in the harem or court. The operation was crudely performed and many fatalities ensued.* The following is indeed a drastic description of castration as practiced by the ancients:

> "When about to be operated on, the patient is placed in a semi-supine position on a broad bench. One man squatting behind him grasps his waist, and another is told to look after each leg. Bandages are fastened tightly around the hypogastric and the inguinal regions, the penis and the scrotum are three times bathed in a hot decoction of pepper pods, and the patient, if an adult, is solemnly asked, whether he repents or will ever repent his decision. If he appears doubtful he is unbound and dismissed, but if his courage has held out, as it usually does, all the parts are swiftly swept away

---

* Castration was a common procedure in Europe (16th to 18th centuries). It was performed on young boys to preserve their alto voices for the choir; on adults during inguinal herniorrhaphy, and specifically to prevent such diseases as varices, leprosy, gout and psychoses. Ambroise Paré was greatly opposed to this practice, arguing that one should preserve carefully these organs "which keep peace in the home" but he was unable to influence its popularity.

Fabricius d'Agnapendente of Italy writes about Horace Norsia (early 17th century) who claimed to have performed an average of 200 castrations yearly. Louis XIV's physician, Pierre Dionis denied that eunuchs were exempt from gout, leprosy or sudden death. Dionis taught operative surgery at the Jardin du Roi, Paris, a famous school for surgeons. In 1776, the Royal Society of Medicine of France, officially condemned this practice, after discovering that in a single diocese more that 500 young men had been castrated.

by one stroke of a sickle-shaped knife, a pewter-plug is inserted into the urethra, and the wound is covered with paper soaked in cold water and is firmly bandaged. The patient supported by two men, is then walked about the room for two or three hours, after which he is then permitted to lie down. For three days he gets nothing to drink nor is the plug removed from the urethra. At the end of this period the dressings are changed, and the accumulated urine is allowed to escape. The parts generally heal in about one hundred days —about two percent of all cases prove fatal, some by hemorrhage, some by extravasation, and some doubtless by sepsis. . . . For a long time there is incontinence of urine."[168]

* * *

Although hydrocelectomy to the modern urological surgeon presents few problems, to the ancients it presented many taxing and often insurmountable problems. According to Landes and Lemhardt,[169] who have written a most delightful narrative entitled *History of Hydrocoele:* "The origins of the surgical treatment of hydrocoele are lost in the dimness of antiquity. But one need not strain his imagination to see, in the darkness of the jungle, a dejected, slant browed aborigine, with a massive hydrocoele, sadly hindered in his flight from enemies and in his search for food and women. In desperation he cuts through the offending flesh with a sharp flaked stone until, to his surprise and relief, there ensues a sudden gush of fluid—and a new-found freedom."

Rathbun believes that the Romans noted hydrocoele. This is confirmed by an ancient stone image of a man with a large scrotal swelling, evidently a hydrocoele. The Romans also wrote of what might be interpreted as extravasation of urine into the scrotal tissues.

Of particular interest to the urologist is Paré's method of treatment for hydrocoele. His comments are singularly intriguing: "The signs (of hydrocoele) are a tumor increasing slowly without much pain, heavy and almost a glassy clearness, which you may perceive by holding a candle on the other side. . . . The cod (scrotum) and membranes wherein the water is contained must be thrust through with a Seton, that is with a large pointed needle, thread with a skeane of silke . . . the skeane of thread must be left there, or moved twice or thrice a day, that the tumor may drop down and be evacuated by little and little. Some practitioners use not a Seton, but with a Razor . . . they open the lower part of the cod . . . penetrating even to the contained water; . . . and they keep the wound open until the water seems evacuated. . . ."[169]

John Hunter* took a keen interest in diseases of the genito-urinary organs, and made many keen clinical observations. With regard to hydrocoele, Hunter in his *Principles of Surgery* wrote: "No disease affecting the human body and requiring an operation for its cure has called forth the opinions and pens of surgeons so much as this disease. Each finds that every mode of operating except his own has failed."

There were ten major methods utilized. All had the usual modifications and temporary popularity. These methods were: a) incision, b) actual cautery, c) caustic, d) acupuncture, e) packing of tunica, vaginalis, f) seton, g) injection, h) excision, i) eversion of the tunica vaginalis.

William Fergusson,[168] Professor of Surgery in Kings College, London, in his popular text of 1845 recommends that when the hydrocoele reforms several times that the following procedure be accomplished: "The serum being drawn off in a manner already directed, a small syringe, provided with a movable stop-cock nozzle, is applied to the end of the canula, and the tunica vaginalis is again distended nearly to its full extent by a fluid of a different quality from that which has previously been present. A mixture of part wine and water (two-thirds of the former to one of the latter) has been generally used

* John Hunter ranks as one of the greatest surgeons of all times and considered with Ambroise Paré and Joseph Lister, in his contributions to medicine. John Hunter found surgery a highly developed art, and left it a true science. For this reason, he is known as the founder of scientific surgery in England. At a very early age, he studied the descent of the testes in the foetus and wrote *"A description of the situation of the testes in the foetus, with its descent into the scrotum.* His great interest was the study of comparative anatomy in man and in lower animals. He dissected more than five hundred different species of animals, many of them more than once, and left records of three-hundred and fifteen dissections. Thus, he is distinguished as a surgeon, comparative anatomist and as a physiologist.

since it was so strongly recommended by Sir James Earle; but the wine will do by itself, and also the water, although the former would perhaps be too stimulating for the generality of the cases, and the latter too little so . . . whatever fluid is selected, it is allowed to remain in the cavity for the space of four, six or ten minutes, or until the patient feels some pain in the testicle, extending perhaps, up the cord and into the loins, when it is allowed to pass away by withdrawing the stop-cock nozzle; then the canula itself is removed and so the operation is completed." Fergusson then advises that the patient should keep his couch for a few days as considerable inflammation will ensue—a statement no one could deny.

Eversion of the sac was first described by Jaboulay of France, but called Winkelmann's method[172] in Germany. It consists of suturing the bivalved tunica vaginalis behind the epididymis. During and after the First World War, every paper written in English dwelt on Winkelmann's false claim to priority and implied "this was a heinous offense in which the entire German people shared the guilt."

Subsequently, many techniques of injection of sclerising substances ran the gamut of popularity but only for a comparatively short time. In 1907, Willys Andrews[170] recommended the so-called "bottle operation." As of today, excision with hemostatic suture of the margin of the tunica vaginalis or simple eversion around the epididymis, without resort to giving the procedure a proper name, seems to be the recommended method of treatment.

Varicocoele does not appear in the old literature as frequently as does hydrocoele. As mentioned above, Arculanius, professor of medicine at Padua, in the fifteenth century, wrote many manuscripts on diseases of the scrotal contents. He clearly described varicocoele and outlined a ligature operation for its cure. Paul of Aegina is said to have performed the operation of castration and is also said to have recognized hydrocoele and varicocoele and performed operations for these conditions (seventh century).

In 1550, Ambroise Paré defined a varicocoele "as a compact pack of vessels quite filled with melancholic blood." For over 300 years, little additional information was available. In 1918, Ivanisevich first explained the dual venous drainage (deep and superficial) of the scrotum which ultimately led to a better understanding and more complete therapy of this annoying disorder.[167]

Cryptorchidism

"Until the approach of birth, the testes of the foetus are lodged within the cavity of the abdomen, and may therefore be reckoned among the abdominal vescira. They are situated immediately below the kidneys, on the forepart of the psoas muscles, and by the side of the rectum, where this intestine is passing down into the cavity of the pelvis, for in the foetus, the rectum which is much larger in proportion to the capacity of the pelvis than in the full-grown subject, lies before the vertebrae lumborum as well as before the os sacrum. . . . From this original situation within the abdomen the testes afterwards descends to its destined station in the scrotum; but it becomes difficult to ascertain the precise time of this descent, as we hardly ever know the exact age of our subject (prior to modern embryological studies). According to the observations which I have made, it seems to happen sooner in some instances than in others; but generally about the eighth month. . . .

"When one or both testicles remain through life in the belly, I believe that they are exceedingly imperfect, and probably incapable of performing their natural functions, and that this imperfection prevents the disposition for descent from taking place. That they are more defective than ever these which are late in passing to the scrotum, is to be inferred from what is very evident in quadrupeds, the testicle that has reached the scrotum being in them considerably larger than the one which remains in the abdomen. . . .

"The testicle, in changing its situation, does not always preserve a proper course towards the scrotum there being instances of its taking another direction and descending into the perinaeum. How this is brought about is difficult to say; it may possibly be occasioned by something unusual in the construction of the scrotum. . . ."

Thus wrote John Hunter in the middle of the eighteenth century. Little has been added to this clinical story other than a better understanding of genes, hormones, embryology and perhaps surgical anatomy, but more particularly microscopic anatomy (electron-microscopy).

Cryptorchidism is a phase of urological surgery that cannot be attributed to antiquity but it is one form of modern surgery that has been subjected to many changes since Bevan,[175] in 1898, described his operation for undescended testicle. The late Harvey Cushing said: "No idea is wholly new; what is new is getting people to adopt it and act upon it." This is strikingly true when applied to the numerous technical plans recommended for orchiopexy.[176] All are essentially based upon bringing a healthy testicle into its true environment, the scrotum, and keeping it there.

Hermaphroditism

According to legend, Aphrodite, as a result of a celestial union with Hermes, had an extraordinary child, in that the offspring was endowed with the attributes of both father and mother. Because of this confusion they decided to name the child with both their names, and thus the child has been recorded in history as Hermaphroditus.

Ovid (43 B.C. to 17 A.D.), the master story teller of the Romans, found the tale of Hermaphroditus an attractive subject for his "Metamorpheses." The following mythical story is found in Book IV of the compendium:[177]

> "Listen, and I will tell you how the fountain Salmacis acquired its ill repute and why its enervating waters weaken and soften the limbs they touch. This property of the fountain is well known, but the reason for it has remained obscure.
>
> "Once a son was born to Mercury and the Goddess Venus, and he was brought up by the naiads in Ida's Caves. In his features, it was easy to trace a resemblance to his father and to his mother. He was called after them, too, for his name was Hermaphroditus. As soon as he was fifteen he left his native hills, and Ida where he had been brought up, and for the sheer joy of travelling visited remote places, and saw

strange rivers. His enthusiasm made him count the hardships as nothing. He even went as far as the cities of Lycia, and on to the Carians, who dwell nearby. In this region he spied a pool of water, so clear that he could see right to the bottom. There were no marshy reeds around it, no barren edges or sharp-spiked rushes. . . . A nymph dwelt there: not one skilled in hunting or practiced in the art of drawing her bow; nor yet a swift runner. She was the only naiad unknown to the fleet-footed Diana . . . often she would gather flowers, and it so happened that she was engaged in this pastime when she caught sight of the boy, Hermaphroditus. As soon as she had seen him, she longed to possess him. But, eager as she was to approach him, she did not do so until she had composed herself, taking pains with her attire, assuming a charming expression, and seen to it that she was at her loveliest. Then she addressed him: 'Fair boy, you surely deserve to be thought a god. If you are perhaps you may be Cupid? Or if you are mortal, blessed are your parents, happy your brother, most fortunate your sister, if you have a sister, and happy too the nurse who reared you. But far and away more blessed than any of these is the maiden, if such there be, who is engaged to you, whom you will deign to make your wife. If there is such a girl, let me enjoy your love in secret, but if there is not, then I pray that I may be your bride, and that we may enter upon marriage together.' The naiad said no more; but a blush stained the boy's cheeks, for he did not know what love was. Even blushing became him: his cheeks were the colour of ripe apples, hanging in a sunny orchard, like painted ivory, or like the moon, when in eclipse, she shows a reddish hue beneath her brightness, and bronze instruments clash vainly in attempts to aid her. Incessantly the nymph demanded at least sisterly kisses and tried to put her arms around his ivory neck. 'Will you stop,' he cried, 'or I shall run away and leave this place and you?' Salamacis was afraid, 'I yield the spot to you stranger, I shall not intrude,' she said, and turning from him, pretended to go away. Even then she kept glancing back till, slipping into the thick clump of bushes, she hid there, kneeling on the ground. The boy, meanwhile, thinking himself unobserved and alone, strolled this way and that on the grassy sword, and dipped his toes in the lapping water—then his feet up to the ankles, then, tempted by the enticing coolness of the water, he quickly stripped his young body of its soft garments. At the sight, Salmacis was spellbound. She was on fire with passion to possess his naked beauty, and her very eyes flamed with a brillance like that of the dazzling sun, when his bright disc is reflected in a mirror. She could scarcely bear to wait, or to defer the joys which she anticipated. She longed to embrace him then, and with difficulty restrained her frenzy. Hermaphroditus, clapping his hollow palms against his body, dived quickly into the stream. As he raised first one arm then the other, his body gleamed in the clear water, as if someone had encased an ivory statue of white lilies in transparent glass. 'I have him, he is mine!' cried the nymph, and flinging aside her garments, plunged into the heart of the pool. The boy fought against her, but she held him, and snatched kisses as he struggled, placing her hands beneath him, stroking his unwilling breast, and clinging to him now on this side, and now on that.

"Finally, in spite of all his efforts to slip from her grasp, she twined around him, like a serpent when it is being carried off into the air by the king of birds, for as it hangs from the eagle's beak, the snake coils around his head and talons and with its tail hampers his beating wings. She was like the ivy encircling tall tree trunks, or the squid which holds fast the prey it has caught in the depths of the sea, by wrapping its tentacles around on every side. Atlas' descendent resisted stubbornly, and refused the nymph the pleasure she hoped for; but she persisted, clinging to him, her whole body pressed against his. 'You may fight, you rogue, but you will not escape. May the gods grant me this, may no time to come ever separate him from me, or me from him!' Her prayers found favor with the gods, for, as they lay together, their bodies were united and from being two persons they became one.

". . . When he saw that the clear water into which he had descended as a man had made him but half a man, and that his limbs had become enfeebled by its touch, Hermaphroditus stretched out his hands and prayed—even his voice was no longer masculine—'O my father and my mother, grant this prayer to your son, who owes his name to you both: if any man enter this pool, may he depart hence no more than half

> a man, may he suddenly grow weak and effeminate at the touch of these waters!' Both his parents were moved with compassion and granted this request of their child, who was now but half male, and half female. They infected the pool with this horrible magic."

Hermaphroditism was encountered long before the age of Greek mythology. Indeed in the first chapter of Genesis, some of the great Hebrew writers, give authority for believing that Adam himself was the first hermaphrodite.

It would indeed be premature to assume that all the problems of intersexuality have been solved, but it can surely be said that within the past quarter of a century great strides have been made. This has been made possible by experimental embryology which has contributed a great deal of information. Cytology had also made possible the ability to establish sex by chromosomal arrangement (in true hermaphroditism this is at times confusing). The combined disciplines of endocrinology, psychiatry, gynecologic and urologic surgery has enabled the modern physician to treat this problem formerly obscured in the mists of antiquity, mythology and ignorance.

Chapter XVI

Urologic Surgery from Antiquity to the 20th Century

Part II

The Stone Cutters

Cutting for Stone

SPACE does not permit complete narration of those who "cut for stone." The role played by these pioneers of lithotomy is indeed important and one that had great influence on urological surgical progress. Chronologically, we will first review the history of lithotomy bearing in mind that such priority permits a better understanding of subsequent surgical techniques perfected for bladder and prostatic pathology.

The operation for stone was performed by the ancients and certainly prior to the days of Hippocrates. All historians are in agreement that the first description of lithotomy was written by Celsus, and accurately described by him in the seventh volume of his *De Medicina*. The approach was perineal and was employed for about fourteen hundred years, only being modified by deviations in the site of the incision.[178]

Paul of Aegina, who lived in the Byzantine period, described a procedure similar to Celsus' technique. Significantly, he advised that the patient be shaken or made to jump from a height to encourage migration of the stone to the neck of the bladder. Well does the the author recall, that as a medical student, his Professor of Urology recommended a ride on top of a Fifth

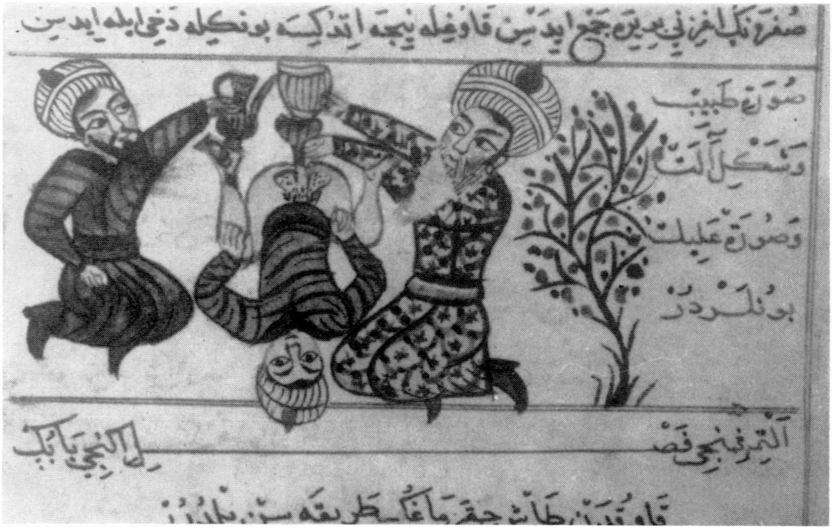

FIGURE 30. Bladder lavage as practiced by the ancients. (Photograph courtesy Rare Book Room, New York Academy of Medicine.)

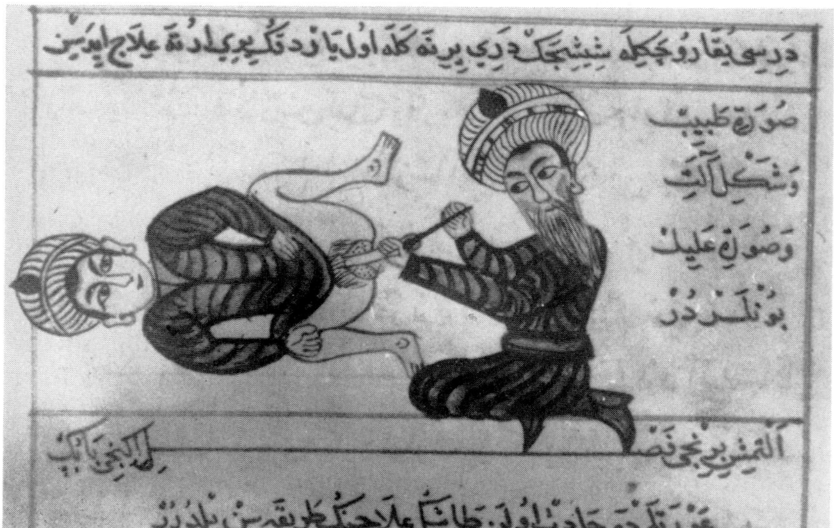

FIGURE 31. Removal of vesical calculus by means of lithotrite. (Photograph courtesy Rare Book Room, New York Academy of Medicine.)

Avenue double decker bus, noted for its lack of springs, to encourage migration of small ureteral stones. Alas, New Yorkers no longer can rely on this form of therapy since these buses are no longer available.

Little change in the technique of perineal lithotomy first described by Celsus occurred until sometime during the Renaissance. Around 1531, Marianus Sanctus recommended the utilization of certain instruments and the procedure subsequently was referred to as the "Marian Operation."* In this change of technique, a grooved staff was introduced into the bladder, upon which the urethra was opened in its membranous portion by carrying the incision down to the groove of the staff. This was followed by gorgets and dilators passed along the groove of the staff into the bladder stretching the prostatic urethra and vesical neck which would then allow forceps into the bladder for ultimate extraction of the calculus.

Barney[178] writes, "Although this operation was destructive, it was a great improvement over the old method of Celsus, and was done in accordance with the aphorism of Hippocrates, that to cut the bladder was fatal; hence not daring to cut it they tore it. The post-operative complications of this method in the way of extravasation of urine, abscesses and incontinence may easily be imagined."

The first suprapubic approach for removal of vesical calculus was performed by Franco† in 1556. However, as vividly portrayed by Cumston,[179] Franco performed this operation in despair. In his *Traité des Hernies,* Franco writes:

---

* The Marian Operation was often called "the method of the great apparatus" so-called because of the great number of instruments required. It continued to be the chosen method operation for quite some time.

† Pierre Franco (1500-1561) was a religious refugee from France to Switzerland, where he became a salaried surgeon of the Republic of Berne, assigned to practice in Lausanne. In 1556, he published his first book, *Petit Traité.*[180] He followed this with a more learned text, *Traité des Hernies.*[181]

Because of the publication of these two books, Bush and Bush[182] believed Franco's importance must be assessed and that he be given a more significant role in medical history. These authors also believe that Franco did considerable surgery and had a long and extensive experience, as well as having a solid foundation of human anatomy.

> "It once happened to me that I desired to remove a stone from a child of about ten years of age, but all my efforts to bring it down were vain. Seeing this, and as the patient was extremely insistent, and the parents still more so, desiring that the child should die rather than live in such agony, I did not wish to be reproached for not having removed it, so much so that foolish as I was I decided to open the bladder on the penile a little to the left. This I accomplished by cutting on the stone, by raising it up with my fingers introduced into the rectum, having it held in place by the hands of an assistant who compressed the little belly, and by this means I withdrew it. The said stone was the size of an egg. And, nevertheless, the wound closed and was cured. However, I do not advise resorting to this means, rather employing the method that we have invented and which we have spoken of previously."

The technique referred to by Franco and which he invented was a two stage perineal section; viz., incision on a sound introduced into the urethra, and then several days later, when the patient is found in good condition, and without fever, the stone is withdrawn. Because of Franco's enthusiasm for the perineal approach, little change occurred in the surgical technique during the sixteenth and seventeenth centuries.

Nevertheless, as so well documented by Cumston,[179] Rousset of France, in the late sixteenth century, advocated the suprapubic route for vesical calculus. He believed this route to be far superior and more practical than the perineal route. Undoubtedly, he came to this conclusion because of his extensive experience with the Caesarean operation, of which he was a master. "Rousset was one of the most ardent partisans of the Caesarean operation, and perceiving that the latter was easy to perform, he was of the opinion that the bladder could be reached by the abdominal route without danger. From his comparison between an incised uterus and section of the bladder in cases of calculus, he in the first place refers to the objectionable points of the perineal incision: 'In the ordinary incision of the bladder by the perineum one only proceeds by groping either in the cutting or in finding the calculus, one or several, and still more when withdrawing them; in such a way that often the most dexterous operators know well that they have often been constrained to leave their work imperfectly performed or to grab, tear away and bring along with their instruments a good portion of the bladder with the calculus. . . . Why, then, should one submit to this danger of incision without need?' "[179]

Our scene now moves to England where, in 1718, James Douglas presented a paper in which he demonstrated the advantages of the suprapubic operation. The operation was actually performed by John Douglas, brother of James. Unfortunately, the lithotomists of England rejected the procedure but Cheselden, surgeon to St. Thomas Hospital, took up the idea and others followed so that soon Douglas' teachings were spread not only in England but on to the continent.

Dahl,[183] in writing of Cheselden,* vividly portrays the setting of lithotomy in the late seventeenth and early eighteenth centuries. "Seventeenth century accounts of lithotomy evoke shudders from the modern urologist. One imagines a trembling patient, bound wrist to ankle, held down upon a much-stained table while the surgeon cuts into the perineum, tears apart muscle and fascia, and finally gouges the stone from the depths of the wound."

Although Cheselden is best known for his accomplishments in the field of surgery, he did write two important books on anatomy. His text, *The Anatomy of the Humane Body* published in 1713 was for many years a textbook of the English medical schools, and ran through thirteen editions. In 1733, he wrote, *Osteographia, or the Anatomy of the Bones*. It contained full and accurate descriptions of all the human bones as well as many of animals. The illustrations are beautifully executed by Van der Gucht, and the whole is a work of permanent value.

In 1723, Cheselden first wrote about vesical calculus, "A treatise on the high operation for stone." In this paper, he describes his method of performing suprapubic lithotomy, a

---

* Contemporary opinion of William Cheselden is reflected in Poe's couplet:

I'll do what Mead and
Cheselden advise
To keep these limbs,
and to preserve these eyes.

method which he abandoned in 1727 for the lateral operation (see below). In 1720, John Douglas wrote, *Lithotomia Douglissiana, or; an account of a new method of making the high operation, in order to extract the stone out of the bladder.* Douglas accused Cheselden of plagiarizing his work even though Cheselden acknowledged his indebtedness to Douglas. Some believe this disagreement prompted Cheselden to abandon the high route for the lateral route.

Cheselden's description of his method of cutting the lateral way is as follows:

> I tie the patient as for the greater apparatus but lay him upon a blanket several doubles upon an horizontal table three foot high, with his head only raised: I first make as long an incision as I can, beginning near the place where the old operation ends, and cutting down between the musculus accelerator urinac, and eractor penis, and by the side of the intestinum rectum. I then feel for the staff holding down the gut all the while with one or two fingers of my left hand, and cut upon it in that part of the urethra which lies beyond the corpora cavernosa urethrae, and in the prostate gland, cutting from below upwards to avoid wounding the gut; and then passing the gorget very carefully in the groove of the staff into the bladder . . . I first feel for the stone with the end of them (forceps) which having felt, I open the forceps and slide one blade underneath it, and the other at top; and if I apprehend the stone is not in the right place of the forceps, I shift it before I offer to extract it, and then extract it very deliberately, that it may not slip suddenly out of the forceps . . . lastly, I tie the blood-vessels by the help of a crooked needle, and use no other dressing than a little bit of lint besmeared with blood, that it may not stick too long in the wound, and all the dressings during the cure are very slight, almost superficial, and with any bandage to retain them; because that will be wetted with urine, and gall the skin.

Cheselden thus brought back to the fold, a new and better technique for perineal lithotomy. It appealed to many lithotomists who were fearful of the peritoneum and equally fearful of violating tradition. Dahl[183] speculates ". . . that Cheselden's success was due in part to the destruction of obstructing lesions resulting from the division of the bladder neck and prostatic urethra." Regardless, his degree of success at a time of limited medical knowledge is incredible.

All are agreed that surgery progressed farther in the nineteenth century than in the two thousand years preceding it. Urology as a surgical specialty emerged and developed. Much of this acceleration could be attributed to the introduction of anaesthesia, to antiseptic and later aseptic methods, and development of endoscopic instruments and x-ray. As far as vesical lithiasis is concerned, the opening of the nineteenth century is definitely epoch-making.[185] Thus, many began to see the advantages of suprapubic cystotomy over perineal lithotomy and with the dawn of the nineteenth century still another method (lithotrity) for the removal of vesical calculus became available.

The instrument used, which was primarily for drilling holes in the stone, and which evolved into our present lithotrite, had several names at first: Lithoprine (Le Roy), Lithontripteur (Civiale) Pierce-Pierre (Heurteloup).[186a] By the middle of the nineteenth century, almost two thousand years had elapsed before serious attention was given to breaking up vesical calculi within the bladder. The open operation had progressed and improved greatly but the surgeon was still confronted with the serious post-operative complications of impotence, incontinence and persistent draining sinuses. Convalescence was prolonged and the general attitude was to postpone the operation until the pain became unbearable and became more disabling than the operation itself and its complications. It follows that intravesical destruction of bladder stones (lithotrity) would meet with great appeal and this it did.*

---

* According to Shelley,[186] the idea of intravesical destruction of bladder calculi was not entirely new. He quotes Albucasis (936-1013) as suggesting such a possibility and mentions such an instrument but gave no adequate description of it.[187] It is known that the Egyptians had dilated the urethra to facilitate the passage of small urethral and bladder stones. Several accounts of vague techniques and grotesque instruments for removal of vesical calculus are to be found in the literature. But the true pioneer is Jean Civiale of Paris, who placed the procedure on a sound basis.

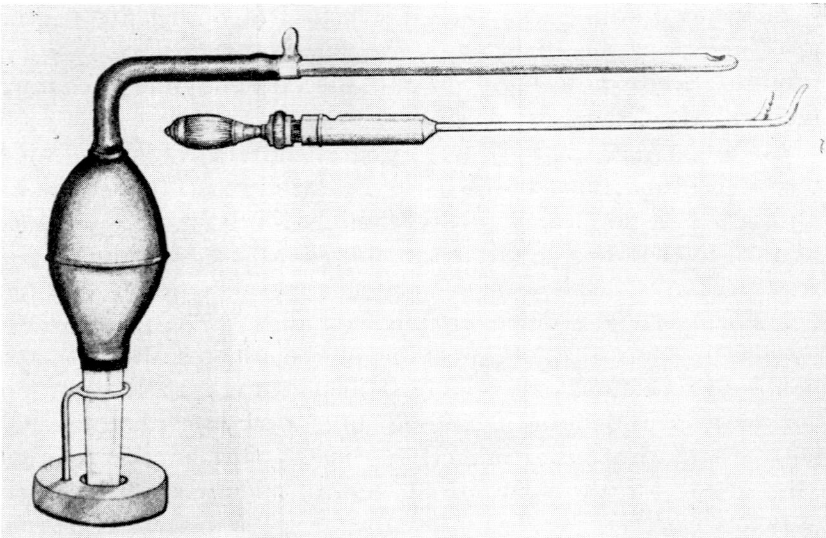

FIGURE 32. Henry J. Bigelow's lithotrite. After grasping the stone the screw could be engaged by a slight twist and the crushing forceps applied. The glass trap below the evacuator bulb prevented fragments from being washed into the bladder. The operation lasted about 2 hours. Circa 1870.

Jean Civiale* first devised an instrument in 1824, which he called a litholabe. He had bitter opposition by Larrey, Sanson, Velpeau and others, but in 1829 he succeeded in having a special service in Hôpital Necker, limited to him for calculus cases. When Civiale died, he left to the French Academy a complete assortment of all his types of lithotrites and a collection of calculi which came from 2200 patients he had treated

* The operations introduced by Jean Civiale soon displaced the time-honored cutting for stone. Lithotrity, or lithotripsy, is an ancient procedure, attempted by the Byzantines and the Arabs, and revived sporadically many times. Its perfection required the forging of a precise and well-tempered instrument that could be passed through the urethra into the urinary bladder, there to seize and crush a stone into tiny fragments. In the hands of a skilled operator, this procedure was safer and less subject to complications than cutting for stone (lithotomy). The great drawback was evacuating the bladder of the bits of stone, for one fragment left behind became the nidus (nucleus) for the formation of a new stone. Dr. Henry Bigelow of Boston devised an apparatus for washing out crushed stones. He christened the procedure litholapaxy.

between 1824 and 1864, of whom 1600 were operated upon by lithotrity.

In America, the procedure was further developed by Henry J. Bigelow of Boston, who in the 1870's introduced his operation of litholapaxy, a name which some believe was coined by Oliver Wendell Holmes. Bigelow advised that after crushing the stone the fragments be immediately evacuated through a separate large calibre, using a rubber bulb and equipped with a glass trap or reservoir under the bulb to catch fragments and keep them from washing back into the bladder. Bigelow was a conscientious, slow and deliberate operator and greatly aided by the use of anaesthesia was quite successful in his attempts to remove vesical calculi. Hugh H. Young, using Bigelow's lithotrite as a model, in 1908 first introduced a lithotrite in which the stone could be viewed as it was grasped—the first lithotriptoscope to be followed by many more accurate and easily manipulated instruments.

Shelley[186] concludes his interesting review of intravesical destruction of bladder stones as: Thus developed litholapaxy. Dreamed of as litholysis, born and fought over as lithotresis, it grew into lithotrity and, wedded to lithocenosis, blossomed into litholapaxy.

Chapter XVI

Urologic Surgery from Antiquity to the 20th Century

Part III

Surgery of the Prostate and Further Advances in Bladder Surgery

OBSTRUCTIVE uropathy due to enlargement of the prostate undoubtedly existed among a large percentage of elderly men since time immemorial, or at least since the time men lived long enough to reach the so-called prostatic age.

In acute urinary retention, the ancients spoke of such victims as suffering from *excrescances* or carnosities at the neck of the bladder. Although they must have known of prostatic obstruction, we have no records of same. The finding of metal sounds and catheters in the ruins of Pompeii does not mean they were used specifically in obstructive uropathy due to prostatic enlargement. It is more likely they were used to overcome stricture formation. The Romans as well as others at this time rarely lived to the age of prostatism, and those who did were few in number.

Faulty and erroneous knowledge of the prostate can be traced to inadequate anatomical knowledge of the human body. Unfortunately, the ancients relied upon animal dissection for their anatomical information. Galen based his anatomical knowledge chiefly on the dissection of apes and the Rhesus monkey.

Reference has previously been made to Herophilus who is credited with being the first to mention the prostate. His description of the prostate is more suggestive of the seminal vesicles. In lower domestic animals and in the monkey, the prostate is a bifid organ and resembles the seminal vesicle of the human. Indeed, even Vesalius' description of a bifid prostate is highly suggestive of it being that of a dog rather than of a human male adult.

Morgagni referred to the middle lobe of the prostate as *caruncle*. For many years thereafter, the prostate was referred to as Morgagni's caruncle. In his discussion of retention of urine by an enlarged prostate, Morgagni writes: ". . . you will observe that they were all from old men: and in like manner, if you examine all my observations in which there was the beginning of a caruncle, you will find that this was found to grow out in the very middle of the internal and upper circumference of the gland, posteriorly; but whether all these things happened by chance, or otherwise, future observations will show."

Almost two hundred years earlier, Leonardo da Vinci (Chapter X) fails to make any drawings of the prostate, despite his many sketches of the remainder of the genito-urinary system. This is probably explained by the fact that most of Leonardo's anatomic drawings were made from the study of the bodies of oxen. Since these animals are castrates, they have small atrophic prostates, which could easily be overlooked or mistaken for the seminal vesicles (see sketch—Vesalius). Human cadavers for dissection were hard to obtain and like Galen, Leonardo frequently transposed knowledge from his animal dissections directly into his sketches aimed to present the anatomy of man.

The clinical picture of benign prostatic hypertrophy has been known since the days of Morgagni and even earlier. The problem of an enlarged prostate with obstructive uropathy was little understood and challenged surgeons for many years. Its final triumph had to await the advent of endoscopy, anesthesia, antiseptics and a thorough understanding of the electrolytic balance of the body. Urologists of the present generation no longer fear this procedure (prostatectomy), and are now trained not in one procedure, but to four methods of removal, all well established and accepted.[189]

Very little progress was made in the treatment of prostatic obstruction from the middle of the sixteenth century, when the gland was first described, until sometime after the middle of the eighteenth century when surgical procedures were instituted for lithotomy of vesical calculus (see preceding section). When obstruction to the vesical neck did occur, the route of primitive attempts to overcome same was by way of the perineum. This route was probably chosen since perineal lithotomy was one of the first widely practiced procedures in the early days of surgery. Definitive approach was not made until the beginning of the twentieth century. Of historical interest are the various procedures recommended for the relief of prostatic obstruction without removal of the gland. For example, Bier in 1893 ligated the internal iliac arteries to diminish the blood supply to the enlarged prostate and thereby hoping to cause it to shrink. Loze, in 1898, recommended removal of the venous plexuses around the bladder. Both methods failed.

John Hunter, realizing that removal of the testes arrested the growth of the prostate in young animals, advocated castration for shrinking the obstructing prostate. Unfortunately, the high mortality rate associated with this procedure led to its abandonment. Had this procedure been continued it might have led to discovery of its beneficial effect in carcinoma of the prostate, at least fifty years earlier. Subsequently, vasectomy was proposed but this too was soon discarded.

Axilrod and Deming[190] have given an excellent historical analysis of cases of prostatism, covering an era when the disease was poorly understood. These authors write: "The ideas concerning the treatment of prostatism, prevailing in the minds of the early Connecticut physicians, leave no doubt of the seriousness of the disease and illustrate vividly the advances made in this special field of medicine in the past seventy years. In the latter half of the 19th century, bladders distended with urine were still being catheterized with the flexible catheter, invented many years before by Benjamin Franklin. Cystitis was recognized and treated with chemotherapeutic agents, some of which are still in good use today. Anodynes, especially opium and belladonna, in the form of suppositories, were freely given and have no equal at the present time for relief of pain and control of bladder spasms." Compare this description with that written by Whately[191] in 1804 and one can readily appreciate the confusion about cystitis and prostatitis. Whately in writing about the treatment for strictures of the urethra adds the following to his appendix: "I add a few remarks on an affection of the bladder, frequently met with in elderly people, which resembles, in some of its symptoms those of the complaint which is the subject of the foregoing treatise, but from which it may be clearly distinguished.

"In the decline of life, the bladder is apt to retain a part of the urine after the act of making water; the frequent efforts made to expel this remainder inflame its inner coat, and bring on a very painful and distressing disease. This complaint generally comes on slowly. One of the first symptoms of it is a more frequent desire to make water than usual, by night as well as day, and the quantity expelled, at each evacuation, is of course diminished . . . this retention of urine does not seem to be the effect of stricture, as there is commonly no stricture in these cases. A much more probable cause is an enlargement of the prostate gland. . . . On the cure of this complaint I may be concise. The first thing to be done is to empty the bladder by a catheter.* It is almost incredible to say how soon the patient finds relief from this operation. The urine and mucus are no sooner evacuated, then he finds himself as it were perfectly well. Instead of finding a return of the painful effort to make water at the expiration perhaps of every hour, or oftener, he is frequently, though not always free from it for

---

* The history of the catheter goes back to Egyptian writings of approximately 3000 B.C. In later years, the Greeks, the Romans and the Chinese employed similar instruments of metal. It is believed that the Arabians were the first to develop a flexible catheter, as reported by Avicenna in 1036 A.D. No further improvement of significance occurred until the 18th century when silver and woven silk catheters came into usage. With the advent of rubber processing, catheters made of this material were introduced. Subsequently, the availability of soft latex permitted the development of the self-retaining Foley catheter, so useful and effective during the last 15 years. (See Chapter XV on development of Endoscopy.)

several hours, and sometimes nearly for half a day after the operation has been performed. The inclination to evacuate his urine of course returns when the bladder is again distended; but if it be again emptied by the catheter, the relief before obtained is again experienced. By this method I have seen many so much improve in a few days as apparently to be cured . . . the intention of using the catheter should be, to draw off the water as often as is necessary to prevent pain, from the distention of the bladder. When this viscus is highly inflamed, and the symptoms severe, the operation should be repeated every six hours. In ordinary cases, once in twelve hours will be sufficient." After describing the type of catheter to be used he concludes: "I have seen different medicines tried in this disease, but with very little effect. They are of service chiefly where the symptoms are extremely violent. In such cases gentle evacuations by the bowels should be procured daily, and opiates should be given either internally or in the form of clysters. The semicupium, and fomentations to the perineum and region of the pubis, joined to a light diet, should be employed. Abstinence from all heating liquors, and rest, should likewise be enjoined."

In 1902, Albarran* first described the sub-trigonal glands, subsequently referred to as Albarran's glands. He had a great interest in the prostate and is credited as being the first surgeon in France to perform perineal prostatectomy.

One of the first procedures for the removal of the prostate gland was that advocated by Peter Freyer. On December 1, 1900, Peter Freyer (later knighted and referred to as Sir Peter Freyer) operated on a 71-year-old man with long standing symptoms of prostatic obstruction, who in the past year could only empty his bladder with the aid of a catheter. Freyer's notes on his suprapubic prostectomy read:

---

* Albarran, a Cuban, became a teacher of the highest rank and at the age of 46, received the singular honor of being awarded the chair of urology at the Sorbonne. His researches were varied and extensive; his bibliography has been stated to fill eight single-spaced printed pages. His treatises included articles on disease of the kidney and of the prostate. He died at the early age of 52, after nicking his finger with a scalpel he used to divide a kidney he had removed because of tuberculosis.

> "Suprapubic incisions: incision into mucous membrane of bladder onto right prostatic lobe: this shelled out easily. Apparently an adenomatous growth not very hard—more elastic than doughy. Corresponding incision into mucous membrane over left lobe which was treated in the same way. This was smaller but apparently of the same consistency. When the right lobe was removed and got out of the way a small median lobe was felt about the size of a marble; this was removed thirdly through the incision made for the right lobe. This also seemed to be identical in its feel and consistency with the other two. Double drain tube put in."

Freyer subsequently performed more than 1625 suprapubic prostatectomies over the next twenty years with an amazingly low mortality rate (5.3%). Of singular interest is that the operation was pioneered by the work of Belfield[193,194] of Chicago. Present historians give Fuller credit for first accomplishing suprapubic enucleation of the prostate gland, an honor claimed by Freyer in 1900. There is no doubt that Fuller first described the operation, but Freyer must be given credit for popularizing this approach to the prostate. Freyer accomplished this by numerous literary contributions with detailed reports of cases, the technique and obstacles to be overcome. He was the first to abandon the use of scissors to divide the mucous membrane over the prostate gland, advocating instead the method of scoring through the mucous membrane with the sharpened finger nail.

The feud concerning the priority in the adoption of suprapubic enucleation of the prostate by Fuller vs. Freyer[195] is significant of historical rather than of academic interest. In 1905, Eugene Fuller, who was then attending surgeon to the city and to the post-graduate hospitals in New York City, published a comprehensive article entitled, "The Question of Priority in the Adoption of the Method of Total Enucleation, Suprapubically of the Hypertrophied Prostate Gland."[195] This article contains the following letter by Ramon Guiteras, who was indeed a pioneer in prostatic surgery, and which should have soothed the anger of Fuller, but unfortunately did not. The following is a copy of the letter:

February 5, 1905

Eugene Fuller, M.D.
Lexington Avenue and 35th Street
City

Dear Doctor:

I read a paper entitled "The Present Status of the Treatment of Prostatic Hypertrophy in the United States," in the section of Urinary Surgery of the International Medical Congress in Paris, August 4, 1900. In this paper I explained the different methods that are employed in operating on the prostatic gland in this country. An abstract of this paper was published in the transactions, but the paper in full came out in the *New York Medical Journal,* December 8, 1900. I had the pleasure of meeting Dr. Freyer in London, on my way to Paris, and explained to him your method of enucleating the prostate that you had been using for a number of years, and which I had been following, with the exception of introducing my fingers into the rectum for the counter-pressure instead of pressing upon the perineum. Dr. Freyer was very much pleased with the description of the operations, and said he would try the method. Since then he has operated a number of times, but describes his operation as though he had originated the operation of suprapubic prostatectomy which had been performed for so many years previously by other operators. I am sending you the reprint of the Paris paper.

Yours sincerely,
(signed) Ramon Guiteras

The controversy concerning priority of total suprapubic enucleation of the hypertrophied prostate certainly established Fuller as the originator of the method, but priority would not seem to be too important. What is important is that it marked the beginning of a better understanding of prostatic hypertrophy and opened avenues through which clinicians have advanced to our present methods of management.*

* The reader is referred to Immergut's *Classical Articles in Urology* wherein Fuller's and Freyer's original articles are reproduced, as well as *Commentary on Prostatic Surgery* by Edgar Burns.

In 1911, J. Bentley Squier[196, 197] of New York made a further refinement in the methods previously used by Fuller, Freyer, Guiteras and others. Squier advised making the incision in the bladder large enough to admit two or three fingers, as high up on the dome of the bladder as possible, close to the peritoneal reflection. Squier believed that the location of the incision had much to do with the length of time necessary for healing of the sinus, pointing out that a low dependent incision during convalescence encourages persistence of the sinus by facilitating the constant escape of urine. Squier also contributed to the technique by advocating insertion of the finger into the internal urethral meatus (prostatic urethra) and breaking through to the roof of the prostatic urethra and thus obtaining a line of cleavage.

The necessity of drainage prior to prostatic surgery was first advocated by Hugh Young.[198] This came about by the inability to catheterize a patient with subsequent cystotomy for draining purposes. The benefits of cystotomy subsequently became obvious. Shortly thereafter, Cabot[199] presented a paper entitled "The Mechanism of the Protection Afforded by the Drainage of Prostatic as a Preliminary to Operation." The advantages of two-stage suprapubic prostatectomy soon became evidenced by the popularity of this procedure thereafter.[200, 201, 202]

With the introduction of antibiotics and drainage of bladder by means of a Foley urethral catheter, the need of a two-stage prostatectomy diminished and this technique is now rarely used. This change in technique can also be attributed to better understanding and handling of such a formerly dreaded complication as shock, now almost eliminated because of proper control of fluid and electrolyte balance and the more intelligent approach to hemorrhage and its control.[203]

As a rule, American urologists have been trained in all methods of prostatectomy. Nevertheless, it is amusing to note the cynical attitude taken by surgeons of different schools of thought. For example, the surgeon who actually sneers at the resectionist, who in turn belittles the retro-pubic enthusiast; and the perineal enthusiast demurs all techniques including the suprapubic approach. Hess[204] and his associates call this attitude "partisanship." They believe that it has stimulated the rapid advances in the development of the divergent techniques but, "partisanship which tends to gloss over disadvantages, minimize shortcoming and magnify virtues (real or assumed), distorts the literature concerning prostatectomy to a significant degree. The partisan operator, in other words, is in a fine position to advance and refine his own particular technique. His contribution is a major one in clinical and technical research, and we should encourage him. But we should be cautious in listening to him when he departs from his accustomed sphere and starts making comparisons to techniques of which he is not the master."

A word about perineal prostatectomy—a procedure still the subject of varying opinions. Although numerous procedures for perineal prostatectomy had been devised and widely used before and after 1900, it remained for Hugh Young* in 1903 to make many subsequent modifications in the procedure, so that it has now become more or less standard. Throughout the early decades of this century, the perineal operation was still preferred by most surgeons because of its lower mortality rate. Young's first prostatectomy was in 1895, while he was in charge of the Negro wards in Johns Hopkins' Hospital. For seven years, he continued doing suprapubic prostatectomies, because it was a rapid and effective way to remove an enlarged prostate. In October, 1902, Young tried the perineal approach and did the same approach on the next fifty patients without one mortality. This convinced him and others of the advantage of this

---

* Hugh Young, pioneer of Modern Urology, was an extraordinary man. Born in San Antonio, on September 18, 1870, he was educated at the University of Virginia and while editor-in-chief of the varsity newspaper thought he might go into journalism. Fortunately for the medical profession and the world in general he chose medicine. He trained at Hopkins with Halstead. After a superb basic training in general surgery, he entered the field of urology which at that time was in its embryonic stages. His contributions were many. He was a prolific writer and because of the need for a journal devoted to urology, he founded the *Journal of Urology* in 1917. "Hugh Young" writes Crowe, "was an expert clinician, a scientist, an educator, and truly the father of American Urology."

approach, particularly at a time when antibiotics and electrolytic studies were unknown. In 1923, Young reported a 3.4% mortality among 1049 prostatectomies performed over a twenty-year period. Of singular interest is that of these patients, 144 were between seventy-five and ninety-five years of age.

Further Advances in Bladder Surgery

With the advent of an ultimate perfection of the cystoscope, the diagnosis and treatment of tumors and other lesions of the bladder took place. Indeed, with further perfection, such instruments became effective for transurethral resection of the prostate and papillomata of the bladder. In this section, we shall confine our discussions to bladder tumors, a surgical entity which baffled the ancients and even to this day may, at times, tax the surgeon with an unsurmountable burden.

Higgins tells us that "at the beginning of this century, the widespread interest in the then relatively new monopolar an bipolar high frequency currents (which had been introduced during the 1890's by Oudin and D'Arsonval) made it inevitable that this modality would be combined with the operating cystoscope."

Young, in 1941, reviewing *Progress in Urology* speaks of Nitze and his contribution. "In 1896, Nitze introduced his operating cystoscope, an instrument with which he could snare the tumor, burn through the pedicle and cauterize bleeding vessels. He later described one hundred and fifty cases treated with his instruments and reported only twenty recurrences and on death."

In 1910, Edwin Beer was the first to use a monopolar current in the destruction of bladder tumors with a cystoscope. Almost at the same time, Keyes used a bipolar current in a similar procedure. Endovesical destruction of vesical papillomata by the high frequency current through a cystoscope now became universal in use, but unfortunately it soon became evident that many malignant papillomas could not be cured in this manner. New surgical treatments had to be devised and many were devised. Some were combined with irradiation be-

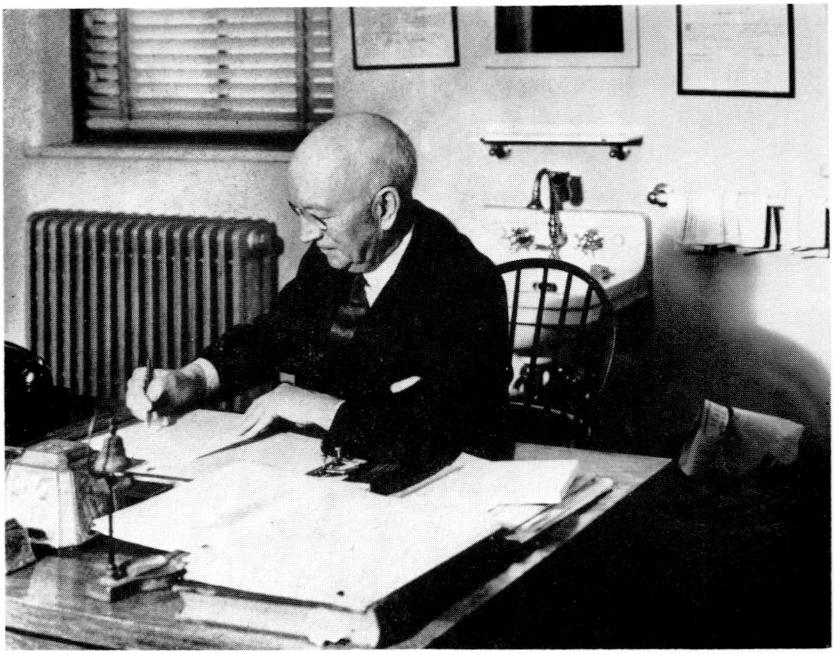

FIGURE 33. Hugh Hampton Young (1870-1945) is universally acknowledged as the "Father of Modern Urology." "Dr. Young's numerous scientific attainments, medical and civic honors, are recorded in *Who's Who in America,* the British *Who's Who,* and in his autobiography, Hugh Young. However, printed words merely tell you that Hugh H. Young was a pioneer member of the American Urological Association and the founder of the *Journal of Urology,* but they cannot portray the humaneness and brilliance of the man. Those who knew him well will always feel that at our meetings, the theoretical seat of honor to the right of the Chairman will be perpetually vacant." (Miley B. Wesson: Obituary, *Journal of Urology,* 57:203-208, 1947. Photograph, courtesy American Urological Association.)

cause therapeutic radiology was then becoming a popular new field. But no advance in therapy could be made until the pathologic differentiation and classification of bladder tumors were made.

The use of roentgen rays, directed through a special cone inserted into a suprapubic incision, was performed by Gray[206] of Richmond in 1906. According to Corbus, Cleaves of Philadelphia was the first to use radium in the bladder in 1903. But according to Higgins, most attempts at radiation therapy prior to 1905 were merely trial and error experiments, but from such steps, data was collected that led to the formulation of Bergonie and Tribondeau's law. This law stated that immature cells and cells in an active state of division are more sensitive to irradiation than those with fixed adult morphologic and physiologic characteristics. This was the dawn of the epoch of radiation therapy primarily associated with the treatment of malignant disease.

In 1913, Pasteau and Degrais,[207] at the International Medical Congress in London read a paper on the use of radium introduced into the bladder with the ordinary rubber catheter. A few years later (1917), Young introduced a cystoscopic radium applicator, the beak of which carried 100 mg radium.

Now followed a period of almost a decade, in which extensive surgical procedures were advocated for the treatment of bladder tumors, but with continuing high mortality and frequent recurrences. It soon became evident that in some cases, it was necessary to remove a portion of the bladder surrounding the tumor and it then followed that complete relief could best be obtained by total cystectomy. Thus, following Coffey's experimental work which demonstrated a method whereby the ureters could be transplanted into the rectosigmoid, cystectomy came into the realm of urologic surgery.

Today, diversion of the urinary stream into some structure other than transplanting the ureters into the rectosigmoid has become popular. In this procedure, a segment of the terminal ileum is isolated and utilized as a substitute bladder. The role of "ilial-loop" has been most gratifying in cases where total cystectomy is indicated.

A complete account of the accomplishments that have made possible modern surgery of the prostate and bladder would encompass the contribution of investigators working in practically every field of medical science. Our purpose is to trace and give a brief sketch of the accomplishments from antiquity to the twentieth century.* In collecting the data for this historical sketch, I have undoubtedly overlooked many important papers, and may have perhaps given others unintentionally unusual prominence, but only to stress the chronological train of events.

---

* For sake of completeness mention should be made of cryosurgical treatment of the enlarged prostate. It is truly modern and cryosurgical techniques are being used successfully in other surgical specialties. In this technique, a vacuum insulated equipment permits the use of liquid nitrogen to freeze circumscribed and well-defined areas.[208] Thus, liquid nitrogen is transported through a conduit to the area to be frozen without damaging adjacent or intervening tissues. The effects of cold on living tissues have been a matter of scientific interest for years. Power,[209] over 300 years ago, carried out experiments in which he froze a jar containing vinegar eels by immersion in ice and salt, and reactivated the eels by thawing. Boyle, 20 years later, carried out a similar experiment with fish and found that after 3 days of freezing followed by thawing the fish did not survive. He concluded that cold was no less effective than heat in the capacity to destroy living tissue.

Of singular interest to the urologist is the application of this technique to the prostate. Kaplan and Kaplan have recently demonstrated that cryosurgical technique can be used to effectively destroy epithelial neoplastic tissue in the bladder. They claim there are many possible advantages that this technique may offer over the accepted modalities used in the treatment of carcinoma of the bladder.[210]

Chapter XVI

Urologic Surgery from Antiquity to the 20th Century

Part IV

Renal Surgery

ACCORDING to Mathé,[211] renal surgery had its scientific beginnings with the chronicling by Hippocrates of the following operations (probably never performed by Hippocrates): drainage of tuberculous and nontuberculous pyelonephritic kidneys, the opening of nephritic and perinephritic abscesses, the incision of swelling in the loin due to renal tumefaction and solidification resulting from stone, and the drainage of kidneys presenting acute congestion caused by nephritis or pyelonephritis. In addition, Hippocrates clearly wrote about and described renal crises, the symptoms caused by kidney disease and the changed appearance (uroscopy) of the urine due to various pathological changes in the kidney.

Hippocrates dominated the beginning of the period of remarkable achievements in medicine; to be followed by Galen whose writings influenced mankind for forty-five generations. It is of singular interest that whereas little is known of Hippocrates as a person, many facts concerning Galen's life are well documented (see Chapter V on Ancient Rome and Galenic Urology).

The medicine and pathology Galen practiced, and about which he wrote, were based mainly on the speculative theories

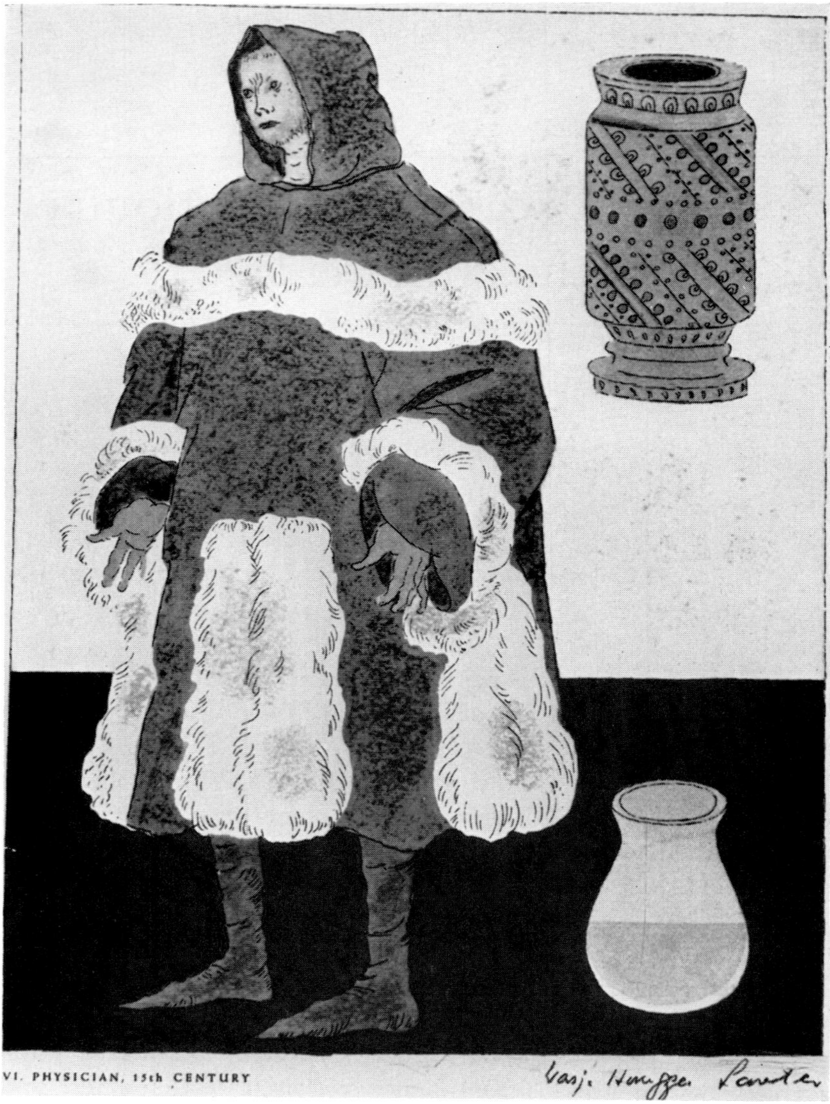

FIGURE 34. Physician—15th Century. (Courtesy of Abbott Laboratories: Collection of Medical Costumes, portrayed by Warja Honegger—Lavater.)

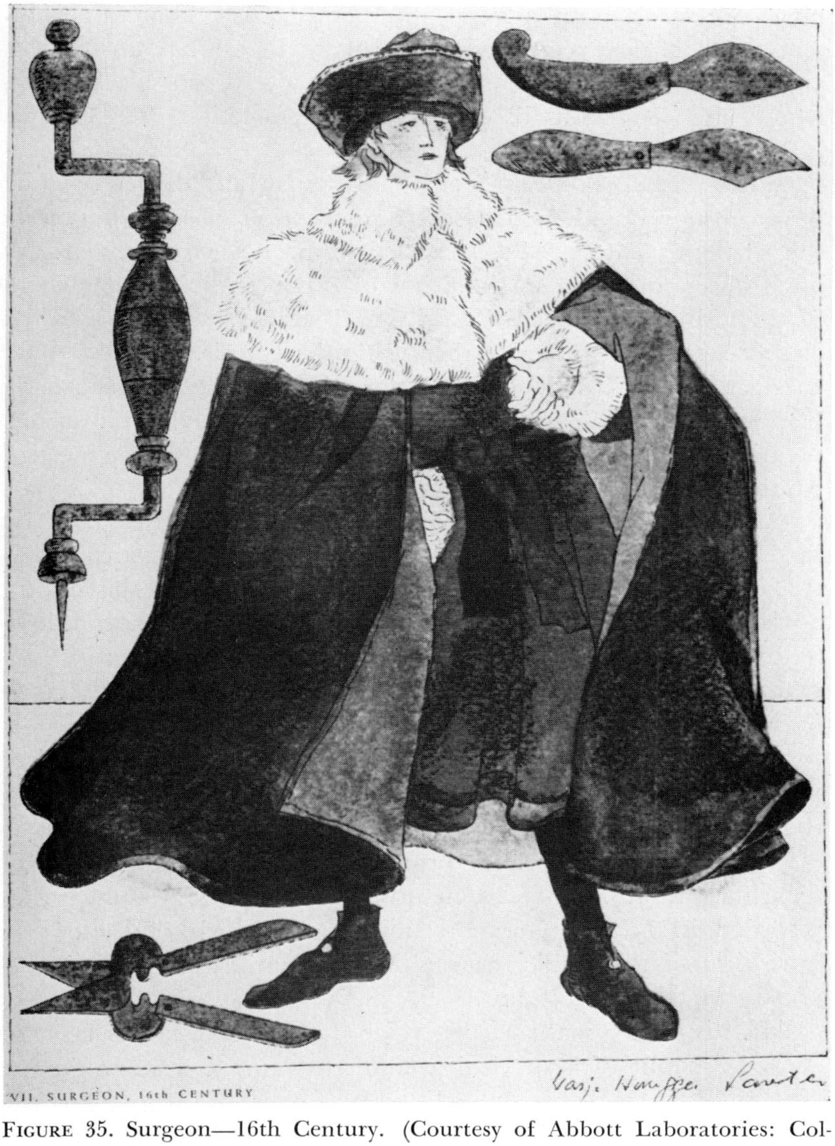

FIGURE 35. Surgeon—16th Century. (Courtesy of Abbott Laboratories: Collection of Medical Costumes, portrayed by Warja Honegger—Lavater.)

of Hippocrates. Galen did not dissect humans, but utilized animals. He cleared up a great number of basic anatomic problems and whatever errors he did make in animal anatomy as applied to humans was subsequently cleared up by Vesalius, whose knowledge was based on human dissection (see Chapter XII).

Galen deserves great credit for opposing theories which were unsound and not based on scientific observation. Like the ancient writers who preceded him, he wrote extensively on lithiasis, omitting any writing of other pathological changes of the kidney. However, he did describe a kidney disease which closely resembles and probably was tuberculosis. He also noted that renal injuries led to bleeding and passage of clots into the bladder, from which they were actually removed by him. He definitely opposed surgery of the kidney since he believed it would only prove to be fatal.

Mathé[211] states that according to Wolfangus Justus, writing in 1556, Serapion, an Arab physician living in Damascus at the end of the tenth and beginning of the eleventh century, advised removal of stone by lumbar incision. He quotes him as follows: *"Quidam antiquorium praeceperunt lapidem renium extrahi cum ferro incidente, retro uper latus duroium iliorum in loco renum."* (Someone among the ancients has prescribed to extract kidney stone from behind by means of cutting iron penetrating through the back at the level of the region of the ileum.)

More adequate accounts began to appear at about the fifteenth century. Numerous manuscripts of stone removal were recorded in France, Germany and England. All of these cases were limited to specific cases with true tumification or evidence of a distinct external tumor.

All historical manuscripts refer to the supposed first recorded account of a surgical attempt to remove a stone from a kidney. This is the so-called "franc-archer of Bagnolet case" the authority of which may be questioned. The account of this case[212] is quoted as follows:

> "The Doctors of the Faculty of Medicine in Paris having learned that an archer fom Bagnolet, who had been afflicted

for a long time with stone, had been condemned to death for his crimes, petitioned the King and the Magistrates to kindly deliver him into their hands in order to prove on him if the kidney could be opened for the removal of stone, without depriving him of his life. Their operation was so successful that this man survived for many years afterwards in excellent health. Unfortunately the surgeons of Paris left no notes or record as to the exact approach, in the extraction of the stone. There are many who do not accept the story as authentic."

However, we do find an authentic record of surgical intervention of the kidney by Cardan, surgeon at Milano, who in the mid-sixteenth century deliberately opened a lumbar abscess containing eighteen stones. Again in 1550, Bauhin observed a tumor mass in the lumbar region followed by total suppression of urine. He first palpated the indurated areas in the center of the tumor, and made an incision over same extracting two stones with immediate relief to the patient.

In 1663, a Mr. Hobson persuaded Dominicus de Marchetti, a famed surgeon of Padua, to perform a nephrolithotomy on him. This interesting facet of early urological surgery is herewith reproduced as it appeared in Charles Bernard's writing of 1696:[213]

"Mr. Hobson, who was consul for the English at Venice, having long been afflicted with stone in the kidney was at length attacked with a fit of such duration and violence, he was reduced almost to desperation. Finding no relief from any means that had been used, he addressed himself to Dominicus de Marchetti, a famed and experienced physician at Padua, imploring him to cut the stone from his kidney. He added that he was not insensible to the danger but that death itself would be infinitely preferable to life and the misery under which he had long suffered. Marchetti seemed very desirous of declining to operate, since the operation represented the extreme hazard, was impracticable and one he had never attempted, and that to proceed to it was in effect to destroy him (Hobson).

"But Mr. Hobson, persisting, said that if he refused he would not desist until he had found someone who would do the operation. His resolution and importunity at length prevailed upon Marchetti to undertake the operation. Having prepared his patient, as he thought convenient, he began with his knife cutting gradually upon the region of the kidney affected until blood disturbed and blinded his work and he could not finish the operation at that attempt. Wherefore dressing up the wound until the next day he then repeated the operation and accomplished it by cutting into the body of the kidney; taking thence three or four stones he dressed it up again. From this instant Mr. Hobson was freed from the severity of his pain and in a reasonably short time was able to walk about his chamber having been in no danger either from the flow of blood or fever. Marchetti continued to dress the wound for a considerable time but was not able to close it up. It soon became fistulous from the continued flowing of urine through the sinus. Being in other respects restored to his former health and vigor, and the matter discharged being little, Mr. Hobson took leave of the professor and returned to Venice under the care and management of his wife. One morning as she was dressing the sore she fancied she felt something hard and rugged as she wiped, and upon examining it a little more closely with her bodkin, which served her instead of a probe, she found it to be a stone of the shape and size of a date stone, which, being removed, Hobson never complained of the least uneasiness in that part.

"About ten years afterwards he returned to London where the learned Dr. Tyson and myself were invited to see him by Dr. Davies, who had known him in Venice. After we had received the foregoing account from himself he gave us the satisfaction of viewing the sore, which remained open. Mr. Hobson, without any complaint permitted me to pass my probe so far into the sinus that we concluded it reached into the kidney. The matter it discharged was but little in quantity, but always diluted with, and smelling strongly of urine. The orifice would sometimes close for three or four days together, and then the matter made its way through the common passages with urine, yet without any difficulty or pain. There was no doubt that there was a coalition of the kidney and the psoas muscles. When we saw Mr. Hobson he was able to perform the functions of life and to undergo fatigue as any man

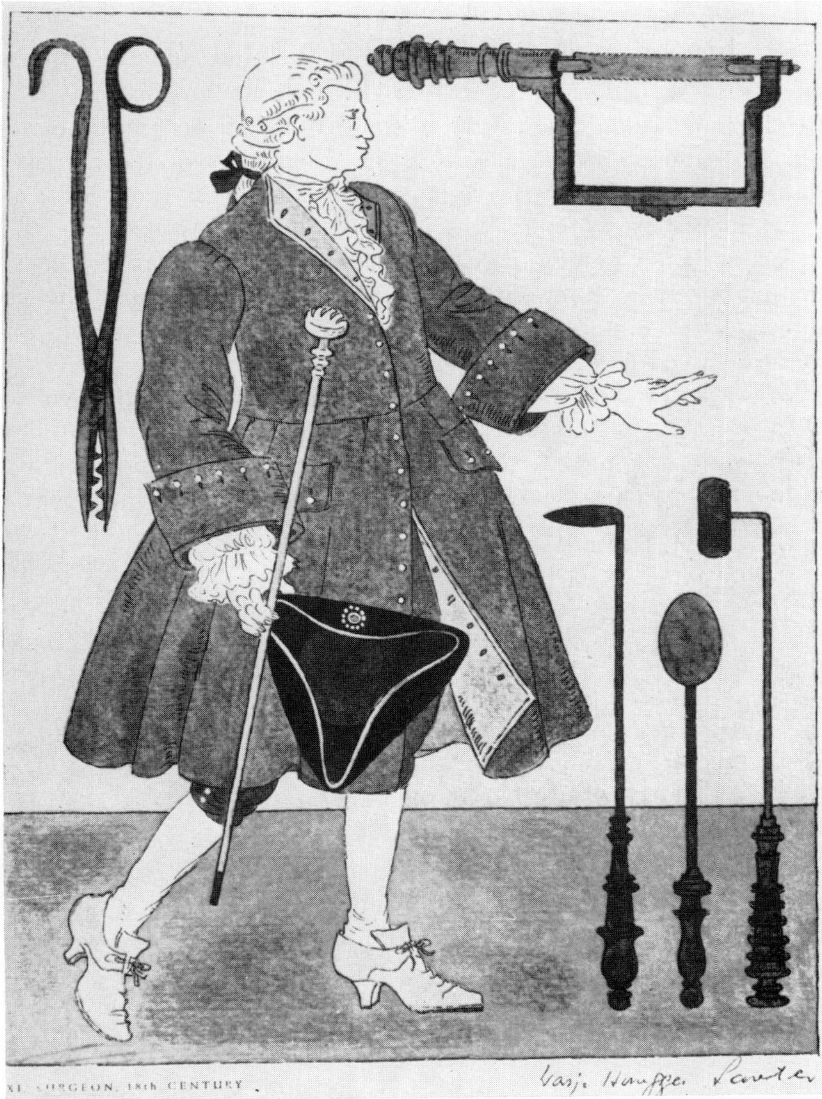

FIGURE 36. Surgeon—18th Century. (Courtesy of Abbott Laboratories: Collection of Medical Costumes, portrayed by Warja Honegger—Lavater.)

> of his years (being then I conceive of fifty) and was the next day to ride post forty or fifty miles."

By the end of the 17th century, most surgeons were more or less in accord that the true indication for nephrotomy was the infected calculous kidney, distended by an accumulation of pus, and those kidneys in which the calculus could be palpated in the organ itself or through a sinus. Based on the results of experiments by Zambeccarius in 1670 and Roonjuyzen in 1672 in which the kidney was successfully removed from experimental animals, Étienne Blancard[214] in 1690 suggested the removal of calculous kidney in man. This proposal, however, was vigorously condemned by contemporary surgeons.

In 1745, Lawrence Heister,[215] who had observed the healing of a number of accidental wounds of the kidney, expressed the opinion, contrary to general belief, that incision of the kidney was not fatal and that this organ could safely be opened. Unfortunately, P. Hevin[216] in a detailed report to the Royal Academy of Surgery, concluded that while such operations on the kidneys were theoretically possible, the associated dangers were of such magnitude, that these operations should only be used as a last resort. In this connection, Hevin had been reproached for retarding the progress of surgical intervention on the kidney for stone, but "we must realize," writes Mathé,[211] "that his conclusions were based on the knowledge of the time and prudence alone influenced his conduct."

The first accurate *recorded* nephrolithotomy on an otherwise healthy kidney was performed by Henry Morris[217] in February, 1880 when he successfully removed a 31-gram stone. The following is the original description of this operation by Henry Morris, in his Hunterian Lecture for 1898.

> "No further advances, however, was made in the operative treatment of renal disorders 'til February 11, 1880, when I successfully removed a renal calculus weighing 30 gr. from the undistended, and to the naked eye, quite normal kidney of a young woman. The kidney was exposed through an oblique lumbar incision, and the stone reached and removed through the renal parenchyma.
>
> "At that time," continues Sir Henry Morris, "I was unfa-

miliar with the attempts of other surgeons, except Durham, whose exploration of the kidney however was not a nephrotomy at all. Nor did I then know that the name nephrolithotomy which I suggested for the operation, I had performed had been used by Hevan more than a hundred and twenty years previously. I was led to undertake the operation in this particular case by the extreme severity and persistency of the symptoms, and by the little fear I felt about hemorrhage from the cut renal parenchyma, on account of my previous experience of the trivial and easily controlled bleeding from the cut surface of the liver in operating for hydrated tumours.

"This case demonstrated for the first time that a stone could be removed by cutting freely upon it through a thick layer of renal tissue. It thus became the starting point of both the development and the conservation of renal surgery which I am persuaded will become more and more conservative in the future."

In 1872, William Ingalls,[218] a member of the surgical staff of the Boston City Hospital, removed a large calculus from the right kidney of Mrs. G. by lumbar approach. Unfortunately, Ingalls did not report the case until 1882 and because of this delay, others have received more credit than he for first popularizing nephrolithotomy. However, it is the first recorded nephrolithotomy performed in America.

The operation of nephrolithotomy, first advocated by Cousinto two hundred and fifty years before, and actually carried out by Morris now rapidly became more popular and recnized as the correct surgical procedure for nephrolithiasis. Seymour,[219] in 1884, and Tiffany,[220] in 1885, used exploratory needles to determine the exact site of the calculus; subsequently made easier by the discovery of the roentgen-ray in 1895. McIntyre,[221] in 1896, demonstrated positive films for stones in five cases with renal calculi removed by surgery. In 1899, Albarran[222] demonstrated three proofs of radiographic evidence of renal calculi and in the same year Abbe[223] collected 22 additional cases from the literature.

The dawn of renal surgery actually took place on August 2, 1862 by Dr. Gustav Simon, Professor of Surgery at the Uni-

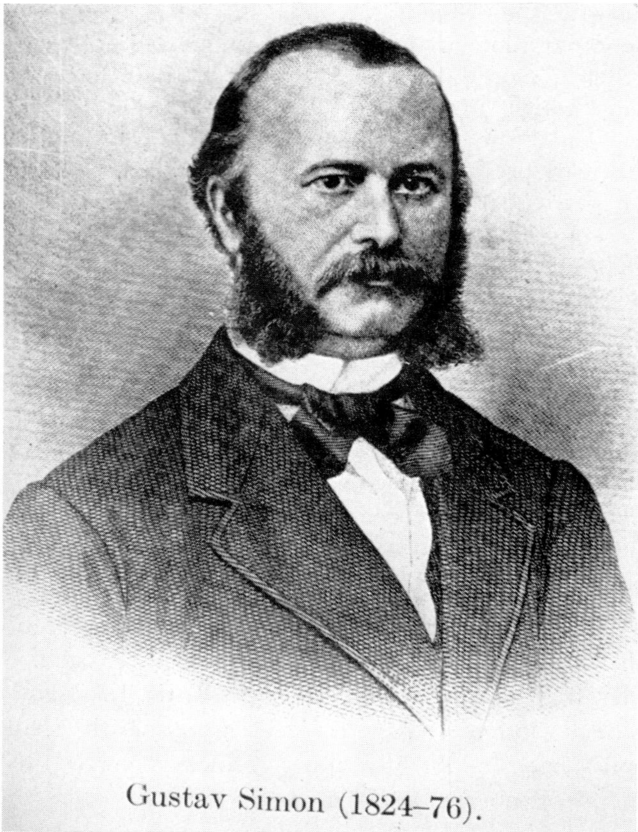

FIGURE 37. Gustav Simon—Pioneer in Renal Surgery.

versity of Heidelberg, when he deliberately and successfully removed a kidney.[224] This was indeed a milestone in the history of urology, for although unintentional nephrectomies had been performed by Wolcott[225] in 1861, this was the first deliberately planned nephrectomy.

The nephrectomy by Simon was a complete success, and firmly established that a single kidney was adequate for the needs of the body and compatible with the support of life. Thus a new era of thought developed which differed greatly from former beliefs. Even as late as 1841, Rayer,[226] in discussing extirpation of the kidney in his *Traite de Maladies des*

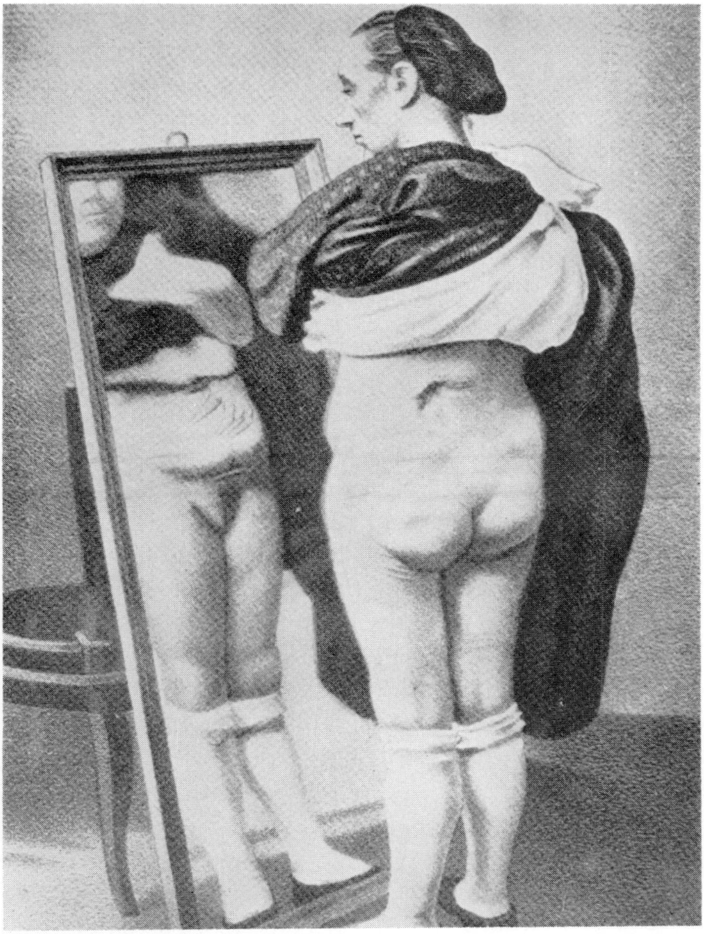

FIGURE 38. Gustav Simon's first successful nephrectomy.

Reins, a book which was believed to include all then known about renal surgery, declared that it would be folly to attempt such an operation.

Although Simon died prematurely in 1876, from an aortic aneurysm, he witnessed the beginning of a new era in kidney surgery. Gilmore,[227] in 1870, repeated Simon's operation successfully removing an atrophied floating kidney from a five-months pregnant woman, who had suffered unbearable pain.

In the following year (March, 1871), Von Bruns removed the left kidney of a German officer who had received a gunshot wound of the flank with resulting left lumbar fistula, pyelonephrosis, and calculus formation. The patient died in a few hours and autopsy revealed the remaining kidney to contain multiple abscesses.

With the development of antisepsis in 1876, and asepsis in 1880 and the improved methods of diagnosis made possible by the invention of the cystoscope by Nitze in 1878 and by the discovery and perfection of x-ray by Roentgen in 1895, nephrectomy no longer was looked upon as a hazardous procedure and subsequently became a daily procedure on all surgical services.

Because of its rich historical background and demonstrations of progress in renal surgery it would be amiss to omit mention of nephropexy. According to Mathé,[211] Francis cus de Pedemontanus in the fourteenth century was the first to describe movable kidney. As a result of the writings of Rayer[226] in 1841 and Dietl[229] in 1864, physicians became aware of a characteristic pain associated with overly mobile kidneys. Surgeons now began to offer their services for the relief of this annoying condition and unfortunately nephrectomy was first offered as a cure for a floating and painful kidney. This procedure soon lost favor because of the then high mortality rate when compared to the more benign procedure of nephropexy.

An American surgeon in Mobile, Alabama, is said to have performed the first surgical suspension of the kidney. Careful search of the literature fails to confirm this belief. In 1875, Dr. Greensville Dowell of Galveston attempted to secure a movable kidney to the walls of the abdomen by passing a tape seton threaded on a needle through the wall of the abdomen, kidney, and out through the lumbar region. The patient, female, aged thirty-five had been suffering from severe pain in the upper abdomen. The seton had pierced the kidney as evidenced by hematuria. Later it broke and came away after it had been retained for three months. In 1879, Dr. A. W. Smyth removed the kidney and found the surface of the lower pole to have been scarred by the seton.

Hahn[230] performed the first two successful nephropexies in 1881 by suturing the capsule into the lumbar fascia and packing the wound with carbolic gauze. Hahn called his operation nephrorrhaphy. Eight years later, Le Dentu[231] in his excellent work entitled *Affections du Rein et des Ureteres* in Chapter VI, devoted to surgical suspension of the kidney, wrote that this term led to confusion as it signified suture of the kidney itself. Therefore, for fixation of the mobile kidney to the posterior abdominal wall by suture he suggested the term "Nephropexy" which comes from the Greek meaning to fix and to coagulate. This term was soon adopted and has been universally employed ever since.

Henry Morris[232] did much to popularize nephropexy. His method consisted of passing silk sutures deeply through the kidney substance and securing them to the transversalis fascia and deeper muscular layers of the wound. He emphasized the importance of not permitting the cellulo-fatty tissue to bulge between the renal surface and the lumbar parietes, thereby impeding the establishment of firm adhesions that would assure lasting fixation.

Trapp and Shelley's[233] more modern comment and thought of nephropexy is interesting: "Since the advent of intravenous urography the actual demonstration of the presence or absence of renal ptosis, ureteral angulation and back pressure changes have been made possible. Today nephropexy is infrequently performed."

Higgins writes, "The changed attitude toward nephropexy has been summed up by Wharton as follows: 'Nephroptosis was once given a significance long since discarded; consequently 50 years ago, in this clinic, nephropexy was the commonest urologic operation. For the past 35 years nephropexy has almost never been performed except when the nephroptosis was perpetuating an infection. Although opinion still varies somewhat as to the value of nephropexy, certainly this conservative attitude is consonant with views of the majority of urologists.' "

With increased knowledge and experience, particularly in controlling hemorrhage, the surgeon now turned to nephrostomy as a means of temporary or even permanent drainage of the kidney. In 1896, the term nephrostomy was first used by Albarran,[234] who placed a drainage tube into the renal pelvis, and suturing the edges of the nephrostomy wound to the skin.

Higgins writes: "In 1905 the kidney operations most often performed were probably nephropexy and decapsulation, but by 1915 many surgeons in this country were attempting more formidable procedures, and contributing, bit by bit, to the technique, so that at present most of the more important operations are quite well standardized." Higgins then includes the following names who made contributions in this direction, namely, Mayo, Young, Lower, Cullen, Burns, Lowsley, Prather, Counseller, Hunt, Cabot, Quinby, Foley, Priestley and Hinman.

Hinman's[235] work on hydronephrosis, which was begun in 1918, is a major contribution to urology and modern urological surgery. Hinman was greatly stimulated by his predecessors in this field. Kuster,[236] in 1891, performed the first successful plastic operation on the kidney pelvis for hydronephrosis. He operated on the solitary kidney of an 18-year-old boy who had a permanent fistula from a previous nephrostomy. He found the upper ureter almost obliterated by stricture. He resected the strictured portion and reinplanted the normal ureter into the dependent renal pelvis. This procedure was then followed by other modifications and techniques.

Mention should be made of renal sympathectomy and denervation of the renal pedicle for the treatment of nephralgia and chronic nephritis. This was first performed in 1920 by Papin.[237] In 1948, Crabtree[238] made a review of the historical and theoretical aspects of this procedure. Crabtree reported on the results of his own case, and gave the opinon that this operation was the procedure of choice in certain selected cases. Suffice it to say that current urologists avoid this form of surgery.

The ancients rarely referred to the adrenal glands other than in anatomical dissections. Indeed, advances in surgery of the adrenal glands represents a recent epochal achievement. "That this development is recent is attested to by the fact that in the *History of Urology* published in 1933, there was no consideration of the adrenal glands, and, although the present trend had its beginnings in the 1930's, Hugh Young's review devoted only a brief paragraph to the earliest adrenal operations."[239] Thus, Young recorded that the first successful operation on the adrenal gland was performed by Gordon Holmes in 1924. Since then, and particularly since the isolation and development of cortisone and ACTH great progress has been made in the diagnosis of adrenal disease and in its treatment. The recognition of the adrenogenital syndrome, chromosomal studies, and a better understanding of genetic disorders have indeed made rapid strides in recent years and is far too great to be included into the scope of this thesis other than to record its progress and status.

Ever since 1898, when Abel first isolated adrenalin from the adrenal medulla, the idea of controlling hypertension by surgical intervention, had always appealed to the surgical researchers. In 1930, George Crile, Sr. became interested and speculated that the future role of surgery would plan an important part of hypertension management.[240]

In 1935, he postulated[241] certain indications and contraindications for adrenal intervention, and in 1937 advocated unilateral adrenalectomy and partial resection of the other gland to control hypertension. This was placed in the background by the more generally accepted surgical procedure of sympathectomy for the control of hypertension. In the post-cortisone era, adrenal surgery received further stimulus and attention was again directed to the possibility of controlling hypertension by bilateral adrenalectomy.

One can well be awed and impressed by the tremendous strides made in the study of urine and diseases of the kidneys since Hippocrates. This is particularly so when one approaches a consideration of the most recent advance in renal surgery, namely renal homotransplantation. Thus from removal of the kidney, as first advocated by Gustav Simon on August 2, 1869, at the University of Heidelberg, to replacement of that organ by transplantation, surgery has indeed made significant progress.

In 1902, the first attempt to perform renal auto-, homo-, and heterotransplantation in animals was performed by Ullmann.[242] Carrel* subsequently developed a new technique of direct suture for anastomosis of blood vessels which was of aid in subsequent organ transplantation. Carrel further pioneered in the basic techniques of renal transplantation and contributed tremendously to this field.

At the beginning, renal transplantation was performed primarily to tide an anuric patient over the acute episode. In 1936, Voronoy[247] transplanted a kidney into a patient who was a victim of bichloride of mercury poisoning. The patient survived 48 hours.

The first successful human renal homotransplantation was performed by Lawler, West, McNulty, Clancy and Murphy in 1950, in Chicago.[248] This was followed by the successful transplantation in 1953 by Hume, Merrill, Miller and Thorne.[249]

---

* Alexis Carrel has often been credited as the original pioneer of organ transplantation. He was born in Sainte-Foyle, Lyons, France on June 28, 1873 and was described as a stocky, trim, broad faced, broad browed, pink complexioned Frenchman with piercing but kindly eyes, who always wore a beret, except when in the operating room. He received his degree of Doctor of Medicine at the University of Lyons in 1900, and since no one seemed particularly interested in vascular surgery[246] and organ transplantation he came to the United States and worked in the Hull Physiological Laboratory in Chicago.

In 1906, Simon Flexner offered him a position at the then new Rockefeller Institute for Medical Research in New York. Here he established new procedures[243, 244] and techniques in vascular surgery and organ transplantation. He contributed greatly to vascular prostheses by using peritoneal grafts. What is most significant is that Carrel recognized the future importance of tissue transplantation and indicated that cadavers would be the ideal source of donor grafts.

In 1938, he, with Charles Lindbergh of aviation fame, designed a sterile perfusion pump and was able to demonstrate continued metabolic activity in most of his perfused organs for various periods of time. Smith[245] writes that Lindbergh described Carrel 'as having one of the most brilliant, penetrating, and versatile minds that he had ever met. He went on to state that Carrel's every action was filled with character, and that the record of his life could not fail to interest anyone who cares about human personality."

Paradoxically, toward the end of World War II this outstanding scientist was charged with aiding the Nazis. That he was sympathetic to the Nazis could not be denied, and it is believed his loyalty was based on similar views on eugenics. Carrel did not believe in the basic democratic ideal that all men are created equal but believed that the stupid and unintelligent had no right to a higher education and certainly not the same voting power as the intelligent. His death on November 1, 1944 cancelled his trial for his obvious misbehavior.[245]

In 1954, Merrill, Murray, Harrison and Guild[250] were the first to successfully transplant kidney between identical twins. More than 240 human kidneys have been transplanted according to Merrill. Twenty-eight monozygotic twins transplants have been reported and up to 1963 seven were still living. Of 211 homotransplants, only nine were living one year after surgery, the longest survivor being two years.

* * *

Despite the many pages of this treatise, it is but a quick glance backward in an attempt to pierce the mists of antiquity. All has not been covered and much has been omitted, but we have tried to stress the historical progress rather than the remarkable advances made in urology making it one of the most exact of all surgical specialties. I am reminded of a statement made to me many years ago by my chief, Dr. Louis René Kaufman who said: "The busy urologist finds in the writings of the past, stepping stones into a more well grounded future."

Bibliography

1. Langer, W. A.: *An Encyclopedia of World History.* Houghton Mifflin Co., Boston, p. 2, 1957.
2. Ackerknecht, F. A.: Primitive medicine and culture. *Bull. Hist. Med.,* 11:503-21, 1942.
3. Sandison, A. T.: Sir Marc Armand Ruffer (1859-1917) pioneer of paleopathology. *Med. Hist.,* pp. 150-155, 1967.
4. Moodie, R. H.: *Paleopathology—An Introduction to the Study of Ancient Evidences of Disease.* Univ. Ill. Press, Urbana, Ill. p. 21, 1923.
5. Brim, C. J.: *Medicine in the Bible.* Froben Press, New York, p. 373, 1936.
6. Dawson, W. R.: The Beginnings—Egypt and Assyria. Hafner Publishing Company, New York, 1964.
7. Montagu, F. A.: Primitive medicine. *New Eng. J. Med.,* 235:43-49, 1949.
8. Puschmann, T.: *A History of Medical Education.* Hafner Publishing Company, New York, 1966.
9. Smith, Homer: De Urina. *Kaiser Found. Med. Bull.,* 6:1, 1958.
10. Castiglioni, A.: Padua in the renaissance from Vesalius to Frucastoro. *Ciba Symposium.* Vol. X, Nov.-Dec. #3, p. 965, 1948.
11. Temkin, O.: Recent publications on Egyptian and Babylonian medicine. *Bull. Inst. Med.,* IV:251, 1936.
12. Sigerist, Henry E.: *A History of Medicine.* Oxford University Press, New York, Vol. I, Primitive and Archaic Medicine, 1955.
13. Morton, L. T.: *Garrison and Morton's Medical Bibliography,* 2nd Edition revised. Argosy Book Stores, New York, 1965.
14. Lutz, H. F.: A contribution to the knowledge of Assyro. Babylonian med. *Am. J. Sem. Lang. Lat.,* 38:74, 1919-1920.
15. Thompson, S.: Assyrian prescriptions for diseases of the urine, etc. *Babyloniaca,* 14:108-9, 1934.
16. Brown, S. A.: *The Physician Throughout the Ages,* Vol. I, Babylonia. Capehart-Brown Co., New York, 1928.
17. Leake, C. D.: *The Old Egyptian Medical Papyri.* Univ. Kansas Press, Lawrence, Kansas, 1952.
18. Personal Communication.
19. Rowling, S.: Paleopathology. In Brothwell, D., and Sandison, A. T.: *Diseases in Antiquity: A Survey of the Diseases, Injuries and Surgery of Early Populations.* Thomas, Springfield, 1967.

20. MOHAMED, AHMED RAGAB: *Lights on the Royal Mummies in the Egyptian Museum*. Cairo, 1964.
21. ISKANDER, Z., and BADAWY, A.: *Brief History of Ancient Egypt*. Cairo, 1965.
22. GRAY, P. H. K.: Radiography of ancient Egyptian mummies. *Med. Radiog. and Photog.*, 43:34-44, 1967.
23. SMITH, G. E., and WOOD-JONES, F.: *The Archaeological Survey of Nubia*. Report for 1907-1908, Vol. 2, Report on the Human Remains. Cairo, 1910.
24. RUFFER, M. A.: *Studies in Paleopathology of Egypt*, edited by R. H. Moodie, University Chicago Press, pp. 49-92, 1921.
25. SANDISON, A. T.: *The Study of Mummified and Dried Human Tissues-Science in Archeology*. London, pp. 413-423, 1963.
26. PETRIE, W. M. F.: *Fiftieth Memoir of the Egypt Exploration Fund*. Published by order of the committee, Egypt Explor. Fund., London, 1898.
27. MOODIE, R. H.: *Roentgenologic Studies of Egyptian and Peruvian Mummies*. Published by the Field Museum of Natural History, Chicago, Ill., 1931.
28. GRAY, P. H. K.: Embalmers restoration. *J. Egypt. Archeol.*, 52:138-140, 1967.
29. GRAY, P. H. K.: A Radiographic Skeletal Survey of Ancient Egyptian Mummies. In abridged Proceedings of the Fourth European Symposium on Calcified Tissues. Leiden, the Netherlands, March 28-April 1, 1966. *Excerpta Medica*, Int. Cong. Series No. 120, Pub. Excerpta Medica Foundation, Amsterdam, the Netherlands, 1966.
30. SMITH, G. E.: Footnote. *Bull. Arch. Survey of Nubia*, 2:56, 1908. Quoted by Moodie.
31. BITSCHAI, J., and BRODNEY, M. LEOPOLD: *A History of Urology in Egypt*. Riverside Press, 1956.
32. BULLOUGH, V. L.: *The Development of Medicine as a Profession*. Hafner Pub. Co., New York, p. 23, 1966.
33. BETTMAN, H. O.: *A Pictorial History of Medicine*. Thomas, Springfield, Third Printing, p. 14, 1962.
34. EDELSTEIN, H.: The distinctive Hellenism of Greek medicine—The Fielding H. Garrison Lecture for 1960. *Bull. Hist. Med.*, May-June, p. 199, 1966.
35. HAGGARD, H. W.: *Mystery, Magic and Medicine*. Doubleday, Doran & Co., Inc. Garden City, N. Y., p. 31, 1933.
36. JAYNE, W. A.: *The Healing Gods of Ancient Civilization*. Yale University Press, pp. 248-249, 1925.
37. BUNN, J. J.: Origin of the Caduceus motif. *J.A.M.A.*, Nov. 13, 1967.
38. FRANKFORT, H.: *The Art and Architecture of the Ancient Orient*. Penguin Books, Inc., Baltimore, Md., pp. 16-17, 1954.
39. BUDGE, F. A. W.: *Egyptian Relations: Egyptian Ideas of the Future Life*. New York Univ. Books, p. 79, 1959.
40. RICHARDS, D. W.: Hippocrates of Ostia. *J.A.M.A.*, 204:12, 1049-1056, 1968.
41. ARCHER, W. H.: The history of anaesthesia. *Proc. Dental Centenary Celebration* (Mar.), pp. 333-363, 1940.
42. KLEINMAN, M.: Histoire de l'anaesthesie. *Anesth. et Analg.* 5:122-138, 1939.
43. KEYS, T. F.: *The History of Surgical Anaesthesia*. Dover Publications, New York, 1963.
44. SIGERIST, H.: *On the History of Medicine*. Edited and with an introduction by

Felix, Mari-Ibanez, M.D., and Foreword by John F. Fulton, M.D., M.D. Publications, New York, 1960.

45. Personal Communication
46. Personal Communication.
47. Polk, H. C.: Notes on Galenic urology—Historical article. *Urol. Survey,* 15:2-6, 195.
48. Green, M. R.: *A Translation of Galen's Hygiene.* Introduction by Henry Sigerist. Thomas, Springfield, 1951.
49. Singer, C., and Rabin, C.: *A Prelude to Modern Science: Being a discussion and circumstances of the "Tabulae anatomical sex" of Vesalius.* Pub. Wellcome Historical Med. Museum, London, 1946.
50. Meyerhof, M.: Pharmacology During the Golden Age of Arabian Medicine. *Ciba Symposia.* Vol. 6, p. 1856, September, 1944.
51. Brody, D. A.: The School of Medicine at Jundeshapur: The Birthplace of Arabic Medicine. *Tr. and Stud. Coll. Physicians, Philadelphia,* 23:39, 1955.
52. Reznikoff, Paul, and Reznikoff, D. G.: Role of Nestorians in preservation of Greek medicine. *New York State J. Med.,* Dec. 15, p. 3263, 1967.
53. Gordon, B. E.: *Medieval and Renaissance Med.* Philosophical Lib., New York, p. 154, 1959.
54. Pope, A. V.: Avicenna and his cultural background. *Bull. N. Y. Acad. Med.,* 31:318, April, 1955.
55. Osler, W.: *Evolution of Modern Medicine.* Yale University Press, 1921.
56. Galdston, I.: Avicenna and Islamic science. *Bull. N. W. Acad. Med.,* 31:305, April, 1955.
57. Castiglioni, Arturo: *A History of Medicine.* A. A. Knopf, New York, 1947.
58. Kruger, C. H.: *Avicenna's Poem on Medicine.* Thomas, Springfield, 1963.
59. Krans, P.: Footnote on Death of Avicenna. *Ciba Symposia,* Vol. 6, 7, p. 1882, 1944.
60. Friedenwald, H.: Moses Maimonides, the physician. *Bull. Hist. Med.,* 3:555-557, 1935.
61. Walsh, J. J.: *Old-time Makers of Medicine.* New York, p. 105, 1911, quoted by Kagan, Solomon R.: Jewish Medicine. Medico-Historical Press, Boston, pp. 66-67, 1952.
62. Gordon, H. L.: *Moses Ben Maimon (Maimonides)—The Preservation of Youth. Essays on Health.* Translated from the original Arabic. Philosophical Lib. New York, pp. 5-6, 1958.
63. Bigelow, G.: *Discourse on Self-limited Diseases.* Boston, 1835.
64. Liebowitz, J. O.: Maimonides on medical practice. *Bull. Hist. Med.,* 31:309, 1957.
65. Melicow, M. J.: Interrelationship of medicine and art. *Bull. New York Acad. Med.,* 33:34-356, 1957.
66. Burroughs, Wellcome & Co.: *Evolution of Urine Analysis. An Historical Sketch of the Clinical Examination of Urine.* London, pp. 92, 1911.
67. Mestler, G. E.: A galaxy of old Japanese medical books with miscellaneous notes on early medicine in Japan. Part III, Urology, syphilology and dermatology. *Bull. Med. Lib. Assoc.,* Vol. 44, No. 2, April, 1956.
68. Nathan, Helmuth: Portrait of the doctor in pre-historic days and antiquity. *Postgrad. Med.,* 32:390-392, 1961.

69. MacKinney, Loren C.: *Medical Illustrations in Medieval Manuscripts.* Univ. Cal. Press, Berkeley and Los Angeles, 1965.
70. Aficanus, C.: *Columbia Encyclopedia,* 2d Ed. Columbia Univ. Press, p. 447, 1959.
71. De Grete, Francesco: The doctors portrait from the fifteenth to the eighteenth century. *Ciba Symposia,* April, p. 1751, 1944.
72. Gerlitt, J.: Cosmas and Damian, the patron saints of physicians. *Ciba Symposia,* Saints in Medicine. Vol. I, No. 4, p. 118, 1939.
73. *Smith, Homer W., His Scientific and Literary Achievements,* Edited by Chasis, H., and Goldring, W. New York Univ. Press. Chapter 8, De Urina, p. 125, 1965.
74. Castiglioni, Arturo: *A History of Medicine.* A. A. Knopf, New York, p. 316, 1947.
75. Sigerist, H.: *History of Medicine.* Ed., Felix-Marti Ibanez, M.D., with Foreword by John F. Fulton, M.D., M.D. Publications New York, pp. 131-134, 1960.
76. Burroughs, Wellcome & Co.: *Evolution of Urine Analysis. An Historical Sketch of the Clinical Examination of Urine.* London, pp. 92, 1911.
77. Leicester, M. H.: *The Historical Background of Chemistry.* John Wiley and Son. Inc., New York, p. 173, 1956.
78. Partington, R. J.: *Origins and Development of Applied Chemistry.* Longmans Green and Co., London, pp. 86-87, 1935.
79. Farbeo, R. J.: *Metallurgy in Antiquity.* Brill, Leiden, p. 22, 1950.
80. Wilson, W. S.: Traditional background of Greco—Egyptian alchemy. *Ciba Symposia,* Vol. 2, No. 7, p. 605, 1940.
81. Stielman, M. J.: *The Story of Early Chemistry.* D. Appleton & Co., New York, p. 24, 1924.
82. Wilson, J. W.: Biographies of early Chinese alchemists. *Ciba Symposia,* Vol. 2
83. Wilson, J. W.: Later developments of Chinese chemistry. *Ibid.,* pp. 610-615. No. 7, p. 615, 1940.
84. Wilson, J. W.: Relation of Chinese alchemy to that of other centuries. *Ibid.,* p. 618.
85. Wilson, J. W.: Leading ideas of early Chinese alchemy. *Ibid.,* p. 600.
86. Goldstein, A. E.: Diagnostic tests and chemicals used in urology. Chapt. IX, p. 223, *History of Urology,* Vol. II. Baltimore, Md., Williams & Wilkins, 1933.
87. Reisman, D.: *Ibid.,* 45.
88. *Encyclopaedia Britannica.* 175th Printing, Vol. II, p. 505b.
89. Willichins: *Urinorin Probationes Basillae,* p. 113, 1582, quoted by Goldstein.
90. Dekkers, Frederik: *Exercitationes Practica Circa Medendi Methodum.* Leyden, 1694.
91. Nixon, J. A.: Bright's disease. In *A Short History of Some Common Diseases* by Divers Authors, ed. Bett, R. W., Oxford University Press, London, 1934.
92. Belt, Elmer: Leonardo the Florentine (1452-1519). *Investigative Urol.,* 3:99, 1965.
93. Giovio, P.: *The Genius of Leonardo on Art and the Artist.* Translation by Andre Chastel. The Orion Press, quoted by Elmer Belt.
94. Belt, Elmer: *Leonardo, the Anatomist.*

95. Da Vinci, Leonardo: *Codice sul volo degli Viccelli.* Publicato de J. Sabachnikoff; transcrizione e note di G. Piumati, con tanduzione francise di C. Ravaisson. Mollien, Paris, 1893.

96. *Garrison and Morton's Medical Bibliography: An annotated check-list of texts illustrating the history of medicine,* Second Edition—Revised edition. Ed. Leslie M. Morton, #365, p. 34, 1965.

97. O'Malley, C. D., and Saunders, C. M. de J. B.: *Leonardo da Vinci on the Human Body.* Henry Schuman, New York, 1952.

98. Binet, L., and Maillant, C.: *Medicine in Art.* Ed., Jean Rousselot.

99. Belt, Elmer: *Leonardo da Vinci—Technical Innovations and Discoveries in Anatomy.*

100. Keele, N. D.: *Leonardo da Vinci on Movement of the Heart and Blood.* Lippincott, London.

101. Belt, Elmer: Personal Communication.

102. Belt, Elmer: *Leonardo, the Anatomist.* Univ. Kansas Press, Lawrence, 1955.

103. Murphy, L.: Leonardo da Vinci and the anatomy of the genito-urinary system. *Med. J. Australia,* Oct. 3, p. 556, 1964.

104. Osler, William: *Ibid.,* #55.

105. Singer, Charles: *Vesalius on the Human Brain.* Oxford University Press, London and Toronto, p. 8, 1952.

106. Sigerist, H. E.: *Primitive and Archaic Medicine,* Vol. I. Oxford University Press, New York, p. 68, 1967.

107. Sigerist, H. E.: *The Great Doctors: A Biographical History of Medicine.* W. W. Norton, New York, p. 109, 1933.

108. Zimmerman, L. M., and Veith, I.: Translation of Paracelsus' *Grusse Wundartznei* by Dr. Michael L. Mason, pp. 174-175.

109. Personal Communication.

110. O'Malley, C. D.: Andreas Vesalius 1514-1564, in memoriam. *Med. Hist.,* 8:229, 1964.

111. Singer, Charles: *A Short History of Anatomy and Physiology from the Greeks to Harvey.* Dover Pub., Chapter IV, p. 111, 1957; Roth, M.: Andreas Vesalius Bruxellensis, Berlin, 1892. In O'Malley, C. D.: *Andreas Vesalius of Brussels.* Berkeley and Los Angeles, pp. 130, 1964.

112. Castiglioni, A.: Padua in the renaissance from Vesalius to Fracastoro. *Ciba Symposia,* Vol. 10, #3, p. 965, 1948.

113. Castiglioni, A.: The origin and development of the anatomical theatre to the end of the renaissance. *Ciba Symposia,* Vol. 3, #2, p. 826, 1941.

114. Gordon, B. H.: *Medieval and Renaissance Medicine.* Philosophical Library, New York, Chapter XX, p. 416, 1959

115. Personal Communication.

116. O'Malley, C. D.: Personal Communication.

117. O'Malley, C. D.: Gabriel Falloppia, c. 1523-1562. *Investigative Urol.,* 4:95-95, 1966.

118. Paré, Ambroise: *The Apologie and Treatise of Ambroise Paré.* Edited and with an Introduction by Geoffrey Keynes. Univ. Chicago Press, 1952.

119. Hamby, Wallace B.: *Case Reports and Autopsy Records of Ambroise Paré.* Thomas, Springfield, 1960.

120. GARRISON, H. F.: The medical literature of France. *Bull. New York Acad.*, May, 1933.

121. Personal Communication.

122. MALGAIGNE, J. F.: *Surgery and Ambroise Paré.* Translated & edited by Wallace B. Hamby. Norman, Okla., Univ. Oklahoma Press, 1965.

123. THORNTON, J. L.: *Medical Books, Libraries and Collectors,* 2nd ed. Andrew Deutsch, p. 109, 1965.

124. SIGERIST, H.: *The Great Doctors.*

125. METTLER, CECILIA CHARLOTTE: *History of Medicine.* Philadelphia, Blakiston, 1947.

126. BOZZINI, P.: Der Lichtleiter oder Beschreibank einer einfachen vorrichtung und ihrer anwendung zur erlenchtung innerer Hohlen und Zwischenraume des lebenden ani-malischen Korpers. Weimar, 1807.

127. BENEDICT, B. E.: *Endoscopy as Related to Disease of the Bronchus, Esophagus, Stomach and Peritoneal Cavity.* Baltimore, Md. The Williams and Wilkins Company, pp. 1-13, 1951.

128. VOLTOLINI, RUDOLPH: Report at a meeting of scientific medicine in Berlin. *Deutsche Klinik,* 12:393-394, 1860.

129. DOSORMEAUX, A. J.: Endoscopy, and its application to the diagnosis and treatment of affections of the genito-urinary passages. *Chicago Medical Journal.* Robert Fergus' Sons, Printers, Chicago, Ill. 1867.

130. BRUCK, J.: *Stomatoskop and Urethroskop.* Breslau, 1867.

131. HAHEN, J.: Dilatorium Urethral zur Urethroscopie. *Wren. Med. Wchnshr.,* 1888.

132. NITZE, M.: Eine neue Belenchtungs und unter-suchungsmethode fur Harnrohre, Hornblase and Rectum. *Wien. Med. Wchnschr.,* 1888.

133. RATHERT, P.: Max Nitze. *Investigative Urol.,* 5:327-330, 1967.

134. NITZE, M.: *Lehrbuch der Kystoskopie.* Wiesbaden, 1889.

135. MARK, E. G.: *An History of Urology,* Vol. I, p. 160. The Williams and Wilkins Company, Baltimore, 1933.

136. NEUMAN, D.: *Glasgow Medical Journal,* 1883.

137. BANDLER, C.: The Semin-Centenary of the New York Society of the American Urol. Association. *J. Urol.*

138. JACOBY, G. W.: *Electrotherapeutic Control of Currents from Central Stations.* Read before the Metropolitan Medical Society, Sept., 1898.

139. OTIS, W. K.: Concerning the new electro-cystoscope. *New York Med. J.,* April, 1909.

140. BROWN, F. T.: New cystoscope. *Med. and Surg. Report Bellevue Hosp. New York,* Vol. I, Jan., 1905.

141. BUERGER, H.: A new indirect irrigating observation and double catheterizing cystoscope. *Ann. Surg.,* Feb., 1909.

142. BUERGER, L.: On methods of posterior urethroscopy with a description of a new cysto-urethroscope. *Am. J. Surg.,* May, 1910.

143. BUERGER, L.: Concerning certain improvements in the optical construction of cystoscopes.

144. Personal Communication.

145. Personal Communication.

146. BROGDEN, B. G.: William Conrad Roentgen (1845-1923). *Investigative Urol.,* 2:200, 1964.
147. MEADOWCROFT, W. H.: The A. B. C. of the x-rays, 1896. Quoted by Thomas, A. B., and Morgan, D. J., in *History of Urology,* Chapter VII. The Williams and Wilkins Co., Baltimore, 1933.
148. CUNNINGHAM, H.: *J. Am. Urol. Assoc.,* 1909. Cited by Brown, P., 1933.
149. VOLKER and VON LICHTENBERG, A.: Pyelographie. *Munich, Med. Wschr.,* 53:105, 1906.
150. KEYES, E.: Cited by Brown, P. (148), 1933.
151. BRAASCH, W. F.: Deformity of the renal pelvis. *Am. Surg.,* 51:534, 1910, cited by Brown, P. (148), 1933.
152. UHLE, A. A., and PFAHLER, G. E.: *Ann. Surg.,* p. 546, 1910.
153. THOMAS, A. B., and MORGAN, D. J.: *Roentgenology in the History of Urology.* Chapter VII, Vol. 11. The Williams and Wilkins Co., Baltimore, Md., 1933.
154. CARELLI and SONDELLA: Un nuevo procedimiento para explorar el rinon. *Rev. As. Med. Argent.,* 1921, 24:424, cited by Brown, P., 1933.
155. ROSENSTEIN: (1921) Cited by Brown, P., 1933.
156. CAHILL, G.: Roentgenography: Perirenal insufflation. In Glasser, O.: *Medical Physics.* Chicago Year Book Publishers, Inc., 1944.
157. CAHILL, GEORGE: Pheochromocytoma. *J.A.M.A.,* 138:180-186, 1948.
158. DOS SANTOS, R., LAMAS, C., and CALDAS, P.: Les recents progress dans la technique de l'arterio-graphic de l'aorte abdominal. *Presse Med.,* 39:574, 1931. Cited by Higgins, 1955.
159. WALLACE, J. F.: Fiber optic endoscopy. *J. Urol.,* 90:324, Sept., 1963.
160. MARSHALL, VICTOR: Fiber optics in urology. *J. Urol.,* 91:110, Jan., 1964.
161. KAUFMAN, J. J.: *Advances in Diagnostic Urology.* Little, Brown and Company, Boston, Chapter 9, pp. 184-191, 1964.
162. PEARMAN, R. O.: Renal photoscanning in urologic disease. Chapter 10, in Kaufman, *Ibid.,* pp. 193-201.
163. RICCI, J. V.: *The Development of Gynecological Surgery and Instruments.* Blakiston, Philadelphia, pp. 1-2, 1949.
164. *Ibid.*
165. *The Odyssey of Homer:* Translated by William Cowper, London, 1855, Book IX, Verses 459-462, quoted by Ricci.
166. Personal Communication.
167. *Medical Classics,* Vol. IV. The Williams and Wilkins Co., Baltimore, Md., pp. 419-420, 1939-1940.
168. FERGUSSON, WILLIAM: *A System of Practical Surgery,* 2nd American Ed. Lea and Blanchard, Philadelphia, Chapter XII, Operations on the scrotum, testicle, prepuce and penis, 1845.
169. LANDES, R. R., and LEMHARDT, K. O.: The history of hydrocoele. *Urological Survey,* pp. 135-146, 1967.
170. ANDREWS, E. WILLYS: The "bottle operation" for radical cure of hydrocoele. *Am. Surg.,* 6:915, 1907.
171. Personal Communication.
172. WINKELMAN, O.: Radical cure of hydrocoele. *Centrablatt, f. chirurgie,* A4:1092, 1898.
173. Personal Communication.

174. Personal Communication.
175. Bevan, D. A.: The surgical treatment of undescended testicle. *J.A.M.A.*, 41:718, 1903.
176. Wershub, L. P.: Orchiopexy: A critique, *J. Urol.*, 60:631, 1948.
177. Jones, W. W., and Scott, W. W.: *Hermaphroditism, Gential Anomalies, and Related Endocrine Disorders.*
178. Barney, J. D.: Lithiasis. Chapter I, Vol. II, *History of Urology*. Williams and Wilkins Co., Baltimore, 1933.
179. Cumston, Charles Green: A short account of the early history of suprapubic cystotomy. *Trans. Amer. Urol. A.*, VI:304-337, 1912.
180. Franco, P.: *Petit traité contenant une des parties principalles de chirurgie.* Antoine Vincent, Lyon, 1556.
181. Franco, P.: Traité des Hernies contenant une ample declaratun de toutes leurs especes, antre excellentes parties de la chirurgie, assavois de la pierre, descataractes des yeux et autre maladies desquelle comme la cure est perilleuse, aussi est-elle de pn d'hommes bien exercel; avec leur causes, signes, accidens, anatomie des parties effectees, etleur entire gueri- son. Thiebauld Payan, Lyon, 1561.
182. Bush, R. B., and Bush, I. M.: Pierre Franco. *Invest. Urol.*, 2:405, 1965.
183. Dahl, S. D.: William Cheselden (1688-1752). *Invest. Urol.*, 5:627-629, 1968.
184. Castiglioni, A.: The dawn of genito-urinary surgery. *J. Urol.*, 50:632, 1943.
185. Churchill, E. D., Editor: *To Work in the Vineyard of Surgery. The Reminiscences of J. Collins Warren (1824-1927).* Harvard Univ. Press, 1958.
186. Shelley, H. S.: Intravesical destruction of bladder stones. *J. Hist. Med.*, XIX:46, 1964.
186a. Heurteloup, Baron: *Principles of Lithotrity*. London, Whittaker, Teacher and Company, p. 11, 1831, quoted by Shelley.
187. Personal Communication.
188. Personal Communication.
189. Weyranch, H. M.: *Surgery of the Prostate*. W. B. Saunders Co., Philadelphia and London, 1959.
190. Axilrod, H. D., and Deming, C. L.: Prostatism then and now in New Haven Hospital. *Conn. State Med. J.*, XIV: 1003-1007, 1950.
191. Whately, Thomas: *An Improved Method of Treating Strictures in the Urethra.* Printed for J. Johnson, St. Paul's Church Yard, London, 1804.
192. Personal Communication.
193. Belfield, W. T.: *Am. J. Med. Sc.*, 434, 1890.
194. Belfield, W. T.: *J. Cut. Genito-Urin. Dis.*, 323, 1892.
195. Fuller, E.: The question of priority in the adoption of the method of total enucleation of the hypertrophied prostate gland. *Am. J. Surg.*, 41:520, 1905.
196. Squier, J. B.: Surgery of the prostate. *Surg. Gynec. & Obst.*, 599, 1912.
197. Squier, J. B.: Surgery of the prostate. *Boston, Med. & Surg. J.*, 911, 1911.
198. Young, H. H.: Prostatic surgery. *Trans. Med. Soe. Virginia,* #160, 1899.
199. Cabot, H.: *The Mechanism of the Protection Afforded by the Drainage of the Prostate as a Preliminary to Operation.*
200. Judd, E. S.: Prostatism. *J.A.M.A.*, 458, 1911.
201. Cabot, H.: *Modern Urology*. Lea and Febiger, Philadelphia, 1924.

202. Thomsch and Walker, J. W.: *British J. Surg.*, 20, 1919
203. Wershub, L. P.: Suprapubic prostatectomy—A critique. *Swiss Med. J.*, Vol. 86, supplement to #20, p. 608, 1956.
204. Hess, E., Roth, R. B., and Kaminsky, S. A.: Prostatic surgery. *J. Urol.*, 67:6, 1952.
205. Personal Communication.
206. Gray, A. H.: Treatment of malignant diseases of the bladder through suprapubic incisions with report of a case. *Am. J. Roentgenol.*, 1:2-53, 1907.
207. Pasteau and Degrais: Cited by Young, H. H.: Progress in urology. *Am. J. Surg.*, 21:140, 1941.
208. Gonder, M. J., Soanes, A. J., and Shulman, S.: Cyrosurgical treatment of the prostate. *Invest. Urol.*, 3:372, 1966.
209. Power, H.: 1663-1664: Cited by Klein, D. *Proc. Roy. Soc. (Biol.)*, 150:149, 1959.
210. Kaplan, J. H., and Kaplan, H.: Cyrogenic electro-coagulative and spontaneous necrosis of bladder neoplasm: A preliminary study. *J. Urol.*, 95:531, 1966.
211. Mathé, C. P.: *History of Urology. Kidney Surgery.* Edited by Bransford Lewis. Baltimore, Md., Williams and Wilkins Co., Vol. 1, pp. 279-385, 1933.
212. Mézeray: L' Abrégé Chronologique de l'Histoire de France, Tome V, p. 113-114, 1687.
213. Bernard, C.: Case of the British Consul Hobson. *Philosophical Trans.*, XIX: 333, 1696.
214. Blancard, Étienne: Lexic. Med. Yenovat., et Prax. Med.-Nephrotomia, Pt. 11, Cap. 13, pp. 252-253, 1690.
215. Heister, H.: *A General System of Surgery.* London, pt. 11, pp. 108-109, 1745.
216. Hévin, P.: Récherches historiques et critiques sur la néphrotomie, ou Taille du Rein. *Mém. Acad. Roy. Chir.*, 3:178-333, 1757
217. Morris, H.: *On the Origin and Progress of Renal Surgery.* Philadelphia, P. Blakiston Son and Company, 1898.
218. Ingalls, W., and Bundy, F. E.: Nephrolithotomy. *Boston Med. and Surg. J.*, 106:843-846, 1882.
219. Seymour, W. W.: A successful case of nephrolithotomy for calculus-pyelitis. *Tr. New York State M.A.*, 1:150, 1884.
220. Tiffany, L. McL.: Nephrolithotomy. *Tr. Am. Surg. A.*, 3:124, 1885.
221. McIntyre, Cited by Mathé, C. P.: *History of Urology. Kidney Surgery.* Edited by Bransford Davis. Baltimore, Md., Williams and Wilkins Co., Vol. 1, pp. 279-385, 1933.
222. Albarran, J.: *Ibid.*
223. Abbe, R.: *Ibid.*
224. Simon, Gustav: *Chir. dev. Nieren, Erlangen,* 1:12, 1871.
225. Wolcott, A.: Cited by Henry Morris.
226. Rayer, P.: *Traite de Maladies des Reins.* 1841.
227. Gilmore, J. T.: A case of successful removal of a kidney from a woman. *Am. J. Obst.*, 4:74, 1871.
228. Personal Communication.
229. Dietl, C.: Wandernde Nieren and deren Eintelemmung. *Wien. Med. Wchnschr.*, 14:363, 1884.

230. Hahn, E.: Die operative Behandlung der bewlglichen mere durch Fixation. *Zentralbe. f. chir.*, Leipsig.

231. Le Dentu, A.: *Affections chirurigicales des reins, des ureters et des capsules surrenales*. G. Masson, Paris, 719, 1889.

232. Morris, Henry: *Surgical Diseases of the Kidney and Ureter*. Casel et cie, London, Paris, New York and Melbourne, 1885, second edition, 11:220, 1901.

233. Trapp, D. J., and Shelley, S. H.: A brief review of the history of renal surgery. *Urol. Survey*, 15:185, 1965.

234. Albarran, J., Cited by Guiterrez, R.: Nephrostomy. *J. Urol.*, 31:307-313, 1934.

235. Hinman, F.: *Principles and Practices of Urology*. Section, Hydronephrosis. W. B. Saunders, Philadelphia, 1935.

236. Kuster, E.: Ein Fal von Resektion des Hornleiters. *Centralbe. f. chir.*, Leipsig, XIX, Suppl. 110-111, 1892.

237. Papin, E.: De l'enervation des reins. *A. Franc. d'Urol.*, 21:527, 1921.

238. Crabtree, F. G.: Renal pedicle sympathectomy. *J. Urol.*, 59:748-50, 1948.

239. Young, Hugh: Fifty years progress in urology. *Am. J. Surg.*, pp. 120-163, 1951.

240. Crile, G. W.: Kinetic system and its control. *South. Surg.*, 1:157-161, 1932.

241. Crile, G. W.: Indications and contra-indications for denervation of the adrenal glands. *Am. J. Surg.*, 100:667-669, 1934.

242. Ullman, E.: Experimentelle Nieren-transplantation. *Wein. Klin. Wchnschr.*, 15:28, 707, 1902.

243. Carrel, A.: Peritoneal patching of the aorta. *J. Exp. Med.*, 12:139, 1910.

244. Carrel, A.: Patching of the abdominal aorta with a piece of rubber. *J. Exp. Med.*, 14:126, 1911.

245. Smith, Robert B.: Alexis Carrel (1873-1944). *Investigative Urol.*, 5:102-5, 1967.

246. Carrel, A.: La technique operative des anastomoses vasculaires et la transplantation des visceres. *Lyon Med.*, 98:859, 1902.

247. Vornoy: Sobre el bloqueo del aparato reticuloendothelial del hombre en alquans formas de intoxicación por el sublimado y sobre la transplación del riñén cadaverico comométodo de tratamiento de la anuria consecutiva a aquella intoxicación. *Sigl o Méd.*, 97:296, 1936.

248. Lawler, R., West, J., McNulty, P., Clancey, E., and Murphy, R.: Transplantation of the kidney in the human. *J.A.M.A.*, 144:844, 1950.

249. Hume, D. M., Merril, J. P., Miller, B. F., and Thorn, G. W.: Experiences with renal homotransplantations in the human: Report of nine cases. *J. Clin. Invest.*, 34:2, 327, 1955.

250. Merril, J., Murray, J., Harrison, J., and Guild, W.: Successful homotransplantation of the human kidney between identical twins. *J.A.M.A.*, 160:227, 1956.

Index

D

E

N

O

P

R

S

W

X

Y

Z